International Perspectives Elder Abuse

Elder abuse has been increasingly recognised over the past ten years in many countries and progress has been made in both understanding and addressing the issue. This volume provides a much-needed international overview of the topic.

Opening with an examination of what elder abuse is, Amanda Phelan sets it in a theoretical context and looks at assessment and approaches to the issue in residential and community care environments. The book then presents a range of country studies, which provide an overview of the context of elder abuse in the country and a discussion of related policy, legislation, research and practice. Countries covered include Ireland, United Kingdom, Spain, China, Australia, Kenya, Israel, Canada and the United States, whilst a regional chapter looks at South America. A concluding chapter draws together cross-cultural comparisons and provides some guidance as to best practice.

The only comprehensive book in this area, *International Perspectives on Elder Abuse* is an invaluable reference for practitioners, academics and researchers from a range of disciplines, including nursing, social work, sociology, public health and social policy.

Amanda Phelan is Subject Head of Older Persons' Nursing in the School of Nursing, Midwifery and Health Systems, University College Dublin and Co-Director of the UCD National Centre for the Protection of Older People. She is also the national representative for the International Network for the Prevention of Elder Abuse and secretary for the All Ireland Gerontological Nurses' Association.

Routledge Advances in Health and Social Policy

International Perspectives on Elder Abuse

Edited by
Amanda Phelan

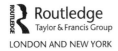

Routledge
Taylor & Francis Group

LONDON AND NEW YORK

First published 2013
by Routledge
2 Park Square, Milton Park, Abingdon, Oxfordshire OX14 4RN

Simultaneously published in the USA and Canada
by Routledge
711 Third Avenue, New York, NY 10017

First issued in paperback 2014

Routledge is an imprint of the Taylor & Francis Group, an informa business

British Library Cataloguing in Publication Data
A catalogue record for this book is available from the British Library

Library of Congress Cataloging-in-Publication Data
International perspectives on elder abuse / edited by Amanda Phelan.
p. cm. -- (Routledge advances in health and social policy)
ISBN 978-0-415-69405-6 (hardback) -- ISBN 978-0-203-38705-4 (ebook)
1. Abused elderly. 2. Older people--Abuse of. I. Phelan, Amanda.
HV6626.3.I577 2013
362.6'82--dc23
2012036188

ISBN 13: 978-0-415-69405-6 (hbk)
ISBN 13: 978-1-138-82337-2 (pbk)

Typeset in Goudy
by Taylor & Francis Books

In memory of my nephew Cian Comerford 1994–2011

Contents

List of tables and figures

Tables

Figures

Preface

The idea for this book began while I was completing my PhD. When reading literature on elder abuse, I became increasingly aware of the different interpretations and understandings of elder abuse in different jurisdictions. However, trying to consider the global issue of elder abuse within a common lens of research, practice, policy and legislation proved a challenge. Consequently, this book allows the reader to examine current international perspectives within a cultural and localised context.

The contributing authors are all leaders in their country's research in the domain of elder abuse and have eloquently articulated indepth insights into the topic. Each author was invited to generate perspectives under the lens of research, practice, policy and legislation. However, the function of each chapter was to provide insights which were not overly superimposed by prescriptive headings, thus allowing the contributing authors the flexibility to develop the discussions as parallel to the country's context. In doing so, the book provides readers with an excellent base in the topic of elder abuse in an international context.

Acknowledgements

This book was a challenging journey for me and I am indebted to many people. Within the UCD School of Nursing, Midwifery and Health Systems, I have received support from many colleagues, but in particular the Dean and Head of School, Dr Martin McNamara, and my friend, Dr Mary Casey. My colleagues, Professors Margaret (Pearl) Tracey and Gerard Fealy, Dr Attracta Lafferty and Ms Nora Donnelly in the UCD National Centre for the Protection of Older People have also inspired my continuing research and interest in the area of elder abuse.

I would like to thank all of the contributing authors for giving their time and craft in each of the chapters. I know academic life has many demands and each contribution required careful reflection and development.

I would also like to thank my family, in particular, my mother Frances, my sisters Mary, Terry, Evelyn and Caroline and my brother Jimmy. Finally, this book would not have been possible without my husband, Gary, and children Aoife and Jack, who patiently tolerated my academic woes!

Contributors

Isabella Aboderin is Senior Research Scientist at the African Population and Health Research Center (APHRC) in Nairobi, Kenya, where she leads the programme on ageing and development in sub-Saharan Africa; and Senior Research Fellow at the Oxford Institute of Population Ageing (OIA), University of Oxford.

Patricia Brownell is Associate Professor Emerita of Social Service at Fordham University. Dr Brownell represents INPEA on the CoNGO Committee on Ageing, UN/New York and also serves on the Executive Committee of the Board of Directors of the (NCPEA) as well as chairing the Public Policy Committee.

Elsie Chau-Wai Yan is an assistant professor at the Department of Social Work and Social Administration. Her research interests include elder abuse, elder sexuality, dementia care, caregiver stress and women's health.

Lía Susana Daichman has worked as a Consultant in Gerontology and Geriatrics at the IADT, Buenos Aires. Lía served as President of INPEA from 2001–2009 and was elected President to the Buenos Aires Gerontological Society (AGEBA) 1994 and has been Chair of the LA Committee for the Prevention of EA (COMLAT - IAGG) since 1995.

Israel (Issi) Doron is the Head of the Department of Gerontology, University of Haifa, and President of the Israeli Gerontological Society. He specialises in the fields of law and ageing, social policy and aging, ethics, ageism and the human rights of older persons.

Yolanda García Esteve is a Professor and the current Secretary-General at the Valencian International University. She is also the Queen Sofía Centre's in-house expert in the field of legislation, where she gathers and comparatively studies legislation on violence from all around the world.

Liliana Giraldo Rodriguez is a researcher in Medical Sciences, Institute of Geriatrics, Mexico (Instituto de Geriatría, México) and holds a Master's Degree on Demography, El Colegio de Mexico. Current research interests are aging, elder abuse, mistreatment, violence, and discrimination.

Ester Grau Alberola is a Professor at several universities: the Valencian International University, the University of Valencia and the University of Salamanca (special courses). She has over 12 years' professional experience in gerontology and social psychology.

Nesta Hatendi is HelpAge International Regional Representative for East, West and Central Africa. Nesta works alongside HelpAge International country offices and their teams in Kenya, Uganda, Ethiopia, Tanzania and DRC, and leads on strategic programme development to influence policy related to older people.

Isabel Iborra is a Professor at the Valencian International University. She is the current National Representative of the INPEA in Spain, a member of the National Security Council Working Group on Elder Abuse (Ministry of the Interior) and the former Scientific Coordinator at the Queen Sofia Centre.

Susan Kurrle is an academic geriatrician in hospital and community practice at Hornsby Ku-ring-gai Hospital in northern Sydney, Australia. She holds the Curran Chair in Health Care of Older People in the Faculty of Medicine at the University of Sydney.

Margaret Lee is a member of the Young Nursing Academic Programme (YNAP) at the University of Hong Kong School of Nursing. Margaret is working with the HKU Domestic Harmony Research team; elder mistreatment is one of the research foci of the team.

Ariela Lowenstein is Acting President, Yezreel Valley College. Lowenstein developed and established in 1999 Haifa University's Graduate Department of Gerontology, heading it for its first five years. In 1990, she established the Center for Research and Study of Aging, which she headed until October 2011, creating a wide network of global collaborations with top researchers and institutions.

Lynn McDonald is a professor in the Faculty of Social Work, where she is the Coordinator of the social work Gerontology Program and Director of the Institute for the Life Course and Aging at the University of Toronto. She is the Scientific Director of a National Centre of Excellence, the National Initiative for the Care of the Elderly (NICE) dedicated to the inter-professional knowledge transfer about and for older adults.

Bridget Penhale is currently Reader in Mental Health of Older People at the University of East Anglia (UEA), UK, and has specialised in work with older people since 1983. In 2010 she received the International Rosalie Wolf Award for her work in the field of elder abuse research and practice.

Amanda Phelan is Subject Head of Older Persons' Nursing in the School of Nursing, Midwifery and Health Systems, University College Dublin, and is also a Co-Director in the UCD National Centre for the Protection of Older People.

Astrid Sandmoe is an Associate Professor at the Department of Health Studies, Faculty of Health and Social Studies, Telemark University College, Norway. She is currently working on a multi-disciplinary elder abuse project in Telemark County to enhance the quality of care to older people exposed to abuse.

Joy Swanson Earnst Ph.D., MSW, is an associate professor and the director of the undergraduate social work programme at Hood College, Frederick, Maryland. Her research focuses on elder neglect and Adult Protective Services.

Agnes (Aggi) Tiwari is Professor and Head of the School of Nursing, Li Ka Shing Faculty of Medicine, University of Hong Kong. She has published extensively on family violence prevention and intervention and also conducts her faculty practice in three shelters for abused women and provides consultancy to victim support services.

1 Elder abuse: an introduction

Amanda Phelan

Introduction

Abuse of older people is a growing challenge in all societies. This is particularly pertinent as demographics demonstrate a global ageing population. For example, Leeson and Harper (2008) indicate that approximately 8 per cent of the world's population was aged 60 years and over in 1950, but by 2006 this figure had increased to 11 per cent, with projections of a rise to 22 per cent by 2050. Elder abuse can occur in any setting that includes older people and in any socio-economic group. The topic of elder abuse has a relatively recent history in public discourse, but there are challenges in definition, understandings and constituent elements. As with other forms of interpersonal violence, elder abuse is an unpalatable taboo subject often shrouded in secrecy and shame and can be considered a 'hidden problem' in society (Baker and Heitkemper 2005). However, elder abuse has serious consequences. Apart from the immediate effects of abuse, such as possible bruises, fractures, distress and financial loss (Lindbloom et al. 2007), there are enduring effects such as premature mortality (Lachs et al. 1998), depression and continued psychological distress (Mowlam et al. 2007, Lafferty et al. 2011) as well as a continued experience of fear (Comijs et al. 1998).

In order to provide an assessment of perspectives of elder abuse in our selected countries, this chapter provides a foundation in understanding the topic of elder abuse. As such, it examines issues of old age, the emergence of elder abuse in public discourse, terminological and definitional challenges, prevalence and theoretical frameworks. The reality of elder abuse can differ due to issues of legislative imperatives, mandatory reporting, cultural norms, response systems, policy guidelines and so forth, but this diversity should not be used as a barrier to addressing the topic through a comprehensive, rights based approach.

Old age

The human life cycle has become increasingly demarcated in terms of age-related components as to how an individual is categorised (Boyd and Bee 2004). Old age exists as a definite chronological life stage, but the precise chronological differentiation and meaning of old age can be interpreted differently (Posner 1996, Katz 1996). Consequently, although chronology can be the primary reference for old age, ageing theories are also influential when considering the ageing process itself (WHO 2002a; UN 2004).

The modern classification of older people has reflected Otto von Bismarck's distinction of 'the elderly' from the general population (Carp 2000) by introducing in the late ninteenth century rudimentary pensions for those over 65 years of age as a reaction to a rising interest in socialism in Germany. Sub-sequently, 'over 65 years' became acknowledged in many Western countries as the demarcation of the category 'older person'. For example, 65 years of age is frequently acknowledged as the age of retirement and is employed when calculating age dependency ratios. Older age dependency ratios are based on the number of older people (generally 65 years and older) compared to the number of people of working age (i.e. 15–64 years of age). Projected population statistics suggest that the old age dependency ratios in Europe may double in the next forty years (Lanzieri 2006). However, with increasing dependency ratios, the age of retirement has risen moderately in some countries (WHO 2011, Phelan 2011) with some commentators lobbying for further increases to 70 years of age (Economist 2011).

Other age references must also be acknowledged; for example, the WHO (2002a, 2011) and the UN (2004) both use the standard of 60 years to describe 'older people'. The WHO (2002a) argues that, although the marker of 60 years may appear young, in the developed world and in the developing world, chronological age is not a precise indicator of the changes that accompany ageing. In addition, increased complexity has occurred in classifying older age to subgroups of young old and older old (see Neugarten's 1974 seminal work). The most remarkable demographic increase in older people has been within the older old age group (UN 2004) who are more vulnerable to elder abuse (O'Keeffe et al. 2007, Naughton et al. 2010). As the population of older people increases globally, elder abuse has the potential to increase and thus it is imperative to understand this social challenge so that preventative and ameliorative activities may be implemented within all levels of society from cultural unacceptability to proactive government policy and practice.

Ageism

Ageism has been highlighted as an underlying factor in the emergence of elder abuse (Brandl et al. 2007, Phelan 2008). An examination of elder abuse using an ageist lens has the advantage of incorporating structural, political and social contexts (Kingston and Penhale 1995, Harbison 1999). Ageist attitudes contribute to the non-identification and non-recognition of elder maltreatment as well as the passive tolerance of abuse of older people. First identified in 1969 (Butler 1969), ageism is a relatively new socially constructed concept and can be defined as the systematic stereotyping and discrimination of older people due to their age (Pickering 2001). This may be accompanied by a failure to reflect individualism and a high valuation on youth (Harbison 1999). Ageism may also encompass an obstruction to social participation (Solem 2005) and covertly support the value given to youthfulness and a 'culturally endemic paranoia' of ageing (Schwaiger 2006: 14).

Ageism is an important factor in considering elder abuse in the context of healthcare settings (Herdman 2002). The health system, as an institution of society, may reflect ageist assumptions of society, which can be introjected into healthcare workers' professional activities (Garner 2004). Ageist attitudes of healthcare staff are important contributors to deficient care of older people. Thus, in preventing elder abuse, confronting ageist attitudes is considered central to responding to the perpetration of elder abuse (Biggs et al. 1995, CHI 2002, Phelan 2008).

Theories of the social construction of old age and political economy perspective on elder abuse are based broadly on the concept of ageism and consider the position of an older person in the social and political environment of contemporary Western society. The social construction of ageing considers issues such as how ageing is constituted in society and the challenges faced by an older person in his or her everyday existence. Advocates of the political economy perspective focus on challenges experienced due to age and the contribution of public policy to these challenges and how such policy interprets social problems. For instance, the application of welfarism, in terms of pensions and other benefits for older persons, presupposes financial dependency. Thus, ageism is one consequence of the division of labour and social inequalities rather than as a result of the ageing process per se (Angus and Reeve 2006, Roscigno et al. 2007, Phelan 2008). Society imposes an artificial dependency on older people through mandatory retirement, which restricts the role of older people in society and enforces poverty on them as retirement pensions are not generally linked to industrial wages. Thus, as Biggs et al. (1995) note, abuse can arise covertly from society due to the marginalisation and disempowerment of older people. The political economy perspective gives credence to the idea that wider societal structures influence elder abuse. However, this approach provides limited insight into the micro-environment of dyadic abuse. Moreover, studies recording elder abuse in countries where old age is valued (Kosberg et al. 2003), such as Japan, militate against ageism as an explanatory framework for elder abuse.

The issue of power relations has also been the focus of elder abuse research. The passivity of older people can occur as they accept their situation of powerlessness and resign themselves to this situation as part of 'being old', thus normalising and internalising the ageist care practices (Minichiello et al. 2002). However, Podnieks (1995) argues that powerlessness is not a central issue for abused older people and proposes that older people in the abusive context develop a 'hardiness' which they use to adapt to the experienced mistreatment. Value judgements regarding older people can underpin tolerance of elder abuse, whereas identical abuse in a child context would be a cause of concern. The abuse may also be justified by seeing the older person as causing the negative action. This perspective of blaming the victim is supported by terminology and perceptions such as seeing older people as 'burdens' and lacking function in society.

Tracing the history of elder abuse

Elder abuse is a component of the family violence spectrum, which also includes domestic violence and child protection. Like child protection, elder abuse emerged in the domain of medicine when Baker (1975) and Burston (1975) both published in scientific journals about the physical abuse of older women. This does not mean that elder abuse did not occur prior to 1975, but, rather, it was not recognised as a distinct phenomenon. For instance, in popular mythology and ancient folklore, there are tales which describe particular practices, such as the abandonment of old people in the woods for being non-productive and, therefore, a burden on the family (Reinharz 1986, Carp 2000). The treatment of older people has also been bound up with the history of the poor (Means and Smith 1998), for example in relation to the Poor Laws from 1563 onwards (Driver 2008). Consequently, various forms of abuse have been supported as norms within interpersonal relationships with a notable societal transformation in attitudes following formal recognition of abuse (Biggs et al. 1995).

Formal recognition of elder abuse has stimulated an interest in the areas of legislature, health and social care to a varying degree within differing countries. Although the 'discovery' of elder abuse was in the United Kingdom, most of the subsequent proactive activities occurred initially in the United States, Canada and Australia. For example, 'elder abuse' was first used in congressional hearings in the United States (US) in the late 1970s by the House Select Committee on Aging, also known as the Pepper Commission (Wallace 2003), although the history of adult protective services in the United States can be traced back to 1958 when the National Council on Aging convened an informal committee of social workers due to concerns regarding the growing number of incapacitated and socially isolated older people with inappropriate care-givers (Mixon 1995). In contemporary society, elder abuse is a significant global concern with a defined focus in the context of international agencies (WHO 2011). However, the complexity of elder abuse is apparent in difficulties such as disclosure, the reality of reduced (due to death or illness) or enforced (by the perpetrator) social networks, and the inability to recognise the abuse due to socially acceptable norms. Moreover, unlike younger age groups, time is not on the older person's side, and, often, elder abuse can be complicated by physical and cognitive challenges as well as a fear of transfer to residential care.

Terminology

Early articulations of elder abuse presented fundamental limitations and, similar to the terminological quagmire of child protection (Kempe et al. 1962), were heavily influenced by a medicalised lens. Initial terms such as 'granny bashing' (Baker 1975), 'granny battering', (Burston 1975) and 'granny abuse'

(Eastman 1988) inferred a clear gender distinction and privileged physical abuse of older people. Acknowledging a need for gender neutral terminology, Block and Sinnott (1979) used the term 'battered older person syndrome', which also implied physical abuse, and medicalised elder abuse by suggesting a group of related symptoms.

The debate on terminology has been contentious and not always accep-table to all professionals or scholars (Wallace 2003). Macdonald (1997: 414), for example, views the term elder abuse as a 'horrific phrase' stating that the real issue should be on the abusive act perpetrated against a vulnerable person regardless of age. Johnson (1986) argues that the term 'elder abuse' is a tauto-logical trap as the term is used to both name the phenomenon and define it, which results in confusion rather than clarification. Furthermore, feminist objections have focused on the gender neutral term of elder abuse, with claims that this neglects to acknowledge the gendered nature of attitudes, expectations and behaviour in elder abuse. Neysmith (1995), for example, argues that the term elder abuse does not make a distinction of how older women's experiences of abuse may differ to those of older men.

A proposed solution to address the terminological problems of elder abuse was to replace the terms 'abuse' and 'neglect' with less incriminating, non-judgemental ones such as 'mistreatment' and 'inadequate care' (Quinn and Tomita 1997) or adult protection or protection for vulnerable adults (Brammer and Biggs 1998). However, different terminology, such as that cited above, does not appear to be less accusatory or does not resolve the complexity of definitional difficulty (Carp 2000).

Other terminological concerns have focused on the interpretation of neglect within elder abuse. While neglect, as a distinct phenomenon, has often been mentioned in abuse definitions (Krug et al. 2002), it has been analysed to a much lesser extent (Bennett et al. 1997). A further complicating issue is the uncertainty regarding neglect by omission (passive) or commis-sion (active). Such uncertainty regarding the position of neglect is also reflected in various approaches to self-neglect, which is also termed Diogenes Syndrome or Senile Breakdown Syndrome. Self-neglect, as defined by Pavlou and Lachs (2006), is the profound inattention to hygiene or health due to an inability, unwillingness or both to access potentially ameliorative services. Self-neglect in older people may be due to lifestyle choices and personality traits and is not necessarily related to a psychiatric disorder (Reyes-Ortiz 2001). In the United States, self-neglect is considered under the term elder abuse and constitutes the highest ranking referral issue in adult protective services (Pavlik et al. 2001). This contrasts with countries such as Ireland and the United Kingdom where self-neglect is not considered the remit of elder abuse activities although in Ireland the Health Service Executive (HSE 2012) has recommended that cases of serious self-neglect are handled according to the general elder abuse guidelines. Consequently, due to this dual interpretation of the term neglect, standardised understanding of elder abuse appears to have been further hindered.

Definition

Defining elder abuse has been a contentious issue (Bonnie and Wallace 2003, Fulmer et al. 2011). Some fundamental elements such as environmental factors (elder abuse in the home or institution) and basic types (physical, psychological, sexual, or financial abuse and neglect) are generally agreed upon but difficulties present beyond this point. Further exacerbating issues are the differences in definitions between older people, carers and professionals, such as health-care workers (Mowlam et al. 2007). Depending on the definitional source, the emphasis can change, yet each of these sources claim an elder abuse definition based on the 'objective statement of fact' (Brammer and Biggs 1998: 301). Definitions are also complicated by complex interpersonal relationships, a lack of discrimination between interpersonal conflict and abuse, and scant attention to wider social forces such as ageism, culture and social circumstances (Mowlam et al. 2007, Phelan 2008). However, as McDonald and Collins (2000: iv) have highlighted, 'definitions determine who will be counted as abused and who will not, what the legislation does and does not cover, and who is and is not eligible for service'. Thus, although definitions are important in elder abuse, in reality their standardisation can be problematic, which can lead to difficulties in interpretation.

Cultural definitions of elder abuse

Understandings and definitions of elder abuse are generated within a cultural context (Ruf 2006). The variations in interpretations are important insofar as they represent elder abuse as grounded in general conceptions of cultural representation, values and historicity. Although Kosberg and Garcia (1995) state that elder abuse is a problem in both developing and developed countries, many studies tend to homogenise results to portray a uniform position. This standardised approach often fails to articulate the variations of cultural and ethnic backgrounds of the population leading to a limited conceptualisation of elder abuse. Such challenges have contributed to the topic's emergence, particularly in terms of the under-development of definitions and interpretations which are culturally sensitive (Brammer and Biggs 1998). In addition, McDonald and Collins (2000) speculate that race and ethnicity may be risk factors for abuse. However, this proposition requires much additional research.

In relation to elder abuse, knowledge generation has been predominantly drawn from white populations (Brandl et al. 2007) and minority groups. The focus has been on the general nature of abuse rather than the particular circumstances of such abuse in specific cultures (Ward Griffin 1998). Understandings of elder abuse can vary discretely within differing populations (Hee-Han 2004). For example, in Norway 'family disharmony' (Johns and Hydle 1995) is seen as abusive, in Hong Kong 'elder dumping' (Kwan 1995), that is, placing an older person in a nursing home, is considered abusive, whilst in India 'disrespect by a daughter in law' is viewed as abusive (Anme 2004). In Asian countries, the Confucian aspect of filial piety particularly influences perspectives on social affiliations (Biggs 2007). In Japan, group survival and respect are important societal considerations and precedence is given to the rights of the collective even if such decisions deny the individual rights of some members of the community (Ignatieff 2001).

Legitimised definitions of elder abuse

Contemporary definitions of elder abuse centre on the principle of an 'expectation of trust' (WGEA 2002, WHO 2002b, UN 2004). A commonly used understanding of elder abuse is:

> A single or repeated act or lack of appropriate action, occurring within any relationship where there is an expectation of trust, which causes harm or distress to an older person.
>
> (Action on Elder Abuse 1995)

However, definitions are in a constant state of flux. The Action on Elder Abuse definition has been considered over inclusive (Brammer and Biggs 1998). In addition, Mowlam et al. (2007) express concern at the lack of definitional clarity wherein there is a lack of distinction between elder abuse and other forms of conflict, challenges in using typologies to classify experiences, exclusion of difficulties related to elder abuse, difficulties with the notion of 'expectation of trust' and inclusion or exclusion of age-related experiences.

In examining the definitions of elder abuse in the literature, Stones (1995) noted three basic approaches to the meaning and understanding of elder abuse: connotative, structural and denotative. Connotative concepts imply that an attempt has been made to delineate the full meaning of elder abuse using the variable of unmet needs and positive actions, and it is assumed that 'a conceptual base for the construct validation of tools' (Stones 1995: 111) is provided. Connotative definitions of elder abuse describe behaviour as abusive due to its unnecessary outcome. In this way, problems which emerge as negative actions are not clearly operationalised. Consequently, attempts have been made to articulate what the term 'unmet needs' means as connotative definitions do not focus on the actual abusive action but rather its negative consequences. In addition, connotative definitions fail to address the question of perpetrator's intent, though the use of structural definitions can provide a logical resolution to this problem (Stones 1995).

Structural definitions focus on criteria against which behaviour is judged to be abusive. When such criteria are not uniform, a miscommunication may result. Definitional confusion is due predominantly to the variation in interpretations amongst vocational and/or interest groups. For example, a legal definition is used by the police and judicial system and focuses on violations against criminal law. In contrast, health and social care personnel use concepts of abuse guided by government and agency policy definitions. Such concepts include evaluative criteria for action plans and the eligibility of older people to access services in response to abuse. Consequently, a broad definition of elder abuse is used in order to cover a myriad of contingencies (Selwood et al. 2007). The widest frame of reference for abuse is used by researchers and interest groups. These structural definitions transcend both criminal law and professional ethics and focus primarily on what the constructs do and/or should do (Stones 1995). Some commonality exists across disciplines, wherein specific cases can fall under the rubric of all of the categories. Elder abuse 'can overlap but is not synonymous with, criminal actions' (Perel-Levin 2008: 5). For example, kicking or hitting an older person is recognised as a legal offence and is classified as abusive by health and social care services, researchers and interest group advocates for older people. In contrast, there is a lack of consensus on psychological abuse, particularly in relation to thresholds of harm and acceptable levels of conflict within relationships.

Denotative definitions are those that provide examples, empirical indicators or classifications of elder abuse which can assist the development of screening or survey tools (Stones 1995). In the early literature on elder abuse, there was a predisposition towards the development of taxonomies or typologies (Pillemer and Finkelhor 1988) or to articulate broad, inclusive, conceptual definitions in order to capture the multi-dimensional nature of abuse (Fulmer and O'Malley 1987). In the 1990s, a concerted effort was made to standardise conceptualisations of elder abuse. Most countries acknowledge six manifestations of elder abuse: physical, sexual, psychological/emotional, financial/material abuse, neglect, (by omission or commission) and discriminatory abuse. Table 1.1 outlines the currently accepted typologies, possible manifestations and potential indicators.

Table 1.1   Elder abuse typologies, possible manifestations and potential indicators

Type of abuse	Possible manifestations	Potential indicators
Physical	Hitting, slapping, pushing, kicking, spitting, medication misuse, restraint, force feeding or inappropriate sanctions, restraint.	Bruising, cuts, lacerations, scratches, sprains, hair loss, missing teeth, fractures, slap marks, kick marks, eye injuries, burns.
Sexual	Rape, sexual assault or acts the older person has not consented to or has not the ability to consent to, or was compelled to consent.	Trauma around the genitals, breasts, rectum or mouth.
Psychological	Humiliation, intimidation, threats of abandonment, ridicule, causing fear/anxiety, bullying, blaming, controlling, coercion, harassment, verbal abuse, lack of acknowledgement, isolation/withholding social contact, denial of basic rights, over protective.	Demoralisation, depression, withdrawal, apathy, feelings of hopelessness, insomnia, appetite change, unexplained paranoia, agitation, tearfulness, excessive fears, confusion, ambivalence towards the perpetrator.

Table 1.1 (continued)

Type of abuse	Possible manifestations	Potential indicators
Neglect[1]	Ignoring physical, medical needs, failure to provide access to appropriate services (health, social, educational) of life and/or aids for activities of daily living (such as medication, heating).	Dehydration, malnutrition, inappropriate clothing, poor hygiene, unkempt appearance, over/under medication, unattended medical needs, exposure to risk/danger, absence of aids (zimmer frame, reading glasses), pressure sores.
Financial	Sudden reduction in financial funds, removal of material property, coerced signing over of property/funds/material goods or change of will.	Sudden/unexplained inability to pay bills or to buy necessities, uncharacteristic withdrawal of funds, diverted funds for another's use, damage to property, disappearance of property, absence of required aids or medication, refusal to spend money, disparity of assets and living conditions, extraordinary interest by others in older person's assets, dramatic financial decisions.
Discriminatory	Negative actions towards older people, individual/group.	Ageism, sexism, racism.

Source: Phelan 2010

Note:
1 Passive neglect represents acts of omission by lack of knowledge. Active neglect represents deliberate acts of omission.

The development of such descriptive lists can be problematic due to the lack of uniformity in defining the specific constituents within the categories themselves (Fryling et al. 2006). For instance, some researchers present abuse as a violation of human rights while others do not (Perel-Levin 2008, WHO 2011).

Older persons' definitions of elder abuse

Older people's subjective accounts of elder abuse can differ from the powerful discourses which have emerged from medicine and science. Consequently, the interpretations of older people were marginalised in constructing the definition of elder abuse apart from some studies such as Hidden Voices (WHO and INPEA 2002), Erlingsson et al. (2005), Mowlam et al. (2007) and Age Action Ireland et al. (2011). These studies have demonstrated some fundamental differences in older people's interpretation of elder abuse as the traditional, accepted understandings excluded issues such as the complexity and diversity of elder abuse cases.

When articulating understandings of elder abuse, older people made firm links to issues of social exclusions, rights violations and compromised decision-making (WHO and INPEA 2002, Erlingsson et al. 2005). Family changes such as unstable family units, lax childcare practices and apathy towards older people were identified as underpinning abuse (Erlingsson et al. 2005). Most importantly, findings from the studies point to the advantages of placing elder abuse within the myriad of related challenges experienced by older people. Thus, revised definitions of elder abuse should be able to identify similar experiences of abuse, negotiate clarity on the relevance of age in elder abuse while concurrently distinguishing such experiences in a meaningful way. In this way, the diversity of older people's experience of elder abuse could be articulated rather than the current abuse categories which are generally based on the descriptions of perpetrators' actions (Mowlam et al. 2007). Similar to other research, findings in the Age Action Ireland et al.'s (2011) study demonstrated the limitations of current definitions of elder abuse. Issues related to the wider societal treatment of elder abuse could become marginalised or even absent in traditional understandings leading to 'personhood abuse'. Personhood abuse was seen to disempower older people and marginalise their rights within society.

General prevalence and incidence

Some countries have attempted to enumerate the extent of elder abuse through prevalence studies (O'Keeffe et al. 2007, Acierno et al. 2010, Naughton et al. 2010, Amstadter et al. 2011, Lifespan of Greater Rochester et al. 2011) and incidence studies (DHHS 1998, Lifespan of Greater Rochester et al. 2011). When reviewing the studies through a comparative lens, the statistical sample source must be considered, for example, whether data are sourced from self-reports by older people or figures identified by professionals in practice. In addition, data collection methods vary and include telephone random digit dialing (Lifespan of Greater Rochester et al. 2011, Amstadter et al. 2011), face to face interviews (O'Keeffe et al. 2007, Marmolejo 2008, Lowenstein et al. 2009, Naughton et al. 2010) as well as a review of documented case studies (Lifespan of Greater Rochester et al. 2011). The operational definition of elder abuse is important as well as the item assessments survey, the age range assumed for older people (i.e. 60 years, 65 years) and the mistreatment types included in the study (Amstadter et al. 2011). Furthermore, some studies include variables such as abuse within the preceding year, or since the older age reference (i.e. 60 years or 65 years) or both (O'Keeffe et al. 2007, Naughton et al. 2010, Amstadter et al. 2011, Lifespan of Greater Rochester et al. 2011) and lifetime abuse (Amstadter et al. 2011). Another distinction focuses on whether abuse offenders were defined within a framework of someone in a position of trust (i.e. spouse, daughter, son), familiars (neighbours, etc.), formal care service employees or any other person who perpetrated abuse. Variations in prevalence figures may, therefore, be due to methodological choices in individual studies.

Most elder abuse prevalence figures are between 2–5 per cent of community-dwelling older people (O'Keeffe et al. 2007, Naughton et al. 2010, Lifespan of Greater Rochester et al. 2011) though some studies have indicated higher rates, for example 18.4 per cent in Israel (excluding neglect; Lowenstein et al. 2009), 10 per cent in South Carolina (Amstadter et al. 2011) and 11.4 per cent in the United States (Acierno et al. 2010). The National Elder Abuse Incidence Study (NEAIS) (DHHS 1998) identified a 1 per cent incidence of abuse (excluding self-neglect) and when combined with such self-neglect, the incidence rate was 1.2 per cent. This contrasts with a recent study in New York (Lifespan of Greater Rochester et al. 2011) which suggests an incidence rate of nearly 24 times higher than cases referred to the health, social, legal and police services. While prevalence or incidence studies seek to enumerate the nature of elder abuse in society, many of these studies represent 'impressionistic estimates' (Bonnie and Wallace 2003: 21) as they underestimate the true reality of elder abuse (DHSS 1998, Rhodes 2005). This supports the iceberg theory, wherein many cases are undetected and are 'under the radar' (Lifespan of Greater Rochester Inc. et al. 2011). Thus, findings are considered as a partial representation of true incidence and prevalence as such figures can be difficult to enumerate (Rhodes 2005).

Most abuse occurs in the home environment and is perpetrated by known perpetrators, generally a family member (O'Keeffe et al. 2007, Naughton et al. 2010, Amstadter et al. 2011). The most prominent form of abuse can vary slightly, with psychological abuse (O'Keeffe et al. 2007, Amstadter et al. 2011) being the most common in some studies, while in others financial abuse has been identified as the highest ranking typology (Naughton et al. 2010, Acierno et al. 2010, Lifespan of Greater Rochester et al. 2011). However, it should be noted that clustering of typologies occurs. For example, in an Irish prevalence study, 25 per cent of participants reported more than one type of abuse, while 14 per cent detailed three or more types (Naughton et al. 2010). In general, studies indicate that females were more likely to be abused than males (O'Keeffe et al. 2007, Naughton et al. 2010, Lifespan of Greater Rochester et al. 2011), although some studies demonstrate gender being an insignificant variable (Amstadter et al. 2011). Increasing age can also be a variable which amplifies risk, with those over 80 years of age being most vulnerable, whilst age in a 2007 UK report (O'Keeffe et al. 2007) showed an increased susceptibility to abuse for males but a decrease for females when correlated to increasing age (excluding neglect). Studies also demonstrated that a decline in the older person's health status and social isolation and low levels of social support increased the perpetration of abusive activities (Naughton et al. 2010, Amstadter et al. 2011). Marital status impacted on abuse perpetration, with respondents who were divorced or separated being at a higher risk of mistreatment than those who were widowed or single, although it is acknowledged that the numbers in the former categories were small. Abuse was also identified as having an inverse relationship with socio-economic group and educational status, thus the higher the educational status and socio-economic group, the lower the prevalence of abuse (Naughton et al. 2010).

Dementia and elder abuse

Dementia refers to a progressive loss of cognitive function due to changes in the brain caused by disease or trauma. As age increases, the prevalence of dementia increases and this can impact decision-making, judgement, memory, spatial orientation, thinking, reasoning, problem solving and verbal communication, as well as behavioural or personality changes. Dementia may manifest in Alzheimer's disease, vascular dementia, dementia with Lewy bodies or fronto-temporal dementia. There are approximately 35 million people in the world living with dementia (Cahill et al. 2012).

Older people with dementia are particularly prone to abuse (Cooper et al. 2008, Wiglesworth et al. 2010). Possible factors which contribute to this include a higher care-giving role and a compromised cognitive status of the older person (Miller et al. 2006). In particular, the agitated behaviour associated with dementia can influence negative interactions. Furthermore, family care-givers may be unaware of actions that are abusive (Beach et al. 2005). In a Hong Kong study (Yan and Kwok 2011) of care-givers to older people with dementia, 62 per cent of the sample of 122 family care-givers reported verbal and physical abuse of older people in the preceding month. A separate study, Caring for a relative with dementia (CARD), demonstrated that over half of the participants reported physical or psychological abuse and one-third met the criteria of significant abuse (Cooper et al. 2009).

For family members, it can be difficult to cope with a change in personality in the older person with dementia, which can mark the 'loss of the person'. Studies show that a depressed effect in carers for frail older people may be related to abuse and a resentment of care-giving (Beach et al. 2005, Shaffer et al. 2007). Carers of older people with dementia demonstrate a great degree of anxiety and may employ dysfunctional strategies (Cooper et al. 2006, 2010). A further complicating issue is that the complexity of interpersonal dynamics as abuse can be reciprocal (Choi and Mayer 2000).

Mental capacity

One of the confounding issues in elder abuse is that of mental capacity. This refers to the ability to make informed choices and to use higher order judgment. Capacity is manifested in being able to make an informed choice, through understanding pertinent information, being able to abstract to one's own context, reasoning in decision making and comprehending the consequences

(Grisso and Appelbaum 1998). It is generally accepted that adults with mental capacity have the right to make decisions, even if these may be considered risky by others. Such decisions may include a reluctance to disclose the abuse or accept any intervention. Many countries are moving from a perspective of a decision of absolute incapacity (generally based on the medical status approach) to a functional approach to capacity. This means that the person is assumed to have capacity unless otherwise proven and all steps are taken to assist the person to make a decision and respect is demonstrated for that decision. A functional approach is time specific and focused on the decision pertaining to the situation as it is. In the event of mental incapacity, actions need to be focused on the principle of 'best interest' of the person which is least restrictive to his or her individual rights (TSO 2005). Even in the event of demonstrating what appears to be competent decision-making capacity, it should be recognised that the older person may be unable to give true consent due to being disempowered through interpersonal dynamics (O'Connor et al. 2009) or may make a decision which is not supported through full comprehension regarding the consequences of that decision.

Concerns regarding capacity can be common in issues of self-neglect as lifestyle decisions may be considered unacceptable to family and professionals. This leads to a conflict between respecting autonomy and self-determination and a paternalistic approach to ensuring the safety of the older person. Careful consideration of cases is required which takes into account possible health decline, cultural beliefs, lifelong personality traits and the right to make risky decisions. Care should promote autonomy while balancing risk to the older person and possible impact of such decisions on others, for example environmental hazards. A refusal of intervention should not lead to a closure of communications and links to external society.

Nursing homes

Empirical research on elder abuse in the environment of nursing homes remains scant (Goergen 2001, Zhang et al. 2011) even though the issue appears to be a significant challenge in this setting (Hawes 2003, Ben Natan et al. 2010). Furthermore, older people who live in residential care homes are more vulnerable to abuse as they tend to be in the older old age group (McDonald et al. 2012) and their dependency levels are generally high (Malmedal et al. 2009). Although elder abuse can be perpetrated within the general typologies (physical, psychological, etc.), there are differences. Firstly, perpetrators may have a formal contract to care for older people and, secondly, abuse may be perpetrated through the systems of practises within care delivered in nursing homes. Resident-to-resident mistreatment may also constitute elder abuse (Lachs et al. 2007, Rosen et al. 2010), as can abuse by visitors to the facility (Bennett et al. 1997). Elder abuse in nursing homes can also be influenced by issues such as the physical conditions of the nursing home (Millard and Roberts 1991), staff-resident ratios (Sandvide et al. 2004,

Goergen 2001, Shinan-Altman and Cohen 2009), profit or not-for-profit facilities (Jogerst et al. 2006, Clarfield et al. 2009), staff burnout (WHO 1995), intrinsic managerial failings (Bennett et al. 1997, DOHC 2009) and resident-to-staff aggression (Goergen 2001), as well as work stressors, role ambiguity and role conflict (Shinan-Altman and Cohen 2009). Comparison between studies can be complicated by issues of culture, staffing complements, sample focus and definition (Saveman et al. 1999).

Most studies of abuse in nursing homes detail acts of physical abuse, psychological abuse and neglect (Pillemer and Moore 1989, Goergen 2001, Malmedal et al. 2009). Neglect may be considered as having a strong correlation to a limitation in the older person's activities of daily living (Post et al. 2010, Zhang et al. 2011). Financial abuse, through theft, was identified as occurring at a rate of 20 per cent in one study of nursing homes (Harris and Benson 2006) with material exploitation being identified in a separate study (Griffore et al. 2009). Paternalistic attitudes to older people were considered abusive, particularly when the care-giver infantilised the older resident (Goergen 2001) or where a lack of privacy was experienced (Cohen et al. 2010). Although sexual abuse is not recorded often in the literature, the most common perpetrator of sexual abuse was a co-resident in the nursing home (Teaster and Roberto 2003, Rosen et al. 2010). Females were disproportionately the victims of such abuse. Studies have demonstrated that older men may also be subject to sexual abuse (Roberto et al. 2007). The perpetration of resident-to-resident sexual abuse may be due to a hypersexualised, disinhibited behaviour which may occur in older people with dementia (Rosen et al. 2010).

Staff may be reluctant to report abuse in nursing homes (Pillemer and Moore 1989, Meddaugh 1993, Saveman et al. 1999, Goergen 2001, Cooper et al. 2009a) and reporting patterns can differ. For example, in Sweden a study indicated that 11 per cent of staff had observed abuse with 2 per cent admitting they themselves perpetrated the abusive activity (Shinan-Altman and Cohen 2009). This contrasts with an Israeli study which pointed to 54 per cent of staff reporting abuse in the preceding year (Ben Natan et al. 2010) and a study in Germany which reported that 70 per cent of staff had perpetrated or observed abuse.

The importance of elder abuse in nursing homes is likely to become heightened as global population ageing occurs, particularly within the older old age group. Acknowledging this, it is important that elder abuse in nursing homes is approached in a comprehensive way and uses a framework, such as the ecological perspective (Schiamberg et al. 2011), to understand risk factors and consequently delivering effective interventions.

Theories of elder abuse

An examination of elder abuse theoretical frameworks is important as meanings and understandings shape thinking and subsequent actions (Hughes 1995). Theories of elder abuse must be underpinned by data which is systematically theory driven, consisting of both qualitative and quantitative evidence and which reflects the changing dynamics of older person relations and risk inherent in such dynamics (Bonnie and Wallace 2003). Typically, elder abuse theories have focused on two individuals: the abused and the perpetrator. Early theories examined the interpersonal behaviours in this dyadic relationship and the victim and abuser characteristics, as removed from the larger contextual environment. Callaghan (1988) has argued that this erroneous practice served to reduce a complex phenomenon to simple factors, which could attribute cause to the perpetrator and/or the abused person who may be subsequently perceived as mad, bad or sad (Sinclair 2005). More contemporary conceptualisations (Biggs et al. 1995, Penhale and Parker 2003) have encompassed a review of the complexities of elder abuse and situated understanding within the macro level of society (Bennett et al. 1997). Such perspectives can be mediated through societal actions and discourses, which in turn may be influential in group and individual behaviour (Killick 2008).

To date, no theory has been able to provide a comprehensive definition and explanation of elder abuse as there has been limited empirical testing resulting in a blurring of theoretical explanations and individual risk factors, such as stress (Fulmer et al. 2004). The varying constituencies of elder abuse, such as the legislature, social services and the medical community, further complicate emerging theoretical frameworks rendering them elusive, ambiguous and complex. In the literature, elder abuse theories generally emanate from three disciplinary schools of thought: psychological theories, social psychological theories and sociological theories (Biggs et al. 1995). The principal theories are detailed below.

Psychopathology of the abuser

The psychopathology of the abuser theory has been used to explain elder abuse and emanates from the discipline of psychology. This perspective emphasises that the perpetrator's innate characteristics, including psychiatric illness, alcohol/substance abuse or intellectual disability, which may predispose them to abusive acts. An individual's characteristics have been suggested as a possible cause for domestic violence (Rosenberg and Fenley 1991) and psychopathology is a commonly held perspective, as it is easier for public consciousness to accept that family violence is perpetrated by 'sick people' (Gelles 1997).

Some research studies have supported a link between the perpetrator's innate characteristics and elder abuse (Wolf and Pillemer 1989, Harris 1996). Support for this theory has emerged in the intimate partner abuse sphere where the rates of psychological/psychiatric illness among abuse perpetrators was higher than other cohorts (Hamberger and Hastings 1986). More recently, perpetrator characteristics such as alcohol dependence, depression, high anxiety (Campbell-Rhey and Browne 2001), mental illness, hostility and/or substance abuse (Zink and Fisher 2007, Just 2007) and personality disorder

(Dutton and Bodnarchuk 2005) were identified as contributing factors for elder abuse. In a review of the literature, Straka and Montminy (2008) propose that individual pathology for violence can be an important causative agent, such as in organic brain syndrome, cognitive impairments and psychiatric illness, whilst it can also be a risk factor, such as in the case of addiction, attention deficit hyperactive disorder and impulse control problems.

Despite linkages between elder abuse and psychopathology, Straus's (1979) early research indicated that fewer than 10 per cent of all instances of perpetrators of family violence had related psychiatric or mental illness predispositions. Although, there is some empirical support for psychopathology of the abuser (Twomey et al. 2005, Just 2007, Zink and Fisher 2007), it has not attained the status of a theory to explain elder abuse. An additional concern is the failure of psychopathology of the abuser to account for extraneous influences on the abusive situation, where for instance, the social organisation of elder abuse as the causative factor is solely attributed to the perpetrator. Moreover, Anderson and Mangels (2006) argue that the psychopathology of the abuser theory is based on an untestable hypothesis and should be reviewed with caution. Consequently, as a theory, psychopathology of the abuser should be considered as a possible risk factor rather than an overarching, explanatory framework.

Social learning theory and intergenerational abuse

The social learning theory emerged from the work of the classic learning theorists in behaviourist psychology (Pavlov 1927, Skinner 1953, Bandura 1965). In early explanations of family abuse, the idea of learned behaviour being a causative factor provided the cornerstone of etiological explorations, particularly in regard to child abuse (Kempe et al. 1962). The social learning theory suggests that abuse occurs when the perpetrator of abuse uses violence to obtain the victim's compliance and resolve conflict. The early literature suggested that families in which an older person was abused had a history of dysfunction (Quinn and Tomita 1986). Consequently, the abuse is normalised within the family and transmitted through generations (transgenerational violence). The selected abusive activity is underpinned by the anticipated consequences of the behaviour rather than any 'drive like' properties or personality traits (Bandura 1986, Bennett et al. 1997).

Although the argument that abuse can be a learned behaviour seems credible, research has not generally supported this explanation (Bennett et al. 1997). However, it has been acknowledged that these studies were limited by small sample sizes which hindered the sensitive discrimination of complex factors related to elder abuse (Homer and Gilleard 1990, Grafstrom et al. 1992). Furthermore, in a review of social learning theories and intergenerational violence, some commentators have argued that these explanations deny free will and choice due to a benevolent, purist, deterministic, cause and effect attitude (Davenport 2002, Weiten and Lloyd 2009). In relation to trans-generational violence, it appears that a history of abuse and violence may increase the risk of an individual perpetrating abuse, but this hypothesis has not received sufficient empirical support to provide a theoretical status (Gelles 1997). In addition, like the theory of psychopathology of the abuser, the focus is on the individual perpetrator rather than any acknowledgement of the social factors which may impinge on elder abuse perpetration (Bennett et al. 1997).

Symbolic interaction theory

Drawing from the work of George Herbert Mead (1927), Phillips (1986) has proposed that symbolic interactionism is a useful framework in which to examine elder abuse. Elder abuse occurs and is perpetuated due to the difficulties associated with role strain or the inability to renegotiate roles within individual, family or institutional interactions. The abuse activity is facilitated due to the success of the perpetrators' consciously chosen activities in face-to-face interactions and is not simply a learned behaviour. The symbolic interactionist approach offers a non-deterministic, individualist perspective and appears useful due to the consideration of the meaning of acts for individuals (Scott 1995, Bennett et al. 1997). However, symbolic interaction, like propositions such as psychopathology of the abuser and the social learning/intergenerational abuse, also neglects the effect of social structures on the abuse situation as the consequences of actions in a social structure may be outside the influence of the 'actors' involved in the abuse experience. The symbolic interactionist approach emphasises the conscious action of social activities. Unconscious drives and social action that are not explicit are minimalised. As a humanistic approach, symbolic interactionism may undermine the gravity of the abuse situation as this liberal perspective of human understanding can allow negative acts on their own terms to be justified without wider consideration of consequences for other people (Bilton et al. 2002).

Exchange theory

Proponents of the exchange perspective argue that older people become increasingly powerless, vulnerable and dependent on their care-givers as they age and this provides the foundations for abuse as the 'cost' of care-giving increases (Phillips 1986). The imbalance leads to a potential conflict environment and provides the foundations for abuse (Schiamberg and Gans 1999). Exchange theorists highlight the breakdown of reciprocity, in which the perpetrator perceives an unacceptable loss of reward and attempts to regain control through abuse (Biggs et al. 1995). Neglect occurs when the carer responds to a difficult situation by ignoring its presence as reciprocity and the relationship is diminished.

Although the exchange theory has gained some support (Phillips 1986, Jack 1994), it is difficult to assess the costs and benefits in intimate relationships as these can be perceived differently by individuals at various times

(Biggs et al. 1995). The exchange theory may have some explanatory value in terms of relationships which have broken down or where no commitment has existed (Biggs et al. 1995). However, there is some debate regarding its mechanistic underpinnings where such relationships are based on cost and reward. While the exchange theory may provide a useful insight into the wider social factors of elder abuse and neglect (Jack 1994), it has inherent ageist assumptions, for example people do not automatically become powerless and dependent as they grow older. However, it may be that the dependency lies elsewhere, for example the abuser may be dependent on the older person and it is a sense of powerlessness which is the catalyst for abuse (Wolf 1986).

Care-giver stress theory

Although the literature cites varying names for this theory of elder abuse, such as the situational theory and dependency theory, its central premise is that stress of the care-giver results in abuse. Early conceptual frameworks of elder abuse focused on the stressed carer hypothesis due to the dependencies enforced on the care-giver through caring for the older person. Based on child abuse theories (McDonald et al. 1991), the care-giver stress theory suggests that the burden of caring becomes so overwhelming that it creates an environment which leads the carer to abuse (Wolf 1986, Bennett and Kingston 1993, Cullen 1996, Speltz and Raymond 2000, Gilmour 2002). Caring is now recognised as a highly stressful activity (Bennett et al. 1997, Salin et al. 2009) and the carer may assume multiple, competing and complex roles despite a lack of resources in terms of personal ability (Anetzberger 2000). 'Generational inversion' (Steinmetz 1988) may exacerbate stress as adult children who care for their parents may also have families of their own and often have to cope with the responsibility of caring for multiple generations.

The care-giver stress theory proposes that as the stressors associated with situational and/or structural factors increase for the perpetrator the likelihood of abuse towards the older person is simultaneously increased. The situational factors include physical or emotional dependency, impaired mental status or a 'difficult personality', while structural factors refer to economic strain, environmental problems or social isolation. Attributes of the care-giver such as burnout, substance abuse, socio-pathic personality, learning disability or dementia can exacerbate stress levels in care-giving for the older person (Phillips 1986, Wolf 1986, Quinn and Tomita 1997, Kaukinen 2004). Steinmetz (2005) emphasises that it is the care-giver's subjective perception of the stress of care-giving which strongly influences his or her behaviour. If high stress levels are experienced, the possibility of abuse increases.

Although the care-giver stress theory appears credible, empirical support is generally scant. As elder abuse occurs in only a small number of families, a direct correlation between dependency and abuse is questionable (Bennett et al. 1997, Pillemer 2005). Research undertaken in the late 1980s and through-out the 1990s failed to provide evidence to support the view that elder abuse was significantly related to care-giver stress (Pillemer and Finkelhor 1988, Lachs et al. 1996, Phillips et al. 2000). However, carer research has tended to focus on the quality of the relationship (Cooney and Mortimer 1995) and recent research demonstrates a higher abuse prevalence in care-givers of older people with dementia (Cooper et al. 2009, Yan and Kwok 2011). An important limitation of the care-giver stress theory is that it comes dangerously close to blaming the victim (Pillemer 2005). Consequently, care-giver stress may be one of a host of factors contributing to elder abuse, rather than a causative factor (Wolf 2000).

Domestic violence theory

Elder abuse can be conceptualised as domestic violence 'grown old' (Phillips 2000). Domestic violence may be defined as:

> the use of physical or emotional force or threat of physical force, including sexual violence in close adult relationships.
>
> (Task Force on Violence Against Women 1997: 27)

Initially the promotion of the idea that the concept of elder abuse was perpetrated by a 'younger' generation as a way of effectively gaining public attention eclipsed spousal elder abuse. In addition, the image of one older adult hitting another older adult did not have the same pathos as an adult child abusing the older person (Gelles 1997). If spousal elder abuse has been minimalised, it may be due to the more ambiguous moral imagery that this problem conjures up (Pillemer and Finkelhor 1988). Elder victims of domestic violence are often referred to as the 'invisible population' and are frequently marginalised in research and practice (Biggs et al. 1995, Phillips 2000). Despite the scant attention afforded to domestic violence as an explanatory basis for elder abuse, research has highlighted the prevalence of abuse being perpetrated by spouses (Taket 2012). Older women are at greater statistical risk of abuse (Speltz and Raymond 2000, O'Keeffe et al. 2007), which justifies a consideration of elder abuse through the lens of domestic violence theory.

Domestic violence theory emanates from the feminist field of sociological research, and emphasises the social and structural conditions which may predispose one to abusive situations (Jonson and Akerstrom 2004, Yllo 2005). The role of gender is considered crucial in feminist perspectives on violence, particularly within the home environment. Feminists highlight the social and economic processes which can overtly or covertly support a patriarchal society and family structure in which women are suppressed (Jack 1994, Whittaker 1996) particularly by marital dependency (Kaukinen 2004). Although, a negative relationship between age and spousal abuse exists for both genders, spousal abuse represents one of the more common forms of elder abuse (Harris 1996) and is considered as an extreme example of the wider attitudes towards women in society. Thus, abuse is linked to wider social influences such as gender inequality.

In conceptualising elder abuse through a domestic violence lens, the reciprocal nature in abuse situations has emerged as a problematic issue (Phillips et al. 2000). The assertion that there is one dominant abuser (usually seen to be male) is problematic in that a single variable (patriarchy) is used to explain violence while an appreciation of the multiple underpinning factors are minimalised (Bennett et al. 1997). Moreover, feminist theory may be viewed as preserving its own ideology by selecting evidence to support its cause, while research that does not serve its ideological ends is ignored (Dutton and Bodnarchuk 2005) leading to a theoretical 'blindness' (Jonson and Akerstrom 2004). For example, although Muelleman et al. (1996) estimate that women are seven to fourteen times more likely to be physically abused by men, Nelson et al. (2004) points out that women also commit violence against men. According to Dutton (1995), a statistical figure of 8–12 per cent is suf-ficient to warrant spousal abuse as a significant social problem but this fails to meet fundamental criteria for gender analysis or evolutionary criteria. If spousal abuse was due to a 'male' characteristic, male violence should be normally distributed in the population (Dutton and Bodnarchuk 2005). The real issue is power imbalance between partners regardless of gender (Jack 1994, Miller 1994). Power imbalance can explain why both men and women can perpetrate abuse. Thus, the domestic violence theory facilitates some insight into elder abuse, but only when the practical difficulty in its application as an overarching theoretical explanation is acknowledged.

Ecological theory

A more recent elder abuse theory is based on the work of Bronfenbrenner (1979).The ecological theory attempts to integrate the individual, social–psychological and socio-cultural levels of analysis (Gelles 1997) and draws on a broad conceptual framework within which behaviour is viewed as a function of a network of factors, which is called the life matrix. The ecological approach is founded on two assumptions: interdependency of organisms with their environment and a myriad of interaction patterns which are dynamic, adaptive and reciprocal.

Although the ecological model has many applications in the context of family violence, it was first used in an effort to explain the nature of child maltreatment (Dubowitz and Poole 2012) and it has also been used in the domain of domestic violence (Chalk and King 1998) and elder abuse (Schiamberg and Gans 1999, Carp 2000). Schiamberg and Gans (1999) emphasise the imperative of contextually based risk analysis of elder abuse incorporating the dyadic reciprocal relationships involved and the significant contexts of human developmental evolution over the life course. The ecological framework seeks to transcend mere descriptions of elder abuse to systematically explore the interactions within intergenerational relationships and the ongoing and determining factors in abusive relationships. Schiamberg and Gans (1999) have used Bronfenbrenner's (1979) framework, incorporating the micro-system (family), the meso-system (relationship of the family and other principle formal/ informal settings), the exo-system (external factors to the 'focused' person) and the macro-system (broad ideological values and norms of the society). The ecological approach has fundamentally allowed an integration of multiple variables in the individual assessment of the perpetrator and the older person in terms of a developmental life span approach. The ontogenic level considers adult development, ageing and abusive relationships that encompass the particular personal characteristics of the older person and the abuser in terms of health, dependency levels, mental illness or attitude to the actual role of care giving and the receipt of care-giving. Looking at care-giving as a generational event allows the integration of aspects of other elder abuse theoretical frameworks. For example, reciprocity in the exchange theory can be examined over time. This multi-level conceptualisation of intergenerational elder abuse has generally been considered in terms of the adult child care-giver and the older person, but is easily transferable to other intimate relation-ships in domestic elder abuse (Schiamberg and Gans 1999). Risk factors and their interdependence and interrelationships are considered in all levels of the 'ecological context of human development' (Schiamberg and Gans 1999: 98).

In a review of all the theories of elder abuse, the ecological theory offers the most beneficial framework to understanding elder abuse. In particular, it has the potential to provide an explanation which facilitates the changing dynamics of old age, associated relationships and assessment of risk, which are important factors for the development of a comprehensive theory (Bonnie and Wallace 2003). Its ability to focus on multiple dimensions of causative factors and contextual levels allows the integration of complex variables which can contribute to elder abuse. However, as with all the the-oretical propositions to explain elder abuse, supporting empirical data is scant and additional credence for this theory is required (Bennett et al. 1997, Bonnie and Wallace 2003).

Conclusion

This chapter has presented a foundational understanding of elder abuse. Elder abuse is engendered in complex societal perspectives, cultures and in certain taken-for-granted assumptions. Often disclosure of elder abuse by the older person is mired by issues of family allegiance, embarrassment and a fear of perpetrator retribution, yet the consequences of such abuse can be severe and enduring.

In this chapter, 'old age' is examined as a distinct socially constructed phenomenon. Older people do not exist in a vacuum but are subject to particular ways of being through societal expectations, attitudes and prac-tices promoted through culture, policy and legislation. Society can promote both explicit and implicit ageist perspectives, which have an inevitable consequence on the way elder abuse is recognised, tolerated and addressed. Elder abuse, as a unique topic, entered formal discourses though the domain of medicine although the issue transcends boundaries of a single discipline. Moreover, challenges are inherent in the context of terminology, definition and typologies. In attempts to understand elder abuse, theoretical frameworks have struggled to attain empirical support due to the diverse nature of the topic. Thus, understandings of elder abuse remain in a persistent state of flux, constantly changing as new knowledge emerges. The complexity of elder abuse is also apparent in considering environmental settings and a major complicating issue is that of dependency in general and cognitive impairment in particular. However, addressing elder abuse is imperative. Older people do not have time on their side, nor do they have mandatory social networks which can trigger a suspicion of abuse. Moreover, as the global population ages, especially in the older old age group, the potential for elder abuse increases, unless the challenge to address this issue is taken seriously by all members of society.

References

Acierno, R., Hernandez, M.A., Amstadter, A.B., Resnick, H.S., Steve, K., Muzzy, W. and Kilpatrick, D.G. (2010) 'Prevalence and correlates of emotional, physical, sexual, and financial abuse and potential neglect in the United States: The National Elder Mistreatment Study', American Journal of Public Health, 100, 2 : 292–7.

Action on Elder Abuse (1995) 'Action on elder abuse bulletin'. Bulletin 1. Online. Available at <http://www.elderabuse.org.uk/> (accessed 30 March 2006).

Age Action Ireland, University of Ulster, Queen's University, South Eastern Health and Social Care Trust and Social Policy and Ageing Research Centre (2011) 'A total indifference to our dignity': Older people's understanding of elder abuse, Dublin: Age Action.

Amstadter, S.B., Zajac, K., Strachan, M., Hernandez, M.A., Kilpatrick, D.G. and Acierno, R. (2011) 'Prevalence and correlates of elder mistreatment in South Carolina: The South Carolina mistreatment study', Journal of Interpersonal Violence, 26, 15: 2947–72.

Anderson, J. and Mangels, N.J. (2006) 'Helping victims: Social services, healthcare interventions in elder abuse', in R.W. Summer and A.M. Hoffman (eds) Elder abuse: a public health approach, Washington: American Public Health Association.

Anetzberger, G.J. (2000) 'Caregiving: Primary cause for elder abuse?' Generations, 24, 2: 46–52.

Angus, J. and Reeve, P. (2006). 'Ageism: A threat to "aging well" in the 21st century', Journal of Applied Gerontology, 25, 2: 137–152.

Anme, T. (2004) 'A study of elder abuse and risk factors in Japanese families: Focused on the Social Affiliation Model', Geriatrics and Gerontology International, 4: S262–3.

Baker, A.A. (1975) 'Granny bashing', Modern Geriatrics, 8: 20–24.

Baker, M.W. and Heitkemper, M.M. (2005) 'The roles of nurses on inter-professional teams to combat elder mistreatment', Nursing Outlook, 53, 5: 253–9.

Bandura, A. (1965) Principles of behaviour modification. New York: Holt, Rinehart and Winston.

——(1986) Social foundations of thought and action: A social cognitive. Englewood Cliffs, NJ: Prentice Hall.

Beach, S.R., Schulz, R., Williamson, G.M., Miller, L.S., Weiner, L.S. and Lance, C.E. (2005) 'Risk factors for potentially harmful informal caregiver behavior', Journal of the American Geriatrics Society, 53, 2: 255–61.

Ben Natan, M., Lowenstein, A. and Eisikovits, Z. (2010) 'Psycho-social factors affecting elders' maltreatment in long-term care facilities', International Nursing Review, 57, 1: 113–20.

Bennett, G. and Kingston, P. (1993) 'Elder abuse: Concepts, theories and interventions'. London: Chapman & Hall.

Bennett, G., Kingston, P. and Penhale, B. (1997) The dimensions of elder abuse: Perspectives for practitioners. Basingstoke: Macmillan.

Biggs, S. (2007) 'Thinking about generations: Conceptual positions and policy implications', Journal of Social Issues, 63, 4: 695–711.

——, Phillipson, C. and Kingston, P. (1995) Elder abuse in perspective. Buckingham: Open University Press.

Bilton, T., Bonnett, K., Jones, P., Lawson, T., Skinner, D., Stanworth, M. and Webster, A. (2002) Introductory Sociology, 4th edn. Basingstoke: Palgrave Macmillan.

Block, M.R. and Sinnott, J.D. (1979) The Battered Elder Syndrome: An Exploratory Study, College Park, MD: University of Maryland Centre on Ageing.

Bonnie, R.J. and Wallace, R. (2003) 'A theoretical model of elder abuse' in R.J. Bonnie and R. Wallace (eds) Elder mistreatment: Abuse, neglect and exploitation in an aging America. Washington, DC: The National Academy Press.

Boyd, D. and Bee, H. (2004) Lifespan development. Upper Saddle River, NJ: Pearson Education.

Brammer, A. and Biggs, S. (1998) 'Defining elder abuse', Journal of Social Welfare and Family Law, 20, 3: 285–304.

Brandl, B., Bitondo Dyer, C., Heisler, C.J., Marlatt Otto, J., Stiegel, L.A. and Thomas, R.W. (2007) Elder abuse detection and intervention: A collaborative approach. New York: Springer Publishing.

Bronfenbrenner, U. (1979) The ecology of human development: Experiments by nature and design. Cambridge, MA: Harvard University Press.

Burston, G.R. (1975) 'Granny battering', British Medical Journal: 592.

Butler, R. (1969) 'Ageism: Another form of bigotry', The Gerontologist, 9: 243–6.

Cahill, S., O'Shea, E. and Pierce, M. (2012) Future dementia care in Ireland, DSIDC Living with Dementia Programmes, Dublin: Trinity College Dublin.

Callaghan, J.J (1988) 'Elder abuse: Some questions for policy makers', The Gerontologist, 28, 4: 453–8.

Campbell-Rhey, A.M. and Browne, K.D. (2001) 'Risk factor characteristics in carers who physically abuse or neglect their elderly dependents', Aging and Mental Health, 5, 1: 56–62.

Carp, F.M. (2000) Elder Abuse in the Family. New York: Springer Publishing Company.

Chalk, R. and King, P.A. (1998) Violence in families: Assessing prevention and treatment programs. Washington, DC: National Academy Press.

CHI (2002) Investigation into Matters Arising from Care on Rowan Ward-Manchester Mental Health and Social Care Trust. Commission for Health Improvement. London: The Stationery Office.

Choi, N.G. and Mayer, J. (2000) 'Elder abuse neglect and exploitation: Risk factors and prevention strategies', Journal of Gerontological Social Work, 33: 5–25.

Clarfield, M., Ginsberg, G., Rasooly, I., Levic, S., Gindind, J. and Dwolatzky, T. (2009) 'For-profit and not-for-profit nursing homes in Israel: Do they differ with respect to quality of care?' Archives of Gerontology and Geriatrics, 48, 2: 167–72.

Cohen, M., Halevy-Levin, S., Gagin, R., Priltuzky, D. and Friedman, G. (2010) 'Elder abuse in ling-term care residences', Ageing and Society, 30: 1027–40.

Comijs, H.C., Pot, A.M., Bouter, L.M. and Jonker, C. (1998) 'Elder abuse in the community: Prevalence and consequences', Journal of the American Geriatrics Society, 46, 7: 885–8.

Cooney, C. and Mortimer, A. (1995) 'Defining the community context for parent–child relations: The correlation of child maltreatment', Child Development, 49: 604–16.

Cooper, C., Howard, R., and Lawlor, B. (2006) 'Abuse of vulnerable people with dementia by their carers: Can we identity those most at risk?' International Journal of Geriatric Psychiatry, 21, 6: 564–71.

Cooper, C., Selwood, A. and Livingston, G. (2008) 'The prevalence of elder abuse and neglect: A systematic review', Age and Ageing, 37, 2: 157–61.

Cooper, C., Selwood, A., Blanchard, M., Walker, Z., Blizard, R. and Livingston, G. (2009) 'Abuse of people with dementia by family caregivers: Representative cross-sectional survey', British Medical Journal: 338.

Cooper, C., Selwood, A., Blanchard, Z., Walker, R. and Livingston, G. (2010) 'The determinants of family carers' abusive behavior to people with dementia' Journal of Affective Disorders, 121: 136–42.

Davenport, G.C. (2002) An introduction to Child Development, 2nd edn. London: Collins.

DHHS (1998) The national elder abuse incidence study: Final report, US Department of Health and Human Services. Prepared for The Administration for Children and Families and The Administration on Aging by The National Center of Elder Abuse at The American Public Human Services Association in Collaboration with Westat, Inc., New York.

DOHC (2009) The Commission of Investigation Final Report. Department of Health and Children. Dublin: Stationery Office.

Driver, F. (2008) 'Power and pauperism: The workhouse system, 1834–1884', Cambridge: Cambridge University Press.

Dubowitz, H. and Poole, G. (2012) 'Child neglect: An overview', in R.E. Tremblay, M. Boivin and RDeV. Peters (eds) Encyclopedia on Early Childhood Development, Montreal: Centre of Excellence for Early Childhood Development and Strategic Knowledge Cluster on Early Child Development.

Dutton, D.G. (1995) The domestic assault of women. Vancouver: University of British Columbia Press.

——and Bodnarchuk, M. (2005) 'Through a psychological lens: Personality disorder and spouse assault' in D.R. Loseke, R.J. Gelles and M.M. Cavanagh (eds) Current Controversies in Family Violence, 2nd edn. Thousand Oaks, CA: Sage Publications.

Eastman, M. (1988) 'Granny Abuse', Community Outlook, October, 15–16.

Economist (2011) '70 or bust', 9 April, 13. Online. Available at <http://www.economist.com/node/18529505> (accessed 5 April 2012).

Erlingsson, C.I., Saveman, B.I. and Berg, A.C. (2005) 'Perceptions of elder abuse in Sweden: Voices of Older Persons', Brief Treatment and Crisis Intervention, 5, 2: 213–227.

Fulmer, T. and O'Malley, T. (1987) Inadequate care of the elderly: A healthcare perspective on abuse and neglect. New York: Springer Publishing Company.

Fulmer, T., Guadagno, L. Bitondo-Dyer, C. and Connolly, M.T. (2004) 'Progress in elder abuse screening and assessment scales', Journal of the American Geriatric Society, 52, 2: 297–304.

Fulmer, T., Sengstock, M.C., Blankenship, J., Caceres, B., Chandracomar, A., Ng, N. and Wopat, H. (2011) Elder mistreatment in J. Humphreys and J.C. Campbell (eds) Family violence and nursing practice, 2nd edn. New York: Springer Publishing Company.

Fryling, T., Summers, R., and Hoffman, A. (2006) 'Elder abuse: Definition and scope of the problem', in R. Summers and A. Hoffman (eds) Elder abuse: A public health perspective. Washington, DC: American Public Health Association.

Garner, J. (2004) 'The role of the doctor in the institutional abuse of older people: A psychodynamic perspective', Journal of Adult Protection, 6, 4: 16–21.

Gelles, R.J. (1997) Intimate violence in families. Thousand Oaks, CA: Sage Publications.

Gilmour, J.A. (2002) 'Dis/integrated care: Family caregivers and in hospital respite care', Journal of Advanced Nursing, 39, 6: 546–553.

Goergen, T. (2001) 'Stress, conflict, elder abuse and neglect in German nursing homes', Journal of Elder Abuse and Neglect, 13, 1: 1–23.

Grafstrom, M., Norberg, A. and Wimbald, B. (1992) 'Abuse is in the eye of the beholder: Reports by family members about abuse of demented persons in home care – A total population based study', Scandinavian Journal of Social Medicine, 21, 4: 247–55.

Griffore, R.J., Barboza, G.E., Mastin, T., Oehmke, J., Schiamberg, L.B. and Post, L.A. (2009) 'Family members' reports of abuse in Michigan nursing homes', Journal of Elder Abuse and Neglect, 21, 2: 105–14.

Grisso, T. and Appelbaum, P.S. (1998) Assessing competence to consent to treatment: A guide for physicians and other health professionals. New York: Oxford University Press.

Hamberger, L.K and Hastings, J.E. (1986) 'Characteristics of spouse abusers', Journal of Interpersonal Violence, 1: 363–73.

Harbison, J. (1999) 'Models for intervention for elder abuse and neglect: A Canadian perspective on ageism, participation and empowerment', Journal of Elder Abuse and Neglect, 10, 3/4: 1–17.

Harris, S.B. (1996) 'For better or for worse: Spousal abuse grown old', Journal of Elder Abuse and Neglect, 8, 1: 1–33.

Hawes, C. (2002) Elder abuse in residential long-term care facilities: What is known about prevalence, causes and prevention – Testimony before the US Senate Committee of Finance. Online. Available at <http://www.canhr.org/reports/2002/061802chtest.pdf> (accessed 21 March 2012).

Hawes, C. (2003) 'Elder abuse in residential long term care settings', in R.J. Bonnie and R.B. Wallace (eds) Elder mistreatment: Abuse, neglect and exploitation in an aging America. Washington, DC: National Research Council.

Hee-Han, D. (2004) 'A study of the approaching abuse in Korea', Geriatrics and Gerontology International, 4: S264–5.

HSE (2012) HSE policy and procedures for responding to allegations of extreme self-neglect. Health Service Executive. Available at <http://www.hse.ie/eng/services/Publications/services/Older/selfneglectpolicy.pdf> (accessed 12 June 2012).Harris, D.K. and Benson, B.M.L. (2006) Maltreatment of patients in nursing homes: There is no safe place. Binghamton, NY: Haworth Pastoral Press.

Herdman, E. (2002) 'Challenging the discourses of nursing ageism', International Journal of Nursing Studies, 39: 105–14.

Homer, A. and Gilleard, C. (1990) A good old age: The paradox of setting limits. New York: Touchstone.

Hughes, M (1995) 'Abuse of older people: A network approach to service provider training', Australian Social Work, 48, 4: 21–7.

Ignatieff, M. (2001) 'The attack on human rights', Foreign Affairs, 80, 6: 102–16.

Jack, R. (1994) 'Dependence, power and violation: Gender issues in abuse of elderly people by informal carers', in M. Eastman (ed.) Old Age Abuse: A New Persective. London: Chapman and Hall.

Jogerst, G.J., Daly, J.M., Dawson, J.D., Peek-Asa, C., and Schmuch, G.A. (2006) 'Iowa nursing home characteristics associated with reported abuse', Journal of the American Medical Directors Association, 7, 4: 203–7.

Johns, S. and Hydle, I. (1995) 'Weakness in welfare', in J.I. Kosberg and J.L. Garcia (eds) Elder abuse: International and cross-cultural perspectives, Binghamton, NY: Haworth Press Inc.

Johnson, T.F. (1986) 'Critical issues in the definition of elder mistreatment', in K. Pilemer and R. Wolf (eds), Elder Abuse: Conflict in the Family. Dover, MA: Auburn House Publishing Company.

Jonson, H. and Akerstrom, M. (2004) 'Neglect of elderly women in feminist studies of violence: A case for ageism', Journal of Elder Abuse and Neglect, 16, 1: 47–63.

Just, M.M. (2007) 'Issues in caregiving: Elder abuse and substance abuse', Journal of Human Behaviour in the Social Environment, 14, 1: 117–37.

Katz, S. (1996) Disciplining old age: The formation of gerontological knowledge. Charlottesville, VA: University Press of Virginia.

Kaukinen, C. (2004) 'Status incompatibility, physical violence and emotional abuse in intimate relationships', Journal of Marriage and Family, 66: 452–71.

Kempe, C.H., Silver, F., Steele, B.F., Droegmueller, W. and Silver, H. (1962) 'The battered child syndrome', Journal of the American Medical Association, 181: 17–24.

Killick, J.C. (2008) 'Factors influencing judgements of social care professionals on adult protection referrals'. Unpublished thesis, University of Ulster.

Kingston, P. and Penhale, B. (1995) 'Elder abuse and neglect: Issues in the Accident and Emergency Department', Accident and Emergency Nursing, 3: 122–128.

Kosberg, J.I and Garcia, J.L. (1995) Elder abuse: An international and cross cultural perspective. New York: The Haworth Press.

Kosberg, J.I., Lowenstein, A., Garcia, J.L. and Biggs, S. (2003) 'Study of elder abuse within diverse cultures', Journal of Elder Abuse and Neglect, 15, 3/4: 71–9.

Krug, E.G., Dahlberg, L.L., Mercy, J.A., Zwi, A.B., and Lorano, R. (2002) Report on violence and health. Geneva: WHO.

Kwan, A.Y. (1995) 'Elder abuse in Hong Kong', in J.I. Josberg and J.L. Garcia (eds) Elder abuse: International and cross-cultural perspectives, Binghamton, NY: Haworth Press Inc.

Lachs, M.S., Williams, C., O'Brien, S., Hurst, L., and Horwitz, R. (1996) 'Older adults: An 11 year longitudinal study of adult protective service use', Archives of Internal Medicine, 156, 4: 449–53.

Lachs, M.S., Williams, C.S., O'Brien, S., Pillemer, K.A. and Charlson, M.E. (1998) 'The mortality of elder mistreatment', Journal of the American Medical Association, 280, 5: 428–32.

Lachs, M.S., Bachman, R., Williams, C.S. and O' Leary, J.R. (2007) 'Resident to resident elder mistreatment and police contact in nursing homes: Findings from a population based cohort', *Journal of the American Geriatric Society*, 55, 6: 840–45.

Lafferty, A., Treacy, M.P, Fealy, G., Drennan, J., and Lyons, I. (2011) Older people's experiences of mistreatment and abuse. Dublin: National Centre for the Protection of Older People, University College Dublin.

Lanzieri, G. (2006) Statistics in focus: Populations and social conditions. Online. Available at <http://epp.eurostat.ec.europa.eu/cache/ITY_OFFPUB/KS-NK-06-003/EN/KS-NK-06-003-EN.PDF> (accessed 1 November 2011).

Leeson, G.W. and Harper, S. (2008) Some descriptive finding from the global ageing survey: Investing in Later Life. Research Report 108. Oxford: Oxford Institute of Ageing.

Lifespan of Greater Rochester Inc., Weill Cornell Medical Center of Cornell University and New York City Department for the Aging (2011) Under the radar: New York State elder abuse prevalence study. New York: New York Department for the Aging.

Lindbloom, E.J., Brandt, J., Hough, L. and Meadows, S.E. (2007) 'Elder mistreatment in the nursing home: A systematic review', *Journal of the American Medical Directors Association*, 8, 9: 610–16.

Lowenstein, A., Eisikovits, Z., Band-Winterstein, T. and Enosh, G. (2009) 'Is elder abuse and neglect a social phenomenon? Data from the First National Prevalence Survey in Israel', *Journal of Elder Abuse and Neglect*, 21, 3: 253–77.

Macdonald, A.D.J. (1997) 'ABC of mental health: Mental health in old age', *British Medical Journal*, 315: 413–17.

McDonald, L. and Collins, A. (2000) Abuse and Neglect of Older Adults: A Discussion Paper. Ottawa: Health Canada, Family Violence Prevention Unit.

McDonald, L., Beaulieu, M., Harbison, J., Hirst, S., Lowenstein, A., Podnieks, E. and Wahl, J. (2012) 'Institutional abuse of older adults: What we know, what we need to know', *Journal of Elder Abuse and Neglect*, 24, 2: 138–60.

McDonald, P.L., Hornick, J.P., Robertson, G.B. and Wallace, J.E. (1991) Elder Abuse and Neglect in Canada. Toronto, ON: Butterworths.

Malmedal, W., Oddbjørn, I, Britt-Inger, S. (2009) 'Inadequate care in Norwegian nursing homes as reported by nursing staff', *Scandinavian Journal of Caring Sciences*, 23: 231–42.

Marmolejo, I.I. (2008) Elder abuse in the family in Spain. Valencia: Fundacion de la Comunitat Valenciana.

Mead, G.H. (1927) Mind, self and society from the standpoint of social behaviouralism. Chicago, IL: University of Chicago Press.

Means, R. and Smith, R. (1998) From Poor Law to community care: The development of welfare services for elderly people 1939–1971. Bristol: Policy Press.

Meddaugh, D.I. (1993) 'Covert elder abuse in Nursing Homes', *Journal of Elder Abuse and Neglect*, 5, 3: 21–37.

Millard, P. and Roberts, A. (1991) 'Old and forgotten' Nursing Times, 87, 22: 24–8.

Miller, S.L. (1994) 'Expanding the boundaries: Towards a more inclusive and integrated study of intimate violence' Violence and Victims, 9, 2: 183–94.

——, Lewis, M.S., Williamson, G.M., Lance, C.E., Dooley, W.K., Schulz, R. and Weiner, M.F. (2006) 'Caregiver cognitive status and potentially harmful behavior', Aging and Mental Health, 10, 2: 125–33.

Minichiello, V., Browne, J. and Kendig, H. (2000) 'Perceptions and consequences of ageism: Views of older people', Ageing and Society, 20: 253–78.

Mixon, P.M. (1995) 'An adult protective services perspective', Journal of Elder Abuse and Neglect, 7, 2/3: 69–87.

Mowlam, A., Tennant, R., Dixon, J. and McCreadie, C. (2007) UK study of abuse and neglect of older people: Qualitative findings. London: King's College London and the National Centre for Social Research.

Muelleman, R.L., Lenaghan, P.A. and Pakieser, R.A. (1996) 'Battered women, injury location and types', Annals of Emergency Medicine, 28: 486–92.

Naughton, C., Drennan, J., Treacy, M.P., Lafferty, A., Lyons, I., Phelan, A., Quin, S., O'Loughlin, A. and Delaney, L. (2010) Abuse and neglect of older people in Ireland, Dublin: National Centre for the Protection of Older People, University College Dublin.

Nelson, H.D., Nygren, P., McInerney, Y. and Klein, J. (2004) 'Screening women and elderly adults for family and intimate partner violence: A review of the evidence for the U.S. preventative services', Annals of Internal Medicine, 140, 5: 387–404.

Neugarten, B.L. (1974) 'Age groups in American society and the rise of the young-old', Annals of the American Academy of Political and Social Science, 415: 187–98.

Neysmith, S.M. (1995) 'Power in relationships of trust' in M.J. McLean (ed.) Abuse and neglect of older people: Strategies for change. Toronto: Thompson Educational Publishing.

O'Connor, D., Hall, M.I. and Donnelly, M. (2009) 'Assessing capacity within a context of abue or neglect', Journal of Elder Abuse and Neglect, 21, 2: 156–69.

O'Keeffe, M., Hills, A., Doyle, M., McCreadie, C., Scholes, S., Constantine, R., Tinker, A., Manthorpe, J., Biggs, S. and Erens, B. (2007) United Kingdom study of abuse and neglect of older people. London: King's College London and the National Centre for Social Research.

Pavlik, V.N., Hyman, D.J., Festa, N.A. and Bitondo Dyer, C. (2001) 'Quantifying the problem of abuse and neglect in adults-analysis of a state-wide database', Journal of American Geriatrics Association, 49: 45–8.

Pavlou, M.P. and Lachs, M.S. (2006) 'Could self-neglect in older adults be a geriatric syndrome?' Journal of the American Geriatric Society, 54, 5: 831–42.

Pavlov, I. (1927) Conditional reflexes: An investigation of the physiological activity of the cerebral cortex. Oxford: Oxford University Press.

Phillips, L. (1986) 'Theoretical explanations of elder abuse', in K. Pillemer and R. Wolf (eds) Elder abuse: Conflict in the family. Dover, MA: Auburn House Publishing Company.

Penhale, B. and Parker, J. (2003) 'Protecting vulnerable adults', in J. Horwath and S. Shardlow (eds) Making links across specialisms. Bournemouth: Russell House.

Perel-Levin, S. (2008) Discussing screening for elder abuse at primary health care level. Geneva: WHO.

Phelan, A. (2008) 'Elder abuse, ageism, human rights and citizenship: Implications for nursing discourse', Nursing Inquiry, 15, 4: 320–30.

——(2010) 'Discursive constructions of elder abuse: Community nurses' accounts'. Unpublished thesis, University College Dublin.

——(2011) 'Socially constructing older people: Examining discourses which can shape nurses' understanding and practice', Journal of Advanced Nursing, 67, 4: 893–903.

Phillips, L. (1986) 'Theoretical explanations of elder abuse', in K. Pillemer and R. Wolf (eds) Elder abuse: Conflict in the family. Dover, MA: Auburn House Publishing Company.

——(2000) 'Domestic violence and aging women', Geriatric Nursing, 21, 4: 188–195.

——, de Ardon E.T. and Solis Briones, G. (2000) 'Abuse of female caregivers by care recipients: Another form of elder abuse', Journal of Elder Abuse and Neglect, 12, 3/4: 123–45.

Pickering, M. (2001) Stereotypes: The politics of separation. Basingstoke: Palgrave.

Pillemer, K. (2005) 'Elder abuse is caused by deviance and dependence of abusive caregivers', in D.R. Loseke, R.J. Gelles and M.M. Cavanagh (eds) Current Controversies on Family Violence, 2nd edn. Thousand Oaks, CA: Sage Publications.

——and Finkelhor, D. (1988) 'The prevalence of elder abuse: A random sample survey', Gerontologist, 28(1), 51–7.

——and Moore, D. (1989) 'Abuse of patients in nursing homes: Findings from a survey of staff', The Gerontologist, 29, 3: 314–20.

Podnieks, E. (1995) 'Introduction: Education issues related to the abuse and neglect of older Canadians', in M.J. MacLean (ed.) Abuse and neglect of older Canadians. Ottawa: Canadian Association of Gerontology.

Posner, R.A. (1996) Ageing and old age. Chicago, IL: University of Chicago Press.

Post, L., Page, C., Conner, T., Prokhorov, A., Fang, Y. and Bioscak, B.J. (2010) 'Elder abuse in long-term care: Types, patterns and risk factors', Research on Aging, 32, 3: 323–48.

Quinn, M.J. and Tomita, S.K. (1986) Elder abuse and neglect. New York: Springer Publishing Company.

Quinn, M.J. and Tomita, S.K. (1997) Elder abuse and neglect: Causes, diagnosis, and interventional strategies. New York: Springer Publishing Company.

Reinharz, S. (1986) 'Loving and hating one's elders: Twin themes in legend and literature', in K. Pillemer and R. Wolf (eds) Elder abuse: Conflict in the family. Dover, MA: Auburn House Publishing Company.

Reyes-Ortiz, C.A. (2001) 'Diogenes syndrome: The self-neglect elderly', Comprehensive Therapy, 27, 2: 117–21.

Rhodes, W. (2005) 'A model to estimate the prevalence of hard-to-reach populations', Abt Associates, abstracts. Online. Available at <http://www.abtassociates.com/Page.cfm?PageId=16285> (accessed 15 May 2010).

Roberto, K.A., Teaster, P.B., and Nikzad, K.A. (2007) 'Sexual abuse of vulnerable adult men', Journal of Interpersonal Violence, 22, 8: 1009–23.

Roscigno, V.J., Mong, S., Byron, R., and Tester, G. (2007) 'Age discrimination, social closure and employment', Social Forces, 86, 1: 313–24.

Rosen, T., Lachs, M.S. and Pillemer, K. (2010) 'Sexual aggression between residents in nursing homes: Literature synthesis of an under-recognised problem', Journal of the American Geriatrics Society, 58: 1070–79.

Rosenberg, M.L. and Fenley, M.A. (1991) Violence in America: A public health approach. New York: Oxford University Press.

Ruf, P. (2006) 'Understanding elder abuse in minority populations', in R.W. Summer and A.M. Hoffman (eds) Elder abuse: A public health perspective. Washington, DC: American Public Health Association.

Salin, S., Kaunonen, M., and Åstedt-Kurki, P. (2009) 'Informal carers of older family members: How they manage and what support they receive from respite care', Journal of Clinical Nursing, 18, 4: 492–501.

Sandvide, Å, Åström, S, Norberg, A., and Saveman, B.I. (2004) 'Violence in institutional care for elderly people from the perspective of involved care providers', Scandinavian Journal of the Caring Sciences, 18, 4: 351–7.

Saveman, B.I., Aström, S., Gösta, B. and Norberg, A. (1999) 'Elder abuse in residential settings in Sweden', Journal of Elder Abuse and Neglect, 10, 1: 43–60.

Schiamberg, L.B and Gans, D. (1999) 'An ecological framework for contextual risk factors in elder abuse', Journal of Elder Abuse and Neglect, 11, 1: 79–103.

Schiamberg, L.B., Barboza, G.G., Oehmke, J., Zhang, Z., Griffore, R.J., Weatherill, R.P., von Heydrich, L and Post, L.A. (2011) 'Elder abuse in nursing homes: An ecological perspective', Journal of Elder Abuse and Neglect, 23, 2: 190–211.

Schwaiger, L. (2006) 'To be forever young? Towards reframing corporeal subjectivity in maturity', International Journal of Ageing and Later Life, 1, 1: 11–41.

Scott, J. (1995) Sociological theory: Contemporary debates. Aldershot: Edward Elgar.

Selwood, A., Cooper, C., and Livingston, G. (2007) 'What is elder abuse: Who decides?' International Journal of Geriatric Psychiatry, 22: 1009–12.

Shaffer, D.R., Dooley, W.K. and Williamson, G.M. (2007) 'Endorsement of proactively aggressive caregiving strategies moderates the relation between the caregiver mental health and potentially harmful caregiving behavior', Psychology and Aging, 22, 3: 494–504.

Shinan-Altman, S. and Cohen, M. (2009) 'Nurses aides' attitudes to elder abuse in nursing homes, the effect of work stressors and burnout', The Gerontologist. 10: 1093.

Sinclair, T. (2005) 'Mad, bad or sad? Ideology, distorted communication and child abuse prevention', Journal of Sociology, 41: 227–46.

Skinner, B.F. (1953) Science and human behaviour. Basingstoke: Macmillan.

Solem, P.E. (2005) 'Ageism, ageing and social participation', Nordisk Psykologi, 57, 1: 47–63.

Speltz, K. and Raymond, J. (2000) 'Elder abuse, including domestic violence in later life', Wisconsin Lawyer, 73, 9: 1–5.

Steinmetz, S.K. (1988) Elder abuse and family care. Newbury Park, CA: Sage Publications.

——(2005) 'Elder abuse is caused by the perception of stress associated with providing care', in D.R. Loseke, R.J. Gelles and M.M. Cavanagh (eds) Current Controversies on Family Violence. Thousand Oaks, CA: Sage Publications.

Stones, M.J. (1995) 'Scope and definition of elder abuse and neglect in Canada', in M.J. MacLean (ed.) Abuse and neglect of older Canadians: Strategies for change. Toronto: Thompson Educational Publishing Inc.

Straka, S.M. and Montminy, L. (2008) 'Family Violence: Through the lens of power and control', Journal of Emotional Abuse, 8, 3: 255–79.

Straus, M.A. (1979) 'Measuring intra-family conflict and violence: the conflict tactics (CT) scale', Journal of Marriage and the Family, 41: 75–88.

Taket, A. (2012) 'Responding to domestic violence in primary care: We know more about what works but questions remain' British Medical Journal, 344: 1–2.

Task Force on Violence Against Women (1997) Report of the Task Force on Violence Against Women. Dublin: Stationery Office.

Teaster, P.B. and Roberto, K.A. (2003) 'Sexual abuse of older women living in nursing homes'. Journal of Gerontological Social Work, 40, 4: 105–19.

TSO (2005) Mental Capacity Act, London: The Stationery Office.

Twomey, M., Quinn, M.J. and Dakin, E. (2005) 'From behind closed doors: Shedding light on elder abuse and domestic violence in later life', Journal for the Centre for Families, Children and the Courts, 6: 73–80.

UN (2004) 'Modalities for the review and appraisal of the Madrid International Plan of Action on Ageing, 2002'. UN Economic and Social Council: Commission for Social Development. Online. Available at <http://www.un-ngls.org/pdf/Ageing_Ecosoc_Res.pdf> (accessed 21 October 2011).

Wallace, H. (2003) Family violence: Legal, medical and social perspectives, 4th edn. Boston, MA: Pearson.

Ward Griffin, L. (1998) 'Elder maltreatment in the African American Community: You just don't hit your Momma!!!' in T. Tartara (ed.) Understanding elder abuse in minority populations. Philadelphia, PA: Brunner/Manzel.

Weiten, W. and Lloyd, M.A. (2009) Psychology applied to modern life, 8th edn, Florence, KY: Wadsworth Publishing Co. Inc.

WGEA (2002) Protecting our future, Working Group on Elder Abuse, DOHC. Dublin: Stationery Office.

Whittaker, T. (1996) 'Violence Gender and Elder Abuse', in B. Fawcett, B. Featherstone, J. Hern and C.Toft (eds) Violence and gender relations: Theories and interventions. London: Sage Publications.

WHO (1995) 'How to prevent burnout', International Nursing Review, 42, 5: 159.

——(2002a) Active ageing: A policy framework. Online. Available at <http://whqlibdoc.who.int/hq/2002/WHO_NMH_NPH_02.8.pdf> (accessed 4 March 2011).

——(2002b) 'The Toronto declaration on the global prevention of elder abuse', Geneva: World Health Organisation.

——(2011) European report on preventing elder mistreatment. Copenhagen: World Health Organisation.

——and INPEA (2002) Missing voices: Views of older persons on elder abuse. Geneva: World Health Organisation and International Network for the prevention of Elder Abuse.

Wiglesworth, A., Mosqueda, L., Mulnard, R., Liao, S., Gibbs, L. and Fitzgerald, W. (2010) 'Screening for abuse and neglect of people with dementia', Journal of the American Geriatric Society, 58: 493–500.

Wolf, R. (1986) 'Major findings from the three models project on elderly abuse', in K. Pilemer and R. Wolf (eds) Elder abuse: Conflict in the family. Dover, MA: Auburn House Publishing Company.

——(2000) 'The nature and scope of elder abuse'. Generations, 24, 2: 6–13.

——and Pillemer, K. (1989) Helping elderly victims: The reality of elder abuse. New York: Columbia University Press.

Yan, E. and Kwok, T. (2011) 'Abuse of older Chinese with dementia by family caregivers: An inquiry into the role of caregiver burden', International Journal of Geriatric Psychiatry, 26: 527–35.

Yllo, K.A. (2005) 'Through a feminist lens: Gender, diversity and violence: Extending the feminist framework', in D.R. Loseke, R.J. Gelles and M.M. Cavanagh M.M. (eds) Current controversies in family violence, 2nd edn. Thousand Oaks, CA: Sage Publications.

Zhang, Z., Schiamberg, L.B., Oehmke, J., Barboza, G.E., Giffore, R.J., Post, L.P., Weatherill, R.P. and Mastin, T. (2011) 'Neglect of older adults in Michigan nursing homes', Journal of Elder Abuse and Neglect, 23: 58–74.

Zink, T. and Fisher, B.S. (2007) 'The prevalence and incidence of intimate partner violence and interpersonal mistreatment in older women in primary care', Journal of Elder Abuse and Neglect, 18, 1: 83–105.

2 Australia

Susan Kurrle

Introduction

In Australia, acknowledgement that older people were at risk of exploitation and abuse from relatives, friends and the general community first occurred in 1975 in a national government report (Social Welfare Commission 1975), but further recognition of the issue did not occur until the late 1980s when health care workers and police began to talk about cases of abuse in older people that they were seeing in their day to day work. There were a number of different terms used, including 'abuse of vulnerable adults', 'abuse of older people' and 'aged abuse'. These were replaced by the term 'elder abuse' in the early 2000s in keeping with US and international terminology.

Whilst elder abuse had been mentioned in 1990 in government reports from the states of Victoria (Barron et al. 1990) and South Australia (McCallum et al. 1990), the first reference to elder abuse in professional journals was a case series reported in the *Medical Journal of Australia* in 1991 (Kurrle et al. 1991). The publication of this study resulted in a marked raising of awareness of the problem particularly in New South Wales, with later recognition in other states. Taskforces and working parties were assembled to address the problem and develop policies and protocols, undertake research, and implement education and training. These occurred at an individual state level, resulting in a diverse range of responses across Australia, with no nationally integrated system. Several states have developed specific services to respond to abuse, and other states have emphasised the use of existing services and programmes to deal with elder abuse. These are described later in this chapter. At the service level, most agencies or service providers who have older people as clients have developed education and training programs and protocols for responding to cases of elder abuse.

Background to aged care in Australia

Australia is an ageing society with 13.6 per cent of its population of 22.3 million people (in 2010) aged 65 years and over. This is projected to rise to 18 per cent of the population by 2021 (about four million people).

Approximately one-third of Australia's population aged 65 years and over was born overseas (including the United Kingdom), coming from over 160 countries, and speaking more than 100 different languages.

Australia is a federation of six states and two territories. There is a strong national social security and welfare system in Australia which provides means-tested income support to the unemployed, single parents, the disabled and older people. All Australian residents have access to Medicare, the universal health insurance scheme which subsidises all primary health care through general practitioners, and services provided by medical specialists. Pharmaceuticals are also subsidised for all Australians through the Pharmaceutical Benefits Scheme. People who are admitted to a public hospital as a public patient are treated free of charge.

Most Australians prefer to remain in their own homes as they grow older, and those who need care receive it mainly from informal carers such as family members, neighbours and friends. Formal care services in the community are provided through many different organisations with considerable funding from the national government. Services provided include home-delivered meals, home help, nursing care, personal care, community transport, community activity centres, home maintenance or modification, and respite care. Packages of care provided in the community are also available, with Community Aged Care Packages providing up to six hours per week of care, and Extended Aged Care at Home Packages providing up to 18 hours of care per week. Some fees are charged for these services and are usually means tested. Approximately 13 per cent of the older population receive some community care services.

If older people are unable to continue to manage in their own homes, there is a comprehensive residential care system which is available to all older residents of Australia. Currently around 8 per cent of older people live in residential care. Both nursing home care ('high' care) and hostel care ('low' care) are provided as part of residential care. These facilities are subsidised by the national government according to the level of dependency of the resident, with a contribution paid by the resident. This amount is means tested and linked to the age pension.

No older person can enter residential care without an assessment from an Aged Care Assessment Team (ACAT). These are multidisciplinary teams (usually consisting of medical practitioner, nurse, social worker, occupational therapist and other allied health staff) which undertake assessment of the medical, functional and social needs of older people, and make recommendations to assist them to remain as independent as possible. These teams give approval for receipt of packages of care and for admission to residential care and may also make referrals to community services or other service. They are accessible throughout Australia and there is no charge for their assessments or provided services. ACATs are traditionally based with hospital aged care services. This enables close linkages between the community services and hospital-based aged care and assists in improving the continuum of care for older people. ACATs are identified as one of the key services likely to encounter cases of abuse, and ACATs throughout Australia have developed policies and protocols for management of elder abuse.

Definitions of elder abuse and neglect

There are several definitions of elder abuse in current use in Australia. These are:

- Elder abuse: Any act occurring within a relationship where there is an implication of trust, which results in harm to an older person. Abuse may be physical, sexual, financial, psychological, social and/or neglect. (Australian Network for the Prevention of Elder Abuse – ANPEA) (Cripps 2000).
- Abuse of older people: A single or repeated act occurring within a relationship where there is an implication of trust, which causes harm to an older person (WHO 2001).
- Elder abuse: Any pattern of behaviour which causes physical, psychological, financial or social harm to an older person. The abuse occurs in the context of a relationship between the abused person and the abuser. The abuser may be a family member, friend, neighbour, paid carer or other person in close contact with the victim. (Australian and New Zealand Society for Geriatric Medicine – ANZSGM) (Kurrle 2004).

These definitions are similar in concept and emphasise that harm occurs to an older person as the result of behaviour occurring within a relationship of trust. The definitions do not have an age limit as it is acknowledged that age-related conditions such as dementia may occur in younger people rendering them vulnerable to the same forms of abuse as an older person. The definitions also exclude self-neglect and self-harm, and exclude harm from a stranger.

Five main types of elder abuse are recognized:

- Physical abuse: The infliction of physical pain or injury, or physical coercion. Examples include any form of assault such as hitting, slapping, pushing, burning. This category also includes physical restraint and overmedication.
- Sexual abuse: Sexually abusive or exploitative behaviour, ranging from indecent assault and sexual harassment to violent rape.
- Psychological abuse: The infliction of mental anguish, involving actions that cause fear of violence, isolation or deprivation, and feelings of shame, indignity and powerlessness. Examples include verbal intimidation, humiliation and harassment, shouting, threats of physical harm or institutionalisation, and withholding of affection.
- Financial or material abuse: The illegal or improper use of the older person's property or finances. This would include misappropriation of money, valuables or property, forced changes to a will or other legal document, and denial of the right of access to, or control over, personal funds.

- Neglect: The failure of a caregiver to provide the necessities of life to an older person i.e. adequate food, shelter, clothing, medical care or dental care. Neglect may involve the refusal to permit other people to provide appropriate care. Examples include abandonment, non-provision of food, clothing or shelter, under use of medication, and poor hygiene or personal care.

The Australian response to elder abuse

Australia does not have a nationally integrated system to deal with elder abuse, although the national-government-funded ACATs are an important resource across the country. State governments have the primary responsibility for services relating to elder abuse and they have developed a range of responses including:

- individual support, counselling;
- specialist aged care services;
- integrated health and community services;
- information, advocacy and referral services;
- legal interventions including criminal law;
- domestic violence legislation;
- substituted decision-making legislation;
- guardianship legislation;
- information and referral telephone help lines.

The response of the Australian national government to elder abuse

As mentioned above, most developments in elder abuse policy and practice have occurred at the state level. However, in 1994, the national government set up a working party on protection of frail older people in the community with representation from all Australian states and including people from a wide range of backgrounds. The report identified ACATs as key services likely to encounter situations of elder abuse (DHSH 1994). It recommended that protocols and guidelines for addressing elder abuse be developed by these Teams. The report of the working party was successful in placing elder abuse on the national social policy agenda.

In 2006, the national government began to respond to elder abuse in residential care settings with the introduction of an aged care complaints scheme. In 2007 mandatory reporting of physical or sexual abuse in residential care facilities was introduced. This is further discussed in the legislation section below.

The response of state governments to elder abuse

South Australia

In 1990, a research project provided information on the scope and nature of elder abuse in South Australia, and provided the framework for a government response (McCallum et al. 1990). An elder protection programme committee was set up in 1992 with the subsequent development of the elder protection programme in 1994 and funded staff to provide support and assistance to existing service providers dealing with situations of elder abuse.

This programme has been delivered by the Aged Rights Advocacy Service (ARAS) since 1997 (www.agedrights.asn.au). ARAS provides an advocacy service for older people who are at risk of abuse or are actually experiencing abuse. ARAS has also developed a website for staff of residential care facilities called Abuse Prevention: Preventing Abuse of Older People (www.elderabuse. org.au), and provides advice and assistance for indigenous Australians in abuse situations through the Aboriginal Advocacy Programme.

As in all the states and territories, detection of elder abuse has been seen as the responsibility of frontline agencies or services such as general practitioners (family physicians), ACATs, geriatric health services, home nursing services, home care service providers and other aged care service providers. The advocacy model utilised by ARAS has been developed to assist in the individual management of cases of elder abuse once they have been identified. ARAS is a free, confidential, independent, state-wide service which acts as an 'agent of change'. It does this by providing the victim of abuse with information, strategies and options to overcome the abuse, and it gives support to the victim of abuse in decision making. ARAS also provides information and advice to aged care providers working with victims of abuse.

ARAS also provides education on elder abuse to community groups of older people and to aged care organisations and service providers, and this education has resulted in a raising of awareness of the issues around abuse and possible risk factors. The education has focussed on ways to prevent abuse occurring by encouraging older people to plan for the future. It provides information on wills, on enduring powers-of-attorney and on decision making with regards to accommodation. It encourages older people to stay active and involved in their community.

New South Wales

The New South Wales (NSW) government demonstrated leadership in addressing elder abuse in the early 1990s with major contributions to research, policy and programme development. Through the Office on Ageing, it established the NSW Taskforce on Abuse of Older People in 1991. This taskforce conducted extensive consultations throughout NSW with more than 550 organisations and individuals, commissioned research in a number of related areas, and released its report 'The abuse of older people in their homes' (NSWADD 1993).

In 1995 an interagency response to elder abuse was formally developed and released by the NSW government with the publication of 'Abuse of older people: An Interagency Protocol' (NSWADD 1995). This protocol had a primary focus on ways of responding to elder abuse, and was designed to assist frontline agencies in dealing with cases of elder abuse. A set of principles for responding to elder abuse was also developed and released with the protocol. The education that formed part of the promulgation of this protocol and the accompanying principles was very important in the raising of awareness of issues around elder abuse. All health services in NSW and the NSW Police Force have developed protocols for dealing with abuse, and these protocols are reviewed at regular intervals. The NSW Interagency Protocol was last reviewed in 2007 and can be found at: http://www.adhc.nsw.gov.au/__ data/assets/file/0011/228386/InteragencyProtocol1.pdf

Queensland

The start of Queensland's response to elder abuse came from the non-government sector with the formation of a Taskforce on the Prevention of Intimidation of the Elderly by the Queensland Council of Carers in 1990. This taskforce organised a national conference entitled 'Dignity and security: The rights of older people' in 1992 which was the first conference in Australia devoted to the issue of elder abuse.

In 1994, the Project on Abuse of Older People commenced with support from the Queensland Department of Family Services and the Office of Ageing. This Project developed guides to protocol development and legal services and recommended the formation of a specific unit to address elder abuse. This occurred in 1997 with the implementation of the Elder Abuse Prevention Unit (EAPU) and its brief has been to prevent and respond to elder abuse in Queensland (www.eapu.com.au). EAPU is based in Brisbane but also has staff working in three regional centres. It raises awareness of the nature and extent of elder abuse through involvement with community groups and by developing and disseminating resources. It provides education to service providers, seniors' organisations, and other community groups. It also provides a state-wide confidential telephone help line to provide information and advice on elder abuse to older people, families and carers, and the community generally, and advice and support to victims of abuse, family members and service providers. EAPU staff are also available to provide direct advice to victims of abuse and assist aged care service providers in dealing with cases of abuse. They do not provide case management, which remains the role of the aged care service providers.

Victoria

Victoria took a different approach to elder abuse from the other states following the release of the report 'No innocent bystanders' (Barron et al. 1990). In this report, the issue of elder abuse was seen in the context of broader societal explanations such as ageism, sexism and patriarchy, rather than at an individual or family level. As a result the Victorian government took a broader approach to elder abuse and encouraged a generic approach with all services dealing with older people having the knowledge to identify and manage cases of abuse. The government policy recommended that all agencies that deliver services to older people develop protocols and procedures to deal with elder abuse and neglect. Like NSW it did not recommend a specialist agency to respond to elder abuse.

The Victorian government released its guide 'With respect to age' in 1995 (VDHCS 1995) and this contained a flowchart which provided services with a blueprint to assist in developing responses to elder abuse. A number of comprehensive protocols and guidelines were developed which emphasised a multidisciplinary approach and encouraged linkages between health-based services, such as ACATs, geriatric health services and general practitioners, and community-based services, such as home nursing and providers of community aged care packages.

In 2003, the Office of the Public Advocate submitted a report to the Victorian government expressing concern that the issue of elder abuse was not receiving adequate attention or policy action. This resulted in the commissioning of a report by the government into elder abuse. This report titled 'Strengthening Victoria's response to elder abuse' (Office for Senior Victorians 2005) was accepted by the government in early 2006. As a result a second guide on dealing with elder abuse has been developed and released (VDHCS 2009).

Tasmania

Tasmania is one of the last states to respond to elder abuse, and has implemented a whole of government approach to elder abuse with the Department of Health and Human Services as the lead agency (www.dhhs.tas.gov.au/elderabuse). In 2010 it released a report outlining the need for prevention of elder abuse and emphasising awareness, empowerment, action and support for older people (TDHHS 2010).

Aged Care Assessment Teams and other health and community workers continue to manage cases of elder abuse, but there is now an increased awareness of abuse across the community following the release of this report.

Western Australia

The move to develop a response to elder abuse in Western Australia was led by the Council on the Ageing WA (COTA WA) in 1992 with the organising of a conference on elder abuse. Together with the Office of Seniors Interests and the Public Guardian's Office, COTA WA produced an issues paper for policy makers, developed protocols for service providers and published an information pamphlet for older people. Protocols for non-government agencies were available in 1995, and those for government agencies were developed and released in 1996. These protocols for government agencies continue to be revised regularly and provide clear guidelines for ACATs, health services and community services in the detection and management of elder abuse. As part of the introduction of these protocols, training on prevention and management of elder abuse was provided to police, general practitioners and community service providers.

In 2001, Advocare, a non-government organisation, was funded to provide a programme including direct assistance to victims of abuse, an information and referral service, and community education on prevention, detection and management of elder abuse. This service, based on the South Australian model, has continued to be funded and to function as a useful and important resource for older people and service providers (www.advocare.org.au).

In order to promote a whole of government approach, the Alliance for the Prevention of Elder Abuse (http://apeawa.advocare.org.au/) was established by the Office of Seniors Interests in 2002. This engaged all the government agencies involved in responding to abuse, and includes representation from Health, Police, the Aboriginal community, Legal Aid, the Public Advocate, the Public Trustee, the Disability Services Commission and the Office of Seniors Interests. Apart from the development of policy, the Alliance has been successful in finding funding for research projects to inform future work. These projects have included important introductory work into the complex issue of abuse in aboriginal communities, and abuse in culturally and linguistically diverse communities.

Australian Capital Territory

There was no formal approach to elder abuse in the Australian Capital Territory (ACT) until the ACT Office on Ageing convened an Elder Abuse Taskforce in 2003. This brought together service providers, government representatives and older people to discuss the issues around elder abuse. Key workers from Queensland and New South Wales were co-opted to provide information on developments in other parts of Australia, and this information was used to develop recommendations for policies and protocols relating to elder abuse. In 2004, as a result of the Taskforce's work, ACT Health released a resource guide, 'Meeting the challenge of elder mistreatment' (ACT Health 2004), to assist service providers in managing situations of elder abuse. Whilst aimed at home care service providers, it also provides health professionals and others with practical guidance, and information on referral services. The ACT government continues to promote awareness of elder abuse through its Office on Ageing which provides an elder abuse information and referral telephone line, training, and advice (www.ahcs.act.gov.au/wac/ageing).

Northern Territory

The Northern Territory has no specific policy framework for managing elder abuse and most cases of abuse are dealt with by the ACATs. Referrals are mainly from community service providers, and closer linkages are being developed with the police, family violence services, indigenous health services and general practitioners.

Vast distances and scattered populations make education of community groups difficult, but education of aged care service providers has occurred using the NSW training kit (NSWADD 1996). In remote communities, community workers are trained to recognise high risk situations for abuse, and work with the older person's family to improve the care of the older person and prevent abuse occurring.

Legislation relating to elder abuse

There is no mandatory reporting of elder abuse for community-dwelling older people in Australia. In formal consultations with older people as part of the development of policies on elder abuse in the state of New South Wales, older people indicated that they wished to make decisions for themselves in cases of abuse and they were not supportive of mandatory reporting. Many older people felt that mandatory reporting was stereotyping them as incompetent and dependent, and considered it to be an invasion of privacy. Mandatory reporting was also felt to create an expectation that services would be available to respond appropriately to cases of abuse (NSWADD 1997).

In 2007, following the media reporting of incidents of alleged sexual abuse of a resident by a staff member in a nursing home in the state of Victoria, the national government introduced legislation for compulsory reporting of sexual abuse and serious physical abuse occurring in residential care facilities. Incidents are reported to the Complaints Investigation Scheme within the national Office of Aged Care Quality and Compliance, and to the Police in the state where the abuse occurred.

Whilst there is no specific elder abuse legislation relating to older people living in the community in Australia, there is guardianship legislation in all Australian states which allows for the appointment of a substitute decision-maker for those older people who are no longer able to make decisions for themselves because of mental or physical disability. The appointment of a guardian or a financial manager for an older person who is at risk of abuse may prevent that abuse occurring. In cases of confirmed abuse, these appointments may allow action to be taken to address the abuse by arranging services or the removal of the abuser from the situation. In cases of financial abuse, the misappropriated assets or property may be restored to the abused older person.

Practice response

The following cases illustrate practitioner responses to situations of elder abuse in several different states.

Case 1

Mr Black was a 79-year-old widower who lived alone in his own home in a town in South Australia. Some months following the death of his wife he was befriended by a younger woman who paid him a lot of attention and cooked meals for him. Initially Mr White was flattered by the attention and the woman eventually moved in with him to provide housekeeping assistance. Mr White was not happy with this arrangement but felt powerless to ask her to leave as the woman had allegedly been a friend of his wife. The woman then brought her teenage daughter to live in the house.

Mr White's general practitioner (GP) was concerned with his patient's domestic situation, and with Mr White's permission made a referral to the Aged Rights Advocacy Service (ARAS) and a staff member from this service visited Mr White. He advised Mr White of his rights regarding unwelcome visitors and assisted Mr White in accessing a lawyer to arrange for a letter requesting that the woman and her daughter leave his home. The woman became aggressive and threatening and an apprehended violence order was taken out by Mr White with the assistance of ARAS and the South Australian Police Force. Mr White was very distressed by the whole experience and required several months of counselling from ARAS and his GP.

Case 2

Mrs Brown was an 84-year-old widow with moderate Alzheimer's disease who lived alone in her own home in New South Wales. She had been seen by the local Aged Care Assessment Team after her diagnosis of dementia was made, and a number of services were arranged for her. She had been managing quite well with regular assistance with housekeeping and shopping from community services and her GP visited her regularly. Then Mrs Brown's daughter moved in with her, ostensibly to care for her. Her daughter cancelled all community services and suggested to the GP that his regular visits were unnecessary. Three months later one of Mrs Brown's neighbours contacted her GP. He was concerned that Mrs Brown appeared to have lost a lot of weight and was often seen crying in her back garden. The GP visited and was reluctantly admitted to the house by Mrs Brown's daughter. The GP noted that Mrs Brown had indeed lost weight, and she appeared unkempt and had facial bruising. She was unable to use her right arm and her mental state had markedly deteriorated.

Arrangements were made for Mrs Brown to be admitted to hospital where she was found to be malnourished, to have an untreated wrist fracture and to have bruising over her trunk and face. As she recovered, unsuccessful attempts were made to involve her daughter in discussions about future care. As it was understood that previously Mrs Brown had been a woman with considerable resources, an application was made by the hospital social worker to the Guardianship Tribunal for Financial Management, and also for Guardianship. It transpired that Mrs Brown's daughter had organised a Power of Attorney for her mother, and the daughter had moved a large amount of money into other accounts for her own use. The case was heard by the Guardianship Tribunal who noted that this was a case of physical and financial abuse. With the making of Guardianship and Financial Management orders, much of the money was retrieved, and Mrs Brown's daughter was ordered to leave her mother's house. Mrs Brown was able to return home and afford to have a live-in carer.

Case 3

Mrs White was an 84-year-old lady who had moderate dementia. She lived in a rural Queensland town with her husband. He was very intolerant of her memory loss and shouted at her often. He would occasionally push her if she was slow to do something and on several occasions had pushed her over. He gave her large amounts of sedation in an attempt to manage her repetitive questioning and she often appeared very drowsy. Mrs White's daughter, who lived nearby, was very concerned by her father's behaviour and she rang the Queensland Elder Abuse Prevention Unit's Helpline. They talked to her about elder abuse and gave her the contact details for the local Aged Care Assessment Team so she could make a referral, and also arranged for her to speak to an Alzheimer's Australia counsellor for advice.

Mr White initially refused to allow the ACAT-registered nurse into their home, saying that there was nothing wrong with him or with his wife. The ACAT nurse arranged a visit with their daughter present, and she was able to ascertain that Mrs White appeared scared of her husband and said very little. She also appeared to have lost weight, according to her daughter. The nurse arranged for a geriatrician to visit, but Mr White took his wife out at the time of the visit, and declined to allow his wife to go to a clinic appointment. He also declined to speak to the ACAT social worker and refused any offers of assistance with in home respite for his wife.

After further advice from the EAPU Helpline, Mrs White's daughter made an application to the Queensland Guardianship and Administration Tribunal. Before this could happen, however, Mrs White fell over in the kitchen and sustained a fractured hip and a traumatic brain haemorrhage, necessitating admission to hospital, where she subsequently died several days later.

Elder abuse research in Australia

The extent of elder abuse in Australia has been difficult to estimate because of the lack of awareness of the problem and its subsequent under-reporting. There is also a high level of sensitivity around the issue with many barriers to its identification. The first definite attempt to measure prevalence was in a one-year retrospective study of all clients referred to an Aged Care Assessment Team in New South Wales (Kurrle et al. 1992) which showed that 4.6 per cent of all community dwelling older people referred to the service were victims of abuse. Psychological and physical abuse were most commonly seen. A further prospective study in Queensland, Western Australia and New South

Wales gave a prevalence rate of 2.3 per cent across the four aged care assessment teams surveyed (Kurrle et al. 1997), but definitional issues meant that not all identified cases of elder abuse were actually included. A similar study performed in a large regional aged care service in New South Wales found that 5.4 per cent of referred clients were victims of abuse (Livermore et al. 2001).

There has been one study of prevalence of elder abuse in the general population performed in Australia. In 2000, a telephone survey in a randomly selected community-dwelling population in urban and rural South Australia identified that 2.7 per cent of the older population (65 years or older) were victims of abuse (Cripps 2000). The most common form of abuse reported was psychological, with financial being the next most common, followed by physical abuse and neglect.

There have been a number of qualitative studies examining older people's experiences of elder abuse and these have provided important insights into attitudes towards abuse, and towards the appropriateness of available services. Schaeffer (1999) described the experience of a number of older women who were not believed when they talked about abuse, and consequently remained in abusive situations for years. The support of friends and families was very important, and the attitudes and knowledge of service providers and professionals (particularly medical practitioners, ministers of religion and the legal profession) were critical in allowing older women who were victims of abuse to access assistance. Accurate information about available services, financial support and alternative accommodation was also important.

In a large national study, Disney and Cupitt (2000) found similar results. They also explored the reasons for older people remaining in abusive situations and relationships. They found that the tolerance of violence within society (such as the use of corporal punishment in schools, and within families) that occurred in the 1920s and 1930s influenced how older women viewed abuse. With the changing societal attitudes towards abuse, it is likely that the coming generation of older people will be more likely to speak out about abuse.

A more recent study looked at the time taken by ACAT staff in dealing with cases of elder abuse compared with the time involved in matched cases where abuse had not occurred (Kurrle 2009). This study showed that staff spent at least twice as much time with abuse cases, and at least three different staff members were required. It was clear that the involvement of experienced senior staff members was essential, and debriefing for staff was also an important component.

Conclusion

Over the past 20 years, Australia has gone from having no awareness of elder abuse to having a reasonable understanding of the problem. It has developed responses to elder abuse which have hopefully resulted in improved outcomes for older people who are victims of abuse. The following two case studies encapsulate the progress that has been made in this important area.

The first case is a man who was seen in early 1989. He was 78 years old and had been living alone and coping quite well until his daughter moved in with him. Over several months his GP noticed weight loss and bruising, and friends at the local club noticed withdrawal from social activities. He was investigated by his GP for depression and a possible underlying cancer. His social situation was not considered, and no one asked any questions about the home situation or his relationship with his daughter. The possibility of elder abuse was not considered. His daughter moved him into an aged care facility and continued to live in his house.

The second case is similar. He is a man who was seen in late 2011. He was 81 years old when his middle aged son moved in with him in late 2010 after the son's divorce. In mid 2011, he was noted to have had weight loss, depression and a change in personality, withdrawing from playing bowls and stopping visits from several old friends. He had also presented to his GP with bruising on several occasions which he said was due to bumping into objects. He was referred to the local Aged Care Assessment Team. His relationship with his son was explored and he eventually admitted that his son shouted at him a lot, occasionally hit him and demanded money on a regular basis. The father said that he loved his son and felt that he could not refuse him anything. The son basically denied that any of this had happened, but agreed that his father needed assistance.

The existence of possible elder abuse was documented. A referral was made by the ACAT social worker to the Guardianship Tribunal for the appointment of a Financial Manager to protect this man's finances and property and this occurred, so that there was no possibility of the son misappropriating more money. Assistance with housekeeping and shopping was arranged on a weekly basis, and the GP visited regularly. His friends resumed their visits and he returned to the bowling club. The son has recently moved to another state.

These two cases presented in a similar way. However, awareness of elder abuse and existence of the mechanisms to manage it resulted in very different outcomes for each man, illustrating how far Australia has come in 20 years.

Acknowledgement

Some of the material in this chapter has previously appeared in a similar form in S. Kurrle and G. Naughtin (2008) 'An overview of elder abuse and neglect in Australia'. *Journal of Elder Abuse and Neglect*, 20(2): 108–25.

References

ACT Health (2004) Meeting the challenge of elder mistreatment: A resource guide for home and community care providers in the ACT. Canberra: ACT Health.

Barron, B., McDermott, J., Montague, M., Cran, A., and Flitcroft, J. (1990) No innocent bystanders: A study of abuse of older people in our community. Melbourne: Office of Public Advocate.

Cripps, D. (2000) 'Australia's first randomised study of the prevalence and effects of elder abuse in the general community'. Proceedings of the Australian Association of Gerontology Conference, Adelaide 25–27 October 2000.

DHSH (1994) 'Working party on the protection of frail older people in the community: Report' Canberra: Commonwealth Department of Human Services and Health, Office for the Aged.

Disney, M. and Cupitt, L. (2000) Two lives – two worlds: Older people and domestic violence. Canberra: Partnerships Against Domestic Violence, Commonwealth Government.

Kurrle, S. (2004) 'Elder abuse: Australian Society for Geriatric Medicine position statement no.1.' Australasian Journal on Ageing, 23, 1: 38–41.

——(2009) 'The costs of assessing and managing elder abuse: The ACAT costing study', Australasian Journal on Ageing, 28, 2: A63–4.

——, Sadler, P., and Cameron, I. (1991) 'Elder abuse: An Australian case series', Medical Journal of Australia, 155: 150–53.

——, Sadler, P., and Cameron, I. (1992) 'Patterns of elder abuse'. Medical Journal of Australia 157: 673–6.

——, Sadler, P., Lockwood, K. and Cameron, I.D. (1997) 'Elder abuse: A multicentre Australian study'. Medical Journal of Australia 166: 119–22.

——, Livermore, P., Bunt, R., and Biscan, K. (2001) 'Elder abuse among clients and carers referred to the Central Coast ACAT: A descriptive analysis', Australasian Journal on Ageing, 20, 1: 41–7.

McCallum, J., Matiasz, S. and Graycar, A. (1990) Abuse of the Elderly at Home: the Range of the Problem. Canberra: National Centre for Epidemiology and Population Health.

NSWADD (1993) Abuse of older people in their homes: Final report and recommendations. Sydney: NSW Ageing and Disability Department.

——(1995) Abuse of older people: Inter-agency protocol. Sydney: NSW Ageing and Disability Department.

——(1996) Dealing with abuse of clients and their carers: A training kit. Sydney: NSW Ageing and Disability Department.

——(1997) Mandatory reporting of abuse of older people. Sydney: Ageing and Disability Department.

Office for Senior Victorians (2005) 'Strengthening Victoria's response to elder abuse: Report of the Elder Abuse Prevention Project'. Melbourne: Office for Senior Victorians. Online. Available : at <http: //www.chpcp.org/resources/Elders%20Abuse%20Report%20FINAL2005.pdf> (accessed 16 October 2012)

Schaeffer, J. (1999) 'Older and isolated women and domestic violence project', Journal of Elder Abuse and Neglect, 1, 1: 59–74.

Social Welfare Commission (1975) Care of the aged report. Canberra: Australian Social Welfare Commission.

TDHHS (2010) 'Protecting older Tasmanians from abuse'.Tasmanian Department of Health and Human Services. Online. Available at <http: //www.dhhs.tas.gov.au/__data/

assets/pdf_file/0010/76672/Protecting_Older_Tasmanians_from_Abuse.pdf> (accessed 16 October 2012).

VDHCS (1995) With respect to age: A guide for health services and community agencies dealing with elder abuse. Melbourne: Victorian Department of Health and Community Services.

——(2009) 'With respect to age – 2009: Victorian Government practice guidelines for health services and community agencies for the prevention of elder abuse'. Available at <http: //www.health.vic.gov.au/agedcare/downloads/with_respect_to_age.pdf> (accessed 16 October 2012).

WHO (2001) Ageing and lifecourse. Online. Available at <http: //www.who.int/ ageing/projects/elder_abse/en/index.html> (accessed 24 January 2007).

3 Canada

Lynn McDonald

Introduction

The field of elder abuse has expanded considerably in Canada since the appearance of the first federal discussion paper in 1989 (Gnaedinger 1989). At that time, elder abuse had just been recognized as another form of family violence, similar in status to child abuse "discovered" in the 1960s and wife abuse in the 1970s. Although the first reference to elder abuse was made in Britain in the 1970s (Baker 1975, Burston 1975), the issue received far greater prominence in the United States at that time, with Canada following suit later in the 1980s. The first prevalence studies by Bélanger (1981) and Grandmaison (1988) in Quebec, Shell (1982) and King (1984) in Manitoba, the G.A. Frecker Association on Gerontology (1983) in Newfoundland, Haley (1984) in Nova Scotia, Stevenson (1985) in Alberta and by the Ministry of Community and Social Services (1985) in Ontario, suggested that an appreciable proportion of Canadian older adults were being mistreated at the hands of their caregivers (McDonald and Collins 2000).

During the 1980s the first Canadian textbook on elder abuse by Schlesinger and Schlesinger (1988), was published and served to formally alert the field to some of the more distressing issues faced by practitioners and legislators. The authors unearthed over two hundred North American papers on elder abuse and neglect to provide the first annotated bibliography for Canadians. During the 1980s, the need to respond to the problem prompted an examination of adult protection legislation and the pros and cons of mandatory reporting of abuse. These debates provided the impetus for further reforms to adult guardianship and adult protection legislation that had begun in 1973 in Newfoundland and 1976 in Alberta. At the same time, the federal and provincial governments of Canada began funding various research, educational, and intervention initiatives, all of which supported the drive to produce irrefutable evidence of the existence of elder abuse and neglect (McDonald and Collins 2000, Podnieks 2008).

In 1989 the landmark national prevalence survey by Elizabeth Podnieks revealed that 4 percent of elderly Canadians living in private dwellings experienced some form of abuse and neglect (Podnieks et al. 1990). With the publication of this study in 1990, the first era of Canadian research on elder abuse had come to a favorable conclusion. A small, but important group of enterprising practitioners, aided by an even smaller group of researchers, successfully brought to the attention of Canadians the disturbing social problem of elder abuse and neglect. At this time, the field was in a nascent stage, brimming with optimism about the growing awareness and initial research about this "new" form of violence against older adults. Equally of concern at that time was the huge demand for legal and social remedies – demands that outstripped the creation of cohesive policies to combat the problem, along with the research to inform these policies (McDonald et al. 1991: 1). In response, the 1990s introduced a new generation of studies in Canada which had the potential to guide practice, help formulate some policies, and, to a lesser extent, reform legislation (cf. McDonald et al. 1991, Poirier 1992, Beaulieu 1992, 1994, Pittaway and Westhues 1993, Manitoba Seniors Directorate, 1993, Beaulieu and Tremblay, 1995, Reis and Nahmiash 1995, Stones and Pittman 1995, Sweeney 1995). Beyond the 1990s, studies turned to institutions, albeit in a limited manner (Ens 1999, Hirst 2000, Kozak and Lukawiecki 2001, Bigelow 2007, McDonald et al. 2008). Studies focused on attempts to update estimates of prevalence (Pottie Bunge 2000, Poole and Rietschlin 2008), community development initiatives (Ontario Government 2002, WHO 2002), expanded abuse descriptions (Plamondon and Nahmiash, 2006), and legal issues (Watts and Sandhu 2006, Canadian Centre for Elder Law 2009).[1] Probably the most important driving force behind these developments was the commitment of governments to increased funding for education and small-scale studies (from both psychosocial and legal perspectives) that were designed to help raise awareness among Canadians about abuse and neglect (PHAC 2010).

The field of elder abuse and neglect in Canada has not been idle in the past 20 years, indeed the field has been a hive of activity in its attempt to protect older adults from abuse and neglect. However, much of the current work is recycling what is already known, and sometimes cycling uncorroborated information. More of the public, older adults, professionals, and policy makers are aware of abuse and neglect thanks to the New Horizons for Seniors funding initiative to create awareness of elder abuse across Canada (PHAC 2010). Nevertheless, we still lack fundamental research that is necessary to equitably solve the problem. The purpose of this article, then, is to review some of the developments that have occurred in the field of elder abuse and neglect more recently in Canada. Here, we revisit the issues about the incidence and prevalence of abuse, problems of definitions of elder abuse and neglect, the lack of progress on the theoretical front and the related problem of identifying risk factors for abuse and neglect. Changes in the adult protection legislation and related research are examined as are the state of interventions for mistreatment. The discussion concludes with a look at some ideas for future research.

What we know about elder abuse in Canada

Without wading into the morass of definitional confusion, it is sufficient to note that most researchers would agree on three basic categories of elder abuse: (a) abuse of the older adult in the community, (b) institutional abuse, and (c) neglect. Most would also agree on the major types of abuse – physical, psychological, financial, and sexual abuse, but beyond this classification there is little agreement, especially about neglect which can be intentional, non-intentional, and self-inflicted according to some (Bonnie and Wallace 2003).[2] One of the more important developments since 1991 is the increase in prevalence studies worldwide. Based on an unpublished systematic review about definitions of mistreatment in Canada (McDonald et al. 2008), used four inclusion factors: explicit inclusion and exclusion factors (e.g. studies up to 2011, age of respondents, language, specific prevalence period); probability sampling; standardized data collection (e.g. structured interviews, face-to-face, telephone or mail survey); and standardized abuse measures such as the Conflict Tactics Scale and the Older Americans Resources and Services (OARS).

Overall, 13 community prevalence studies in the research literature met the inclusion guidelines relevant to the research program. The community prevalence research included two studies from Canada (Podnieks 1993, Pottie Bunge 2000), four from the United States (Pillemer and Finkelhor 1988, Laumann et al. 2008, Acierno et al. 2010, Lifespan of Greater Rochester 2011), one from India (Chokkanathan and Lee, 2005), five from Europe (Comijs et al. 1998, Iborra 2005, O'Keeffe et al. 2007, Garre-Olmo et al. 2009, Naughton et al. 2010), and one from Israel (Lowenstein et al. 2009).

The prevalence rates varied widely between countries (2.6 percent in the UK versus 29.3 percent in Spain) and within countries, as is the case for the United States and Spain. This comes as no surprise because the age for inclusion varies, as does the prevalence periods, the types of abuses addressed, the mechanisms for data collection, and the measures used. The most common factor among the studies was the absence of a theoretical model to guide the research except in one instance in which a family violence provided the framework (Pottie Bungie 2000).

The most recent community-based study in Canada – the 1999 General Social Survey on Victimization – interviewed 4,324 randomly selected older adults aged 65 years and older, by telephone. Only 1 percent of this population indicated physical or sexual abuse by a spouse, adult child, or caregiver in the five years prior to the survey, while 7 percent experienced psychological abuse, and 1 percent financial abuse (Pottie Bunge 2000). There was no overall abuse rate presented. The first study in Canada in 1989 by Podnieks et al. (1990) found that 0.5 percent of older persons living in private dwellings had experienced some form of physical violence, 1.4 percent psychological abuse, and 2.5 percent financial abuse. In the Podnieks survey in 1989 only 0.4 percent suffered neglect. Even though the two prevalence studies are often compared, this is misguided because the prevalence periods are different (five years versus one year), the abuse categories are different (sexual abuse was not measured in the Podnieks study) and different measures of financial abuse were used. As a result, little can be said about an increase, decrease, or constancy in abuse rates from 1989 to 1999 because of the differences between the studies.

It wasn't until the early 1990s that the federal government, through the family violence initiative, highlighted the abuse and neglect of older adults in institutions by commissioning a literature review (Ens 1999), several discussion papers (Spencer 1994, Spencer and Beaulieu 1994), and a three-part monograph on abuse and neglect in institutions (Kozak and Lukawiecki 2001). The latter represented the views in publicly funded institutions of residents, staff, and family according to their perspectives of what constituted abuse and neglect, what should be done about it, and a description of what an abuse-free environment would be. In one of the first attempts to establish the prevalence of institutional abuse and neglect in Canada, a random telephone survey of 804 nurses and nurses' aides in Ontario, 20 percent reported witnessing abuse of patients in nursing homes, 31 percent witnessed rough handling of patients, and 28 percent witnessed yelling and swearing at patients (College of Nurses of Ontario 1993). Where the abuse was witnessed, over what time frame, and to whom it was directed was not explained. To date, there continues to be considerable interest in abuse and neglect in care facilities on the part of the public, the media, researchers, and educators, along with myriad organizations (McDonald et al. 2008), but the reality is that the prevalence and incidence of abuse and neglect in institutions in Canada remains unknown.[3]

The institutional abuse studies include three from the United States (Pillemer and Moore 1989, Ramsey-Klawsnik et al. 2008, Griffore et al. 2009), two from Germany (Göergen 2001, 2004), one from Norway (Malmedal et al. 2009), one from Finland (Nurminen, et al. 2009), one from Sweden (Saveman et al. 1999), and one from Italy (Ogioni et al. 2007). There was one reliable pilot study of institutional abuse carried out in the United Kingdom by Purdon et al. (2007). The absence of a Canadian study in the literature is still the norm today.

The increasing research on institutional mistreatment is at least informative for any future study in Canada. The recent growth of institutional studies has demonstrated how methodological issues are amplified when the research focus moves from the community to the institution. The institutional studies indicate that staff members were more likely to be asked about abuse than the older adults themselves, and, if staff were unavailable, families served as proxies. The methodological problems are similar to those found in community studies of prevalence, but there is the added complication of whom to interview: the staff and at what level, or family members and which family members. One of the studies in Germany indicated that 37 percent of staff providing hands-on care self-reported psychologically abusing an older adult, but the number differed in a repeat German study by the same author who reported 53.7 percent of staff self-reported psychological abuse during hands-on care (Göergen 2001, 2004).

Marshall et al. (2000) have argued that abuse is worse in the community than in institutions, but there are no grounds for this observation because the two cannot be compared on the basis of research design, especially since the respondents are different. What is significant about institutions in Canada in 2010 is that:

- the proportion of people aged 65 or older living in institutions has remained stable at 7 percent since 1981 (Ramage-Morin 2005), though the actual number living in health care institutions rose from 173,000 to more than 263,000 residents in 2005 (Ramage-Morin 2005). As a result, even though the latest government policies support "aging-in-place" (Szikita Clark 2008), there will still be a substantial number of older adults who require institutional care (Kozak and Lukawiecki 2001, Ramage-Morin 2005). If the same level of institutionalization is maintained, it has been projected that over half a million (565,000) Canadians will require long-term care by 2031 (Trottier et al. 2000), and the quality of care – including the prevention of abuse and neglect of residents – will become increasingly significant; and
- those aged 85 years and older constitute the largest age group in long-term care settings and are frailer, have more complex needs, and are more likely to have some degree of cognitive impairment, such as dementia, or physical disabilities compared to their community-residing counterparts (Spector et al. 2001).

Only about 12–13 percent of residents are married, and many others lack a close family member who lives within an hour of the facility (Hawes 2002). Without an advocate, older adults in institutions are more dependent on others to provide care that heightens their vulnerability to abuse and neglect. Within this context, a study of institutional mistreatment in Canada would seem reasonable.

Definitional differences

Today, few researchers can discuss the abuse and neglect of older adults without first pausing to describe exactly what words will be used to explain the phenomenon. The discussion of definitions of elder mistreatment is both passionate and sometimes heated: terms that are offensive to some are acceptable to others,[4] ethnic and marginalized groups reportedly have their own definitions which do not match the conventional definitions (Bent 2009, Moon 2000), researchers and practitioners rarely see eye to eye (Payne 2002), practitioners from different professions have difficulties communicating with each other, and older adults themselves are often ignored in the debate (Pillemer and Finkelhor 1988, Bennett 1990, Council of Europe, 1992, Decalmer and

Glendenning, 1993, Kozma and Stones 1995, Sanchez 1996, Wallace 1996, Bonnie and Wallace 2003). In support of the difference in perspectives, a Canadian study found that there was considerable difference between the public's view of physical abuse and that of elder abuse professionals (Geobytes et al. 1992).

As would be anticipated, the definitions of mistreatment reflect the differences in purpose and agendas of the various stakeholders. There is no uniformity of the categories used by the experts, coupled with a lack of uniformity within the categories themselves. Some researchers, for example, include sexual abuse as a category while other researchers omit it (Podnieks et al. 1990, Pottie Bunge 2000). The most common measurement used to evaluate physical and psychological abuse is the Conflict Tactic Scale (CTS), or its later version CTS2, but in some studies the Conflict Tactics Scales is modified to suit each study (e.g. Podnieks et al. 1990, Lowenstein et al. 2009). The categories can also contain such a wide range of abuses that they tend to become ineffectual in application because every act (e.g. spiritual abuse) in effect becomes abusive or neglectful (Spencer and Gutman 2008), which is unrealistic. In addition, some definitions focus on the outcome of abuse while others contain reference to the causal factors, the means, or the outcomes of abuse (Johnson 1991, Stones 1995).

The legal definitions of abuse and neglect are no less challenging. An unpublished work by the Canadian Centre for Elder Law (Canadian Centre for Elder Law 2009) indicates that definitions of elder abuse and neglect in Canada have evolved differently than in other prevalence study jurisdictions. Because of Canada's unique and forward definitions of breach of fiduciary duty, trust relationship breaches have their own more developed area of law, which is argued in addition to other "elder abuse" type torts. As such, definitions found in the common law in Canada are not limited to situations "in a relationship where there is an expectation of trust". Rather, the scope of what is considered "elder abuse" in Canadian common law is significantly broader and can include systemic issues, stranger-targeted elder abuse, and directed exploitative marketing and "grooming" of an elder victim.

According to Watts and Sandhu (2006), within the criminal context, Canada has no specific "elder abuse" code provision, such as those found within some other prevalence study comparator jurisdictions such as the United States. Generally, elder abuse and neglect cases are woven into criminal code charges such as assault and aggravated assault, unlawfully causing bodily harm, murder/manslaughter, forcible confinement, criminal negligence, fraud, extortion, forgery, theft, theft by person holding a power of attorney, unlawful conversion, and sexual assault. However, there is also a growing body of criminal case law which has been using key sections of the criminal code to prosecute "elder abuse and neglect" cases. In particular, there has been a recent expansion of Canada's Criminal Code, R.S., 1985, c. C-46, s. 215, on failure to provide the necessaries of life. Recent decisions of elder abuse and neglect have expanded understandings of failure to provide necessaries and have also broadly interpreted this section. In a recent case, financial abuse was formally connected with this section, paving the way for new elder abuse and neglect cases to more easily be located and prosecuted under this section.

Although it is now 20 years since this problem was identified, Canada has finally agreed upon common definitions of mistreatment as a result of a two-year research project with an international team (McDonald et al. 2011).[5] A consensus-building approach that involved major policy makers, practitioners and research stakeholders was used to develop definitions and measurements of mistreatment. The attributes of the definitions included cross-national comparability, comparability to earlier studies in Canada, adaptability for longitudinal surveys, ability to expand and contract definitions, ability to do statistical analyses, ability to add the definitions to a larger national study, and the ability to frame qualitative work. The definitions and the questionnaires that were developed were subsequently tested for validity and reliability in a pilot telephone survey of 267 community older adults and 32 face-to-face interviews with institutional dwelling Canadians of 55 years of age and over. The recruits were divided between those previously abused and those never abused to test the questionnaires using the 'known group' approach to validity. As one of the first surveys to ever test the validity and reliability of the measures (some common to other studies), the results were somewhat surprising.

For example, during cognitive testing of the survey instrument, some respondents noted that, although they said "yes" to one or several items of abuse, they did not feel they had experienced abuse. Because of this finding, we included a summary question that addressed this issue in the telephone interviews. Respondents were given a definition for each type of abuse. If respondents said "yes" to any abuse item, they were asked if they felt they had experienced that particular type of abuse (e.g. physical abuse). To further understand how they felt, we asked them to describe their experiences. While 122 (46 percent) of respondents said "yes" to one or several abuse items, only two-thirds of them (78) felt they had been "abused." In classifying a series of events as abuse, it became evident that it was relevant to take account of respondents' own perceptions and descriptions of the situation. It may be necessary to make qualitative judgments about whether a specific case constitutes abuse, a unique contribution to the measurement of elder mistreatment in prevalence studies currently not the norm. The issue is that this study has raised the issues of over and under reporting of different types of mistreatment.

Theoretical issues

It has been proposed in other contexts that establishing an explanation for mistreatment could be more important than determining prevalence, because explanations are integral to the development of preventative programs (Hawes 2002). Unfortunately, there has been very little theorizing about abuse and neglect that occurs in the community or institutions (Phillips 1983, Wolf and Pillemer 1989, Ansello 1996, Schiamberg and Gans 1999, Bonnie and Wallace 2003, Harbison et al. 2008). Reasons for this are many (cf. McDonald 2007, 2008, Harbison et al. 2008). All of the theories in the field of elder abuse are well-known and have been critiqued extensively to the point that it is obvious that the theories are not especially useful (McDonald and Collins 2000, Harbison et al. 2008). Theories such as the situational model, learning theory, exchange theory and symbolic interaction are seen as not able to sufficiently distinguish between theoretical explanations and the individual factors related to mistreatment. In the elder abuse literature, particular factors, such as stress or dependency, are often treated as complete theoretical explanations although they are only factors and could be incorporated into any of the theories.

Many scholars have realized that there is a broad diversity in the manifestations of abuse and neglect and so have abandoned their search for a comprehensive, all-inclusive explanation of the phenomena. In the future, new theories of elder abuse may explain different dimensions of abuse and neglect but only a few have thus far been engaged in this undertaking (Shaw 1998). Also, none of the more popular theories can link structural and individual factors for a more complete understanding of abuse and, consequently, it comes as no surprise that there may be different theoretical frameworks required for institutional and domestic mistreatment.

Borrowing from the field of gerontology instead of from family violence, the life course perspective could possibly serve as a new starting point for explaining mistreatment. The complexity of elder abuse and neglect necessitates a longitudinal perspective that integrates the multiple levels that address individual characteristics, contextual factors such as institutional or community contexts, and structural indicators such as ageism in society (Marshall 2009).[6] The utility of a life course perspective is that it can be either be incorporated into existing theories such as the "situation model" with its emphasis on care burden or utilized as a shell-like framework of the life course that can host other theories and concepts about mistreatment at different levels of analysis (George 2003). The life course perspective has been used in a number of ways such as (a) the cohort approach, which focuses on social change from generation to generation (Bengtson et al. 2005), (b) constructionist approaches that consider individual action and social contexts as they interact over the life course (Cohler and Hostetler 2003, Kelley-Moore 2010), and (c) the structural approach that focuses on the interaction between policies and individuals that affects the sequencing and timing of life course transitions (Leibfried 1999, Leisering 2003).

Most life course scholars focus on several of five paradigmatic principles that provide a concise, conceptual map of the life course: (a) development and aging as lifelong processes, (b) lives in historical time and place, (c) social timing, (d) linked lives, and (e) human agency (Elder and Pellerin 1998). If the principles of this framework are considered, abuse and neglect can be treated as a major turning point in a person's life. The benefits of using this perspective include: the inclusion of systematic factors in abuse such as those found in institutions or the law, recognition that the abused older adult is embedded in relationships with others that incorporate professional and informal caregivers, the inclusion of period and cohort effects to show how abuse and neglect may be influenced by the historical times and the cohort with whom the person has traveled through life, and, most importantly, the appreciation that older adults are their own agents who are knowledgeable and capable of making their own decisions.

The life course perspective also opens the theoretical doors to make way for a number of current or new theories to be incorporated into its framework. For example, critical theory (Estes 1999), which focuses on a critique of the existing social order and its treatment of the aged by exposing underlying assumptions such as ageism, could serve as the bridge between the nature of the socioeconomic order (e.g. ageist policies) and the setting where the individual resides. The link between critical theory (macro level) and institutionalization theory (meso level) to explain the setting, ties socioeconomic factors to the institution, and in the schemata of Bonnie and Wallace (2003) links the setting to the individual to more comprehensively explain abuse and neglect. Conversely, if a researcher chooses a theory such as symbolic interaction that is already used to explain elder abuse, the theory could be considered over a life course. This type of analysis focuses on the different meanings that people attribute to violence and the consequences these meanings have in certain situations. Social learning, or modeling, is part of this perspective: the theory holds that abusers learn how to be violent from witnessing or suffering from violence, and the victims, in suffering abuse, learn to be more accepting of it. In short, this theory is already longitudinal, but little research has been collected to support the learning model over an older person's life course.

In the recent Canadian pilot study that developed definitions, a life course perspective was used to frame the research and questions were asked about mistreatment over the life course. Although not a random sample, results suggested that a life course perspective provided a useful framework for understanding elder abuse and neglect. Results showed that a childhood history of abuse had a deciding influence on later mistreatment, over and above what happened later in life. For many older adults, abuse and neglect may be part of a continuing pattern of mistreatment that begins very early in life.

Turning to institutional mistreatment, McDonald (2008) has argued that explanations of elder abuse in institutional settings is a case of the underdetermination of theory and proposed that, to integrate findings, researchers could consider theory from the field of complex organizations. The underdetermination of theory refers to a set of facts that can support any number of theories. The most reported factors from the research today have not changed much from the outset and continue to emphasize staff training and resident aggression (Cassell 1989, Brennan and Moos 1990, Pillemer and Bachman-Prehn 1991, Stilwell 1991, Chappell and Novack 1992, Kingdom 1992, Feldt and Ryden 1992, Whall et al. 1992, Meddaugh 1993, Gilleard 1994, Spencer 1994, Beaulieu and Tremblay 1995, Braun et al. 1997, Göergen 2001). These factors, which have sometimes been referred to as the "blame and train" list, are ineffective as a list of problems because the roots of the problem are in the organization and its environment. Institutional organizational theory (Selznick 1949, Meyer and Rowan 1977, DiMiaggio and Powell 1983, Greenwood et al. 2008), which sees organizations as influenced by institutional logics of getting the job done and their institutional contexts (i.e. regulations, norms, organizational culture, and community environment), is proposed as a possible alternative (McDonald 2008).

Interventions

In 1986, Montgomery and Borgatta (1986: 599) noted the difficulty in understanding "the rapid emergence in the literature of recommendations for practice and policy." Wolf (1997: 81) indicated that the elder abuse research was particularly lacking in "reliable data on the effectiveness of interventions." Bonnie and Wallace (2003: 119) concluded in their chapter on evaluating interventions that "research on the effects of elder mistreatment interventions is urgently needed." In a review of the many strategies for preventing, detecting, and responding to abuse of older adults, Stolee and Hillier (2008: iii) noted, "there is minimal research evidence to support their effectiveness." In a systematic review of the elder abuse research up to 2006, Erlingsson (2007) found that, of the 398 citations, 8 percent were related to program development/evaluation and only 6.5 percent examined detection, assessment, or interventions.

In 2009, Ploeg et al. (2009) conducted a rigorous systematic review of 1,253 interventions for elder abuse, and sifted their findings down to eight studies that met their criteria for inclusion (Scogin et al. 1989, Filinson 1993, Jogerst and Ely 1997, Davis and Medina-Ariza 2001, Davis et al. 2001, Brownell and Wolden 2002, Richardson et al. 2002, 2004, Brownell and Heiser 2006). They found that in the majority of studies, methodological flaws limited the validity of the results. Some of the limitations included (a) few random clinical trial designs, (b) failure to describe randomization procedures, (c) small sample sizes and missing sample size estimations and power analyses, (d) measures with little information about psychometric properties, and (e) biased outcome assessments (Ploeg et al. 2009: 191). They concluded "there is currently insufficient evidence to support any particular intervention related to elder abuse targeting client, perpetrators, or health professionals" (Ploeg et al. 2009: 206).

Why these would be the findings is conjecture since there is limited research that has asked practitioners why practice research is slim (McDonald et al. 2008, Stolee and Hillier 2008). Some of the identified problems include

(a) limited capacity for intervention research in the field of elder abuse, (b) limited targeted funding by governments to the research areas most in need of support like prevalence studies and random clinical trials, (c) limited access to what knowledge already exists, and (d) limited capability to professionally evaluate the quality of the knowledge. Anecdotally, it is evident that if tested knowledge was available – in an easily readable format like pocket tools, coupled with a formal venue for interdisciplinary knowledge exchange for both researchers and practitioners – the opportunity for knowledge exchange increases.[7] Whether knowledge transfer changes outcomes is anyone's guess at this point in the brief history of knowledge transfer, which is itself a field with considerable hype and little evidence to its effectiveness (Graham et al. 2006).

In the 1990s we argued that the practitioner was in a rather thorny spot where he or she must solve a problem but where the definitions of abuse are unclear, where there are no reliable estimates of the people affected, where no one is sure about the cause or causes, and the intervention strategies remain unproven (McDonald et al. 1991: 83). Twenty years later the situation appears unchanged in Canada.

Legal interventions

Canada does not follow a comprehensive elder abuse statute approach as in the United States but pursues different aspects of elder abuse within separate legislative responses to domestic violence, to institutional abuse, and to adults who are incapable or otherwise unable to access assistance on their own. Besides the Criminal Code, the Canadian response to elder abuse continues to be a set of statutes that may apply to older adults but not always to the extent that the applicable legislation falls under domestic violence, adult protection, human rights, and institutional abuse legislation (Hall 2008). For example, in British Columbia, the older adult would receive some redress under the Adult Guardianship Act, R.S.B.C. 1996, c. 6, while both Nova Scotia and Prince Edward Island have specific adult protection laws. In Quebec, Article 48 of the Charte des droits et liberte? de la personne a RSQ c. C-12 and the provisions of New Brunswick's Family Relations Act contain older adult specific provisions (Hall 2008).

The law, ultimately, often refers to adults of all ages, rather than specifically to older adults. This broader terminology may not be a problem if the goal is not to marginalize older adults. Moreover, elder abuse and neglect probably represent many problems that legislation could "mask" (Coughlan et al. 1995). More importantly, the law is frequently directed only to those cases where it is perceived that the older adult is in need of protection. From a research perspective, few attempts have investigated exactly what contribution legislative provisions for adult protection make to the resolution of abuse and neglect of older adults (Harbison et al. 2008). In many instances, the legal enterprise continues to underscore that legislative solutions sometimes come dangerously close to undermining the rights and autonomy of older adults by providing more intrusive solutions to problems that could have been handled by the health or social services systems (Harbison et al. 2005, Harbison et al. 2008). A recent example is the Personal Information Protection and Electronic Documents Act (PIPEDA), implemented in phases over a three-year period that began on January 1, 2001.

PIPEDA is based on balancing an individual's right to the privacy of personal information with the need of organizations to collect, use, or disclose personal information for legitimate business purposes (Office of the Privacy Commissioner of Canada 2008). While the Act maintains that, generally, the individual has to give consent to the business to use personal information, usually at the time the information is collected, in certain sections this is not required, especially if for medical, legal, or security reasons or for the prevention of fraud or law enforcement where seeking consent "may defeat the purpose of collecting the information" (PIPEDA, s. 1 c. 4.3). It is easy to see that this law has the potential to undermine the autonomy and independence of the older person as in the case of a police investigation of financial abuse involving a bank (Parliamentary Committee on Palliative and Compassionate Care 2010).

Debate, which varies across Canada, also continues over mandatory reporting of abuse and neglect (e.g. mandatory reporting in Alberta, Manitoba, and Ontario of institutional abuse and, in the community, in Nova Scotia and Newfoundland). The question remains as to whether elder abuse laws appear to have had an impact on the detecting or reporting of abuse in Canada or the United States (Rodriguez et al. 2006). No new evidence has yet emerged that mandatory reporting is effective in enhancing the treatment of elder abuse: previous research shows that reporting (voluntary or mandatory) is substantially less effective than public and professional education and awareness (Silva 1992), but this data needs to be updated and replicated.

Conclusion

This overview of the situation in Canada clearly indicates that we lack the type of investigations we most greatly need. While we have managed to develop a national consensus about a set of mistreatment definitions that are Canadian-appropriate to meet regional needs (e.g. cultural diversity) and simultaneously expandable or collapsible to make international comparisons, we still require a national prevalence study with a random stratified sample of sufficient size, with a longitudinal component to monitor trends over time both in the community and in institutions. Although most prevalence studies have been retrospective to date, a prospective study of abuse would provide an etiology of the different types of mistreatment and their risk factors.

We desperately need innovative theory development to put an end to how Canada dissipates research resources on studies that are non-accumulative over time. Because the complexity of elder mistreatment spans the societal, contextual, and individual levels on the vertical axis, involves linked lives on the horizontal axis, and likely represents an accumulation of events over time, a life course perspective may offer a framework for theoretical advancement. Earlier on, it was thought that many theories were required to explain abuse, but there was no apparent integrating framework as there is today. Moreover, the life course perspective would recognize the agency of the older person and lessen the tendency of many researchers and clinicians to infantilize older people. That preliminary research supports this approach indicates that further investigation would not be wasted. The theoretical research agenda could also be furthered through qualitative methodologies to construct explanations of mistreatment.

Finally, it is time to use rigorous experimental designs to test our interventions both socially and legally, no matter how challenging. In particular, studies require (a) correct sample sizes, (b) appropriate random sampling and randomization techniques, (c) the use of measurement instruments with solid psychometric properties, and (d) appropriate adjustment for baseline differences between comparison groups. Some of the more pressing interventions would include education of older adults and their caregivers, training of staff in institutions, and crisis interventions that support older mistreated adults. Clearly, the best of all circumstances would be to have more qualitative and more quantitative studies, but when the topic of elder abuse and neglect is not popular and the funds are severely constrained, priorities must be set if we are to move forward.

A first priority would seem to be a prevalence study since everything else falls into place thereafter. Many of the theoretical wars that have been waged for a long time could genuinely be settled by rigorous research conducted with sensitivity and respect for older adults. This has been done in other countries, and it can be accomplished in Canada. Elder abuse and neglect literally increase the rate of mortality, a compelling statistic that should jolt the research community into action.

Notes

1 See Podnieks (2008) for a full version of the history of elder abuse in Canada.
2 Self-infliction of abuse, which is really a case of not looking after one's self due to dementia or other disabilities, is considered to be a failure of the caregiving system, not a case of neglect.
3 There are a number of Canadian qualitative studies of institutional abuse (e.g. Beaulieu and Tremblay 1995, Bigelow 2007, Bond et al. 1999, Hirst 2000, 2002), one recent literature review (McDonald et al. 2008), and a snapshot of what is current in institutional abuse and neglect in Canada (Institute for Life Course and Aging 2008).
4 In Canada in the mid-1990s, a number of researchers, practitioners, and government officials decided to use different labels for the term "elder abuse". The new terms proposed were "abuse and neglect of older adults", terms that could not be confused with those in other ethnic and religious communities. There was also the suggestion that, because "elder abuse" had the potential to be "stigmatizing" and to focus on the "oldest of the old", the proposed terms were more suitable

(Spencer 1995). Most recently, the term "mistreatment" has come into its own. For example, in the UK community prevalence study of elder abuse, the word "mistreatment" refers to all forms of abuse (psychological, physical, sexual, and financial) and neglect, "abuse" refers to all forms of abuse, excluding neglect, "interpersonal abuse" collectively describes physical, psychological, and sexual abuse (Biggs et al. 2009).

5 The overarching goals of this research were to address (a) the main problems associated with the conceptual definitions and measurement of mistreatment of older adults, (b) the difficulties on the theoretical front, (c) the current challenges associated with identifying risk factors for abuse and neglect, and (d) the issues surrounding the collection of reliable and valid data related to the prevalence of abuse and neglect. The international research team consisted of Drs. M. Beaulieu, S. Biggs, T. Goergen, S. Hirst, A. Lowenstein, C. Walsh, Ms. L.Watts, J. Wahl, Drs. C. Thomas and K. Willison, led by Dr. L. McDonald. At a Consensus Meeting (June 2010) of Canadian and international researchers and practitioners, conceptual definitions were decided upon that reflected Canadian law and practice (National Initiative for the Elderly: NICE 2010). Not everyone agreed and changes were made, recognizing that not every definition in the country could be included.

6 Podnieks (1992) first called for a life course perspective in her qualitative follow-up of 42 abused respondents to her domestic prevalence study in 1989 (Podnieks et al. 1989).

7 The National Initiative for the Care of the Elderly (NICE), which is a National Centre of Excellence and knowledge transfer network, has seven Canadian teams and nine international teams that produce pocket tools for policy makers, practitioners, researchers, and older adults. Only information that is evidence-based is utilized and is presented in an easily readable format on cardboard that fits in a pocket or on a handheld device. NICE has one team devoted to elder abuse and neglect, which has developed a number of pocket tools that are requested at the rate of 40,000 per year across Canada, not counting international requests.

References

Acierno, R., Hernandez, M.A., Amstadter, A.B., Resnick, H.S., Steve, K., Muzzy, W. and Kilpatrick, D.G. (2010) 'Prevalence and correlates of emotional, physical, sexual, and financial abuse and potential neglect in the United States: The National Elder Mistreatment Study', American Journal of Public Health, 100, 2: 292–7.

Ansello, E.F. (1996) 'Causes and theories', in A. Baumhover and S.C. Beal (eds) Abuse, neglect and exploitation of older persons: Strategies for assessment and intervention. Baltimore, MD: Health Professions Press.

Baker, A.A. (1975) 'Granny battering', Modern Geriatrics, 5, 8: 20–24.

Beaulieu, M. (1992) 'La formation en milieu de travail: l'expression d'un besoin des cadres en ce qui concerne les abus à l'endroit des personnes agées en centre d'accueil', Le Gérontophile, 14, 3: 3–7.

——(1994) 'Réagir face aux mauvais traitements en institution: une responsabilite? individuelle et collective', Le Gérontophile, 16, 4: 35–40.

——and Tremblay, M.J. (1995) Abuse and neglect of older adults in institutional settings: Discussion paper building from French language sources. Ottawa: Health Canada, Mental Health Division.

Bélanger, L. (1981) 'The types of violence the elderly are victims of: Results of a survey done with personnel working with the elderly'. Paper presented at the 34th Annual Scientific Meeting of the Gerontological Society of America, Toronto.

Bengtson, V.L., Elder, G.H., and Putney, N.M. (2005) 'The life course perspective on ageing: Linked lives, timing, and history', in M. Johnson, V.L. Bengtson, P.G. Coleman and T. Kirkwood (eds) Cambridge handbook on age and aging. Cambridge: Cambridge University Press.

Bennett, G. (1990) 'Action on elder abuse in the 1990s: New definitions will help', Geriatric Medicine, 20, 4: 53–4.

Bent, K. (2009) Literature review: Aboriginal senior abuse in Canada. Ottawa: Native Women's Association of Canada.

Bigelow, B.J. (2007) 'What happens when the wheels fall off? Elders abuse complaints and legal outcomes in residential care facilities in Canada', American Journal of Forensic Psychology, 25, 2: 35–64.

Biggs, S., Erens, B., Doyle, M., Hall, J. and Sanchez, M. (2009) Abuse and neglect of older people: Secondary analysis of UK prevalence study. London: King's College London and the National Centre for Social Research.

Bond, J.B., Cuddy, R., Dixon, G.L., Duncan, K.A., and Smith, D.L. (1999) 'The financial abuse of mentally incompetent older adults: A Canadian study', Journal of Elder Abuse and Neglect, 11, 4: 23–38.

Bonnie, R.J., and Wallace, R.B. (eds) (2003) Elder mistreatment: Abuse, neglect, and exploitation in an aging America. Washington, DC: The National Academies Press.

Braun, K.L., Suzuki, K.M., Cusick, C.E., and Howard-Carhart, K. (1997) 'Developing and testing training materials on elder abuse and neglect for nurse aides', Journal of Elder Abuse and Neglect, 9, 1: 1–15.

Brennan, P.L., and Moos, R.H. (1990) 'Physical design, social climate, and staff turnover in skilled nursing facilities', Journal of Long Term Care Administration, 18, 2: 22–7.

Brownell, P., and Heiser, D. (2006) 'Psycho-educational support groups for older women victims of family mistreatment: A pilot study', Journal of Gerontological Social Work, 46, 3–4: 145–60.

Brownell, P., and Wolden, A. (2002) 'Elder abuse intervention strategies: Social service or criminal justice?' Journal of Gerontological Social Work, 40, 1/2: 83–100.

Burston, G.R. (1975) 'Granny-battering (letter)', British Medical Journal, 6, 592.

Canadian Centre for Elder Law (2009) Definitions of elder abuse and neglect. Vancouver: Canadian Centre for Elder Law.

Cassell, E.J. (1989) 'Abuse of the elderly: Misuses of power', New York State Journal of Medicine, 89, 3: 159–62.

Chappell, N.L. and Novack, M. (1992) 'The role of support in alleviating stress among nursing assistants', The Gerontologist, 32, 3: 351–9.

Chokkanathan, S., and Lee, A.E. (2005) 'Elder mistreatment in urban India: A community based study', Journal of Elder Abuse and Neglect, 17, 2: 45–61.

Cohler, B.J., and Hostetler, A.J. (2003) 'Linking life course and life story: Social change and the narrative study of lives', in J. Mortimer and R. Shanahan (eds) Handbook of the life course. New York: Kluwer Academic/Plenum Publishing Company.

College of Nurses of Ontario (1993) 'Abuse of clients by registered nurses and registered nursing assistants'. Report to council on results of Canada Health Monitor Survey of Registrants, Toronto.

Comijs, H.C., Smit, J.H., Pot, A.M., Bouter, L.M., and Jonker, C. (1998) 'Risk indicators of elder mistreatment in the community', Journal of Elder Abuse and Neglect, 9, 4: 67–76.

Coughlan, S., Downe-Wamboldt, B., Elgie, R., Harbison, J., Melanson, P., and Morrow, M. (1995) 'Mistreating elderly people: Questioning the response to elder abuse and neglect'. (Vol. 2), Legal Responses to Elder Abuse and Neglect. Halifax Canada: Dalhousie University Health Law Institute.

Council of Europe (1992) Violence against elderly people. Strasbourg: Council of Europe Steering Committee on Social Policy.

Davis, R.C. and Medina-Ariza, J. (2001) 'Results from an elder abuse prevention experiment in New York City', National Institute of Justice: Research in Brief: 1–7.

Davis, R.C., Medina, J., and Avitabile, N. (2001) Reducing repeat incidents of elder abuse: Results of a randomized experiment, final report. New York: US Department of Justice.

Decalmer, P., and Glendenning, F. (eds) (1993) The mistreatment of elderly people. Newbury Park, CA: Sage.

DiMiaggio, P.J., and Powell, W.W. (1983) 'The iron cage revisited: Institutional isomorphism and collective rationality in organizational fields', American Sociological Review, 48: 147–60.

Elder, G., and Pellerin, L. (1998) 'Linking history and human lives', in J. Giele and G. Elder (eds) Methods of life course research: Quantitative and qualitative approaches. Thousand Oaks, CA: Sage.

Ens, I. (1999) Abuse and neglect of older adults: A discussion paper. Ottawa: Public Health Agency of Canada.

Erlingsson, C.L. (2007) 'Searching for elder abuse: A systematic review of database citations' Journal of Elder Abuse and Neglect, 19, 3/4: 59–78.

Estes, C.L. (1999) 'Critical gerontology and the new political economy of aging', in M. Minkler, and C.L. Estes (eds) Critical gerontology: Perspectives from political and moral economy. Canterbury: Baywood Publishing Company.

Feldt, K.S., and Ryden, M.B. (1992) 'Aggressive behavior: Educating nursing assistants', Journal of Gerontological Nursing, 18, 5: 3–12.

Filinson, R. (1993) 'An evaluation of a program of volunteer advocates for elder abuse victims', Journal of Elder Abuse and Neglect, 5, 1: 77–93.

G.A. Frecker Association on Gerontology (1983) Summary report on aging and victimization including 1983 St. John's survey results. St. John's, NF: MVN Extension Service.

Garre-Olmo, J., Planas-Pujol, X., Lopez-Pousa, S., Juvinya, D., Vila, A. and Vilalta-Franch, J. (2009) 'Prevalence and risk factors of suspected elder abuse subtypes in people aged 75 and older', Journal of the American Geriatrics Society, 57, 5: 815–22.

Geobytes, R.L., O'Connor, D. and Mair, K.J. (1992) 'Public perceptions of elder mistreatment', Journal of Elder Abuse and Neglect, 4: 151–69.

George, L. (2003) 'Life course research: Achievements and potential', in J.T. Mortimer and M.J. Shanahan (eds) Handbook of the life course. New York: Kluwer Academic Publishers.

Gilleard, C. (1994) 'Physical abuse in homes and hospitals', in M. Eastman (ed.) Old age abuse: A new perspective (2nd edn). London: Chapman and Hall.

Gnaedinger, N. (1989) Elder abuse: A discussion paper. Ottawa: Health and Welfare Canada, Family Violence Prevention Division.

Göergen, T. (2001) 'Stress, conflict, elder abuse and neglect in German nursing homes: A pilot study among professional caregivers', Journal of Elder Abuse and Neglect, 13, 1: 1–26.

——(2004) 'A multi-method study on elder abuse and neglect in nursing homes', The Journal of Adult Protection, 6, 3: 15–25.

Graham, I.D., Logan, J., Harrison, M.B., Straus, S.E., Tetroe, J., Caswell, W. and Robinson, N. (2006) 'Lost in knowledge translation: Time for a map?' The Journal of Continuing Education in the Health Professions, 26, 1: 13–24.

Grandmaison, A. (1988) 'Protection des personnes âgées: étude exploratoire de la violence à l'égard de la clientele des personnes âgées'. Unpublished manuscript. Montréal, Centre de Services Sociaux du Montréal Metropolitain (CSSMM).

Greenwood, R., Oliver, C., Sahlin, K., and Suddaby, R. (2008) 'Introduction', in R. Greenwood, C. Oliver, K. Sahlin and R. Suddaby (eds) The Sage handbook of organizational institutionalism. London: Sage.

Griffore, R.J., Barboza, G.E., Mastin, T., Oehmke, J., Schiamberg, L.B. and Post, L.A. (2009) 'Family members' reports of abuse in Michigan nursing homes', Journal of Elder Abuse and Neglect, 21, 2: 105–14.

Haley, R.C. (1984) Elder abuse/neglect. Halifax, Canada: Department of Social Services.

Hall, M. (2008) 'Constructing elder abuse: The Canadian legal framework'. Paper presented at the HRSDC Expert Roundtable on Elder Abuse, Ottawa.

Harbison, J., Coughlan, S., Karabanow, J., and VanderPlaat, M. (2005) 'A clash of cultures: Rural values and service delivery to mistreated and neglected older people in eastern Canada', Practice–Social Work in Action, 17, 4: 229–46.

Harbison, J., Beaulieu, M., Coughlan, S., Karabanow, J., Van-derPlaat, M., Wildeman, S., et al. (2008) Conceptual frame-works: Understandings of 'elder abuse and neglect' and their implications for policy and legislation. Ottawa: Human Resources and Social Development Canada.

Hawes, C. (2002) 'Elder abuse in residential long-term care facilities: What is known about prevalence, causes, and prevention'. Paper presented at the Testimony given before the US Senate Committee on Finance, 18 June.

Hirst, S.P. (2000) 'Resident abuse: An insider's perspective', Geriatric Nursing, 21, 1: 32–8.

——(2002) 'Defining resident abuse within the culture of long-term care institutions', Clinical Nursing Research, 11, 3: 267–84.

Iborra, I. (ed.) (2005) Violencia contra personas mayores. Barcelona: Centro Reina Sofía para el Estudio de la Violencia.

Institute for Life Course and Aging (2008) A way forward: Promoting promising approaches to abuse prevention in institutional settings, (2005–2007). Online. Available at <http://www.aging.utoronto.ca/node/125> (accessed 10 August 2010).

Jogerst, G.J., and Ely, J.W. (1997) 'Home visit program for teaching elder abuse evaluations', Family Medicine, 29, 9: 634–9.

Johnson, T.F. (1991) Elder mistreatment: Deciding who is at risk. Westport, CT: Greenwood Press.

Kelley-Moore, J. (2010) 'Disability and ageing: The social construction of causality', in D. Dannefer and C. Phillipson (eds), The Sage handbook of social gerontology. Thousand Oaks, CA: Sage, pp. 96–110.

King, N.R. (1984) 'Exploitation and abuse of older family members: An overview of the problem', in J.J. Costa (ed.) Abuse of the elderly: A guide to resources and services. Lexington, MA: Lexington Books.

Kingdom, D. (1992) 'Preventing aggression', Canadian Nursing Home, 3, 2: 14–16.

Kozak, J., and Lukawiecki, T. (2001) Returning home: Fostering a supportive and respectful environment in the long-term care setting. Ottawa: National Clearing-house on Family Violence.

Kozma, A., and Stones, M.J. (1995) 'Issues in the measurement of elder abuse' in M.MacLean (ed.), Abuse and neglect of older Canadians: Strategies for change. Toronto: Thompson.

Laumann, E.O., Leitsch, S.A., and Waite, L.J. (2008) 'Elder mistreatment in the United States: Prevalence estimates from a nationally representative study', The Journals of Gerontology, 63, 4: S248–54.

Leisering, L. (2003) 'Government and the life course', in J.T. Mortimer and M.J. Shanahan (eds) Handbook of the life course. New York: Springer.

——and Leibfried, S. (1999) Time and poverty in western welfare states. Cambridge: Cambridge University Press.

Lifespan of Greater Rochester (2011) Under the radar: New York State elder abuse prevalence study. Final Report. Online. Available at <www.lifespan-roch.org/documents/UndertheRadar051211_000.pdf> (accessed 24 July 2012).

Lowenstein, A., Eisikovits, Z., Band-Winterstein, T., and Enosh, G. (2009) 'Is elder abuse and neglect a social phenomenon? Data from the First National Prevalence Survey in Israel', Journal of Elder Abuse & Neglect, 21, 3: 253–77.

McDonald, L. (2007) 'Abuse and neglect of elders' in J.E. Birren (ed.) The encyclopedia of gerontology (2nd edn). New York: Academic Press.

——(2008) 'Explanations of institutional abuse: A case of the under determination of theory'. Paper presented at the Symposium on elder abuse: The need for theory. Paper presented at the 61st Annual Meeting of the Gerontological Society of America, National Harbor, MD.

——and Collins, A. (2000) Abuse and neglect of older adults: A discussion paper. Ottawa: Health Canada.

——, Hornick, J.P., Robertson, G.B., and Wallace, J.E. (1991) Elder abuse and neglect in Canada. Toronto: Butterworths.

——, Collins, A., and Dergal, J. (2006) 'The abuse and neglect of adults in Canada', in R. Alaggia and C. Vine (eds) Cruel but not unusual treatment, Waterloo, Ontario: Wilfred Laurier.

——, Beaulieu, M., Harbison, J., Hirst, S., Lowenstein, A., Podnieks, E. and Wahl, J. (2008) Institutional abuse of older adults: What we know, what we need to know. Ottawa: Human Resources and Social Development Canada.

Malmedal, W., Ingebrigtsen, O., and Saveman, B.I. (2009) 'Inadequate care in Norwegian nursing homes as reported by nursing staff', Scandinavian Journal of Caring Sciences, 23, 2: 231–42.

Manitoba Seniors Directorate (1993) Abuse of the elderly: A guide for the development of protocols. Winnipeg: Manitoba Seniors Directorate.

Marshall, C.E., Benton, D., and Brazier, J.M. (2000) 'Elder abuse: Using clinical tools to identify clues of mistreatment', Geriatrics, 55, 2: 42–4, 47–50, 53.

Marshall, V.W. (2009) 'Theory informing public policy: The life course perspective as a policy tool' in V.L. Bengston, D. Gans, N. Putney and M. Silverstein (eds) Handbook of theories of aging. New York: Springer.

Meddaugh, D.I. (1993) 'Covert elder abuse in the nursing home', Journal of Elder Abuse and Neglect, 5, 3: 21–37.

Meyer, J.W., and Rowan, B. (1977) 'Institutionalized organizations: Formal structure as myth and ceremony', American Journal of Sociology, 83, 2: 340–63.

Ministry of Community and Social Services (1985) Report of a survey of elder abuse in the community. Toronto: Standing Committee on Social Development, Government of Ontario.

Montgomery, R.J.V. and Borgatta, E.F. (1986) 'Plausible theories and the development of scientific theory: The case of aging research', Research on Aging, 8: 586–608.

Moon, A. (2000) 'Perceptions of elder abuse among various cultural groups: Similarities and differences', Generations, 26, 1: 75–80.

Naughton, C., Drennan, J., Treacy, P., Lafferty, A., Lyons, I., Phelan, A., Quin, S., O'Loughlin, A. and Delaney, L. (2010) Abuse and neglect of older people in Ireland: Report of the national study of elder abuse and neglect. Dublin: HSE and UCD.

NICE (2010) National initiative for the care of the elderly. Online. Available at <http://www.nicenet.ca/> (accessed 12 August 2010).

Nurminen, J., Puustinen, J., Kukola, M., and Kivela, S.L. (2009) 'The use of chemical restraints for older long-term hospital patients: A case report from Finland', Journal of Elder Abuse & Neglect, 21, 2: 89–104.

Office of the Privacy Commissioner of Canada (2008) 'Office of the privacy commissioner of Canada'. Online. Available at <http://www.priv.gc.ca/index_e.cfm> (accessed 12 August 2010).

Ogioni, L., Liperoti, R., Landi, F., Soldato, M., Bernabei, R., and Onder, G. (2007) 'Cross-sectional association between behavioral symptoms and potential elder abuse among subjects in home care in Italy: Results from the Silvernet Study'. American Journal of Geriatric Psychiatry, 15, 1: 70–78.

O'Keeffe, M., Hills, A., Doyle, M., McCreadie, C., Scholes, S., Constantine, R., Tinker, A., Manthorpe, J., Biggs, S. and Erens, B., et al. (2007) UK study of abuse and neglect of older people: Prevalence survey report. London: National Centre for Social Research.

Ontario Government (2002) Ontario government takes action on elder abuse. Online. Available at <www.gov.on.ca/citizenship/english/about/n280302> (accessed 16 September 2003).

Parliamentary Committee on Palliative and Compassionate Care (2010) Toronto elder abuse hearing. Toronto: Sutton Place Hotel.

Payne, B.C. (2002) 'An integrated understanding of elder abuse and neglect', Journal of Criminal Justice, 30, 6: 535–47.

PHAC (2010) 'September 2010: Social media in elder abuse prevention'. Online. Available at <http://www/phac-aspc.gc.ca/ea-ma/EB/eb-Sept-2010-eng.php> (accessed 20 August 2010).

Phillips, L.R. (1983) 'Abuse and neglect of the frail elderly at home: An exploration of theoretical relationships', Journal of Advanced Nursing, 8, 5, 379–92.

Pillemer, K., and Bachman-Prehn, R. (1991) 'Helping and hurting: Prediction of maltreatment of patients in nursing homes', Research on Aging, 13: 74–95.

Pillemer, K., and Finkelhor, D. (1988) 'The prevalence of elder abuse: A random sample survey', The Gerontologist, 28, 1: 51–7.

Pillemer, K., and Moore, D.W. (1989) 'Abuse of patients in nursing homes: Findings from a survey of staff', The Gerontologist, 29, 3: 314–20.

Pittaway, E.D., and Westhues, A. (1993) 'The prevalence of elder abuse and neglect of older adults who access health and social services in London, Ontario, Canada', Journal of Elder Abuse & Neglect, 5,4: 77–93.

Plamondon, L., and Nahmiash, D. (2006) 'Portrait de la vulnérabilité et des risques dans la population âgée vivant en HLM', Vie et Vieillissement, 5, 1: 27–36.

Ploeg, J., Fear, J., Hutchison, B., MacMillan, H., and Bolan, G. (2009) 'A systematic review of interventions for elder abuse', Journal of Elder Abuse & Neglect', 21, 3: 187–210.

Podnieks, E. (1992) 'Emerging themes from a follow-up study of Canadian victims of elder abuse', Journal of Elder Abuse & Neglect, 4, 1/2: 59–111.

——(1993) 'National survey on abuse of the elderly in Canada', Journal of Elder Abuse & Neglect, 4, 1/2: 5–58.

——(2008) 'Elder abuse: The Canadian experience', Journal of Elder Abuse & Neglect, 20, 2: 126–50.

——, Pillemer, K., Nicholson, J.P., Shillington, T., and Frizzel, A.F. (1989) A national survey on abuse of the elderly: preliminary findings. Toronto: Ryerson Polytechnical Institute.

——, Pillemer, K., Nicholson, J., Shillington, T., and Frizzel, A. (1990) National survey on abuse of the elderly in Canada: final report. Toronto: Ryerson Polytechnical Institute.

Poirier, D. (1992) 'The power of social workers in the creation and application of elder protection statutory norms in New Brunswick and Nova Scotia', Journal of Elder Abuse and Neglect, 4, 1/2: 113–33.

Poole, C., and Rietschlin, J. (2008) Spousal/Partner victimization among adults aged 60 and older: An analysis of the 1999 and 2004 General Social Survey. Ottawa: Human Resources and Social Development Canada.

Pottie Bunge, V. (2000) 'Abuse of older adults by family members', in V. Pottie Bunge and D. Locke (eds) Family violence in Canada: A statistical profile. Ottawa: Statistics Canada.

Purdon, S., Speight, S., O'Keeffe, M., Biggs, S., Erens, B., Hills, A., et al. (2007). Measuring the prevalence of abuse of older people in care homes: A development study. (Part of the UK study of abuse and neglect of older people) London: Comic Relief and the Department of Health.

Ramage-Morin, P.L. (2005) 'Successful aging in health care institutions', Health Reports, 16(Suppl.): 47–56.

Ramsey-Klawsnik, H., Teaster, P.B., Mendiondo, M.S., Marcum, J.L., and Abner, E. L. (2008) 'Sexual predators who target elders: Findings from the first national study of sexual abuse in care facilities', Journal of Elder Abuse & Neglect, 20, 4: 353–76.

Reis, M., and Nahmiash, D. (1995) When seniors are abused: A guide to intervention. North York, Ontario: Captus Press Inc.

Richardson, B., Kitchen, G., and Livingston, G. (2002). 'The effect of education on knowledge and management of elder abuse: A randomized controlled trial'. Age and Ageing, 31(5), 335–41.

Richardson, B., Kitchen, G., and Livingston, G. (2004) 'What staff know about elder abuse in dementia and the effect of training', Dementia, 3, 3: 377–84.

Rodriguez, M.A., Wallace, S.P., Woolf, N.H., and Mangione, C.M. (2006) 'Mandatory reporting of elder abuse: Between a rock and a hard place', Annals of Family Medicine, 4, 5: 403–8.

Sanchez, Y.M. (1996) 'Distinguishing cultural expectations in assessment of financial exploitation', Journal of Elder Abuse & Neglect, 8, 2: 49–59.

Saveman, B.-I., Astrom, S., Bucht, G., and Norberg, A. (1999) 'Elder abuse in residential settings in Sweden', Journal of Elder Abuse & Neglect, 10, 1: 43–60.

Schiamberg, L.B., and Gans, D. (1999) 'An ecological framework for contextual risk factors in elder abuse by adult children', Journal of Elder Abuse & Neglect, 2, 1: 79–103.

Schlesinger, B. and Schlesinger, R. (1988) Abuse of the elderly: issues and annotated bibliography. Toronto: University of Toronto Press.

Scogin, F., Beall, C., Bynum, J., Stephens, G., Grote, N.P., Baumhover, L.A., et al. (1989) 'Training for abusive caregivers: An unconventional approach to an intervention dilemma', Journal of Elder Abuse & Neglect, 1, 4: 73–86.

Selznick, P. (1949) TVA and the grass roots: A study of politics and organization. Berkeley, CA: University of California Press.

Shaw, M.M.C. (1998) 'Nursing home residents abuse by staff: exploring the dynamics', Journal of Elder Abuse & Neglect, 9, 4: 1–21.

Shell, D.J. (1982) Protection of the elderly: A study of elder abuse. Report of the Manitoba Council on Aging. Winnipeg: Association on Gerontology.

Silva, T.W. (1992) 'Reporting elder abuse: Should it be mandatory or voluntary?' HealthSpan, 9, 4: 13–15.

Spector, W.D., Fleishman, J.A., Pezzin, L.E., and Spillman, B.C. (2001) Characteristics of long-term care users. Rockville, MD: Agency for Healthcare Research and Quality.

Spencer, C. (1994) Abuse and neglect of older adults in institutional settings: An annotated bibliography. Ottawa: Health Canada.

——(1995) 'New directions for research on interventions with abused older adults', in M.J. MacLean (ed.) Abuse and neglect of older Canadians: Strategies for change. Toronto: Thompson Educational Publishing, Inc.

——and Beaulieu, M. (1994) Abuse and neglect of older adults in institutional settings: A discussion paper building from English language sources. Ottawa: Health Canada.

——and Gutman, G.M. (2008) Sharpening Canada's focus: Developing an empirical profile of abuse and neglect among older women and men in the community. Final report – Expert Roundtable on Elder Abuse in Canada. Ottawa, Ontario, Canada: Human Resources and Social Development Canada.

Stevenson, C. (1985) Family Abuse of the Elderly in Alberta. Edmonton: Seniors Advisory Council for Alberta.

Stilwell, E.M. (1991) 'Nurses' education related to the use of restraints', Journal of Gerontological Nursing, 17, 2: 23–6.

Stolee, P., and Hillier, L. (2008) Best practices in dealing with elder abuse: Identifying, communicating, and adopting processes for prevention, detection, and response. Ottawa: Human Resources and Social Development Canada.

Stones, M. (1995) 'Scope and definitions of elder abuse and neglect in Canada', in M. MacLean (ed.) Abuse and neglect of older Canadians. Ottawa: Thompson Educational Publishing.

——and Pittman, D. (1995) 'Individual differences in attitudes about elder abuse: The Elder Abuse Attitude Test (EAAT)', Canadian Journal on Aging, 14, (2, Suppl. 2): 61–71.

Sweeney, V. (1995) Report on needs assessment for senior women as victims of violence. Kentville, Nova Scotia: Gerontology Association of Nova Scotia Valley Region.

Szikita Clark, C. (2008) Aging at home: Allowing seniors to live safely at home with dignity and independence. Toronto: University of Toronto, Faculty of Social Work.

Trottier, H., Martel, L., and Houle, C. (2000) 'Living at home or in an institution: What makes the difference for seniors?' Health Reports, 11, 4: 49–61.

Wallace, H. (1996) Family violence: Legal, medical, and social perspectives. Boston, MA: Allyn and Bacon.

Watts, L., and Sandhu, L. (2006) 'The 51st state – the "state of denial": A comparative exploration of penal statutory responses to criminal "elder abuse"', Elder Law Journal, 14, 1: 207–11.

Whall, A.L., Gillis, G.L., Yankou, D., Booth, D.E., and Beel-Bates, C.A. (1992) 'Disruptive behavior in elderly nursing home residents: A survey of nursing staff', Journal of Gerontological Nursing, 18, 10: 13–17.

WHO (2002) "Missing voices": Older persons views of elder abuse. Geneva: World Health Organization.

Wolf, R.S. (1997) 'Elder abuse and neglect: An update', Reviews in Clinical Gerontology, 7: 177–82.

——and Pillemer, K.A. (1989) Helping elderly victims: The reality of elder abuse. Irvington, NY: Columbia University Press.

4 Chinese society

Agnes Tiwari, Elsie Chau-Wai Yan, Margaret Lee

Introduction

Older people in Chinese societies have traditionally been well respected and taken care of by their families as part of the Confucian doctrine of filial piety. Yet, in recent years, there have been increasing concerns that Chinese elders are not exempt from the plight of elder mistreatment, partly as a result of the changing social norms and cultural values affecting family relationships. In order to understand Chinese elder mistreatment, an examination of the phenomenon in the prevailing Chinese culture in which the mistreatment occurs is required. In the following sections, the definition of elder mistreatment in Chinese societies will first be introduced, followed by a review of the policy and legislations relating to its reporting and protection of the victims. Practice response to and research on Chinese elder mistreatment will then be described. Finally, implications for practice, policy, and research will be highlighted. Chinese societies, in this chapter, refer to the People's Republic of China (PRC), Hong Kong, and Taiwan.

Definition

The National Research Council (NRC 2003: 40) defines elder mistreatment as:

- intentional actions that cause harm or create serious risk of harm (whether or not harm is intended) to a vulnerable elder by a caregiver or other person who is in a trust relationship with the elder; or
- failure by a caregiver to satisfy the elder's basic needs or to protect him or her from harm.

While the NRC definition has been widely adopted, its relevance for the Chinese population has been questioned. Specifically, whether the NRC definition accurately reflects the meaning of elder mistreatment in Chinese societies has been called into question (Yan 2012). Research findings have fuelled the debate about what constitutes elder mistreatment through the Chinese lens. For example, in a qualitative study involving home care workers, Tam and Neysmith (2006) reported that older Canadian Chinese considered disrespect as a form of elder mistreatment. Wang (2006) in a study of elderly Taiwanese, found that "wishes to see relatives unfulfilled" was the most frequently reported form of elder mistreatment. In Hong Kong, elderly respondents identified "treated by family members as if transparent" as elder mistreatment (Hong Kong Christian Service 2002). Thus, there are concerns that some culturally specific forms of elder mistreatment (such as those reported above) may not be visible if the assessment is derived from a Western cultural perspective (Yan 2012, Tam and Neysmith 2006).

In order to comprehend what may be interpreted as elder mistreatment in Chinese societies, it is necessary to understand the traditional values that have kept Chinese families as a close-knit social unit for thousands of years. Filial piety, or xiao, the highest of all virtues in Confucian teachings, has long regulated the relationship between children and parents in Chinese families (Chow 2001). In return for their parents taking good care of them when they were young, adult children are socialized to practice filial behaviors including showing respect to their parents, being obedient, living with the parents, taking care of the parents in sickness or health, producing a male heir, and carrying on the family line (Yang 1997, Chow 2001). More recently, however, industrialization and urbanization have brought fundamental changes to the structure of Chinese families and disrupted the practice of filial piety (Chan and Lee 1995, Chan and Lim 2004). Specifically, as a result of the change in family structure and the replacement of the extended family with the nuclear family, co-residence of parents and married children has been on the decline (Hsu et al. 2001). Young couples with children who move away from their aging parents may be less likely to visit their parents frequently. Against this background, it is not surprising that the elderly Taiwanese respondents in Wang's (2006) study identified "unfulfilled expectations of seeing their adult children" as psychological mistreatment. Also, studies have found that, with the decline in the practice of filial piety and the erosion of parents' authority, giving absolute deference to parents' wishes and continuing the family line are no longer popular beliefs among younger Chinese (Ho 1996, Kwan et al. 2003, Teo et al. 2003). Thus, discrepancy may occur between aging parents' expectations of filial behaviors and their children's performance of their filial roles. Such filial discrepancy may account for "disrespect" and "treated by family members as if transparent" being identified as forms of elder mistreatment in studies by Tam and Neysmith (2006) and Hong Kong Christian Service (2002), respectively. It is therefore important to incorporate Chinese elders' views about how they want to be treated by their adult offspring into the existing framework of defining elder mistreatment in Chinese societies.

Policy and legislation

In Hong Kong, the Domestic and Cohabitation Relationships Violence Ordinance (Cap. 189) (formerly known as the Domestic Violence Ordinance) was first enacted in 1986. The ordinance allows domestic violence victims to obtain quick and temporary relief from molestation by applying to the court for an injunction order that restrains the perpetrator from molesting the victim; excludes the perpetrator from the matrimonial home; and requires the perpetrator to permit the victim to enter and remain in the matrimonial home.

Under the early versions of the Domestic Violence Ordinance, however, only persons in current spousal or cohabitation relationships could apply for an injunction order for himself or herself or any child living together with him or her. In response to public concerns on the report of domestic violence cases that involve non-spousal familial relationships, for instance, elder abuse, the legislative counsel passed the Domestic Violence (Amendment) Bill in 2008, thereby extending the scope of victims being protected under the Ordinance to include elderly relatives, amongst others.

In the PRC, the interests of any citizens aged 60 or above are protected under the Law of the People's Republic of China on Protection of the Rights and Interests of the Elderly, passed in 1996. Under this legislation, family members have the primary responsibility to provide support for an older person financially, physically, and emotionally. Specifically, Article 4 of this legislation prohibits "discrimination against, insult of, maltreatment of or desertion of the aged." In addition, Article 46 of this legislation deals primarily with elder abuse in general. It states

> whoever, by violence or other means, publicly insults an aged person, or fabricates facts to defame him, or maltreats him, if the circumstances are relatively minor, shall be punished in accordance with the relevant provisions of the Regulations on Administrative Penalties for Public Security, and, if a crime has been instituted, be investigated for criminal liability according to law.

There is also a separate article that focuses on financial exploitation of older persons. Under Article 48,

> where a family member steals, swindles, forcibly seizes, extorts, or intentionally destroys property of an aged person, if the circumstances are relatively minor, he shall be punished in accordance with the relevant provisions of the Regulations on Administrative Penalties for Public Security, and if a crime has been instituted, be investigated for criminal liability according to law.

In Taiwan, the interests of elder abuse victims are protected under the Domestic Violence Prevention Act. enacted in 1998, the Act provides sanctions against any act of infringement, mental or physical, amongst family members. Since 1998, several amendments have been made to the Act. In the latest update in 2002, family members protected under this Act include:

- a person who is identified as a spouse, or ex-spouse;
- a person who has or has ever had an on-going marital, or de-facto marital, parental and/or dependent relationship;
- a person who is or has been related as a lineal-blood or a lineal-blood-by-marriage; and
- a person who is or has been related as a lateral blood or a lateral-blood-by-marriage falling within the relation rank.

Older persons subjected to elder mistreatment, therefore, are protected under this act.

Aside from the Domestic Violence Prevention Act, which protects family members against domestic violence in general, the Senior Citizen Welfare Act, first announced in 1980, focuses more specifically on elder abuse and aims to assert the dignity and health, to maintain the standard of living, to protect the rights, and to facilitate the welfare of elders. In the latest version of the Act, updated in 2002, Article 51 states,

> Legal supporters or contractual supporters of the elders will receive a fine of no less than NT$30,000, but less than NT$150,000, if they violate one of the following: 1. Desertion; 2. Freedom impeding; 3. Abuse; 4. Physical and mental mistreatment; 5. Leaving incompetent elders alone in dangerous places or places where the elders might get hurt; and 6. Deserting the elders in an institution without a proper reason or refusing to take care of the case after a period of being informed by the institution.

Also, the name of the supporter will be made public if he or she violates criminal laws, and he or she will be referred to the judicatory authority.

Reporting of elder abuse

There is no mandatory reporting of elder abuse cases in the PRC or Hong Kong. In Hong Kong, as from 2006, a Central Information System on Elder Abuse Cases has been introduced and human service professionals working with older persons are recommended to report any suspected elder abuse cases to the system. A minimal number of cases, however, have been reported to the system. In 2006, 2007, 2008, 2009, and 2010, only 522, 612, 647, 465, and 319 elder abuse cases were reported. This suggests that many elder mistreatment cases go undetected.

In Taiwan, reporting of elder abuse cases is mandatory. Frontline human service professionals have legal responsibilities to report any suspected case of elder abuse to the appropriate authorities within 24 hours. As stated in Article 50 of the Domestic Violence Prevention Act:

> while performing their duties, medical, social, psychological, educational, and nursing professionals, police, staff of the immigration service, and all personnel involved in the enforcement of the control and prevention of domestic violence shall report any suspicion of domestic violence to local regulating authorities within 24 hours. The methods and matters of report are regulated by the central regulating authorities and the identity of the informant is kept confidential.
>
> Upon being informed, the regulating authorities, when required, shall conduct or cause other agencies, institutions, or groups involved in the control and prevention of domestic violence to conduct visits and investigations. In conducting such visits and investigations, the regulating authorities or the undertaking agency, group, or institution may request assistance from the police, medical center, school, or any other related agency or institution; and said agency or institution shall not deny such requests for support.

Following the enactment of the mandatory reporting system, reporting of cases received by the Social Welfare Administration of the Ministry of the Interior in Taiwan rose from 1,144 in 2002 to 3,044 in 2010.

Practice response

There is a paucity of information relating to practice response to elder mistreatment in the PRC. However, in Hong Kong both governmental and non-governmental organizations provide services in response to elder mistreatment. Governmental bodies, such as the District Elderly Community Centers, Neighborhood Elderly Centers, and Integrated Family Services Centers, provide case work services for elder mistreatment victims and perpetrators. In addition, non-governmental organizations provide services ranging from hotline enquiries and shelters to case management and mediation between the victims and the perpetrators. Government and non-governmental bodies also provide public education to raise public awareness about the prevalence and consequences of elder mistreatment in the community.

A multidisciplinary approach to elder mistreatment is advocated in Taiwan. Article 8 of the Domestic Violence Prevention Act requires a domestic violence prevention center incorporating efforts from police administration, education, health, social administration, household administration, and judicial units concerned to be created and maintained by the government. Services provided by this center include a 24-hour hotline, a 24-hour emergency rescue that largely involves medical care, psychological support, economic support, legal supports, an education service, housing guidance, vocational training, an employment service, and short-, medium-, and long-term shelters for the victim and for minors. As elders are protected under the Domestic

Violence Prevention Act, these services would be available to victims of elder mistreatment. Apart from the services provided for the victims, the centers also provide physical and mental treatment programs and follow-up consultation for the perpetrators as well as education, training, and promotion programs for the community.

In general, practice response to elder mistreatment in Chinese societies is challenged by several factors: rapid growth of the aging population, social changes that threaten traditional family relationships, and under-reporting of elder mistreatment.

Rapid growth of the aging population in Chinese societies

As with their global counterparts, older people in Chinese societies are growing in number and proportion due to the lower fertility and increased longevity in these societies (Harbaugh and West 1993, Joseph and Phillips 1999, Kinsella 2000, Du and Guo 2000). In the 1990s, Harbaugh and West (1993) noted that, compared to the 1950s, life expectancy at birth in Mainland China has increased by about 15 years. More recently, the life expectancy in Hong Kong is 80 years for men and 86 for women (Census and Statistical Department 2011), while in Taiwan it is 76 years for men and 83 for women (Tsui and Hsu 2011). As in other parts of the world, better nutrition and improved health care largely account for the longer life expectancy in Chinese people. Also, there has been a decline in fertility rates in Chinese societies. In Mainland China, the reduction in the fertility rate, from 6.0 in the 1950s to less than 2.0 at the turn of the twenty-first century, is related to a stricter population policy, including the introduction of the "one-child policy" in the late 1970s. As Jones (1993) pointed out, the one-child policy has led to a 4-2-1 family structure: each child will most likely have four grandparents, two parents, and no siblings. In Hong Kong and Taiwan, lower fertility rates are likely to be the result of younger people marrying later in life and having fewer children than their parents (Shen and Dai 2006, Chang and Li 2011). As a result of increased longevity and reduced fertility, the elder population is the fastest-growing group in Chinese societies. For example, elders in Taiwan made up about 10 percent of the total population in 2006 and this figure is expected to rise to over 20 percent by 2050; in Mainland China, the figure was 12 percent in 2010 and will be 21 percent to 24 percent by 2030; in Hong Kong, the figure was about 10 percent in 2010 and is estimated to increase to 28 percent by 2039 (Census and Statistical Department 2011). As with other countries facing a rapidly aging population, the Chinese also have to grapple with the challenges of providing social and health care to a growing number of older people in their communities.

Social changes impacting on traditional Chinese family relationships

Traditionally, under the Confucian principle of filial piety, elders were guaranteed prestige, power, and care in the family. However, social changes brought about by industrialization and urbanization have severely threatened such traditional values (Chan and Lee 1995). With the increase in the number of nuclear families (from 52 percent in 1930 to 56 percent in 2000) and simultaneous decrease of multigenerational families (from 49 percent to 21 percent in the same period) in Mainland China (Zeng 1991, Zeng and Wang 2003), there are increasing numbers of older people living alone. Also, daughters and daughters-in-law, who traditionally would have been assigned the duty of carers, are now more likely to be in paid employment (Chen 2001) thus leaving their elderly parents and parents-in-law with no one to care for them. Contrary to the traditional Chinese belief that old age is one of the five great blessings of life, with the decline of filial piety and rapid social changes, many elderly Chinese can no longer expect "satisfying and well-provided-for lives" (Yan et al. 2002: 172). Furthermore, even when elders relocate to urban cities with their adult children, they may find it hard to develop new social support networks. As their children may be unable to provide care and emotional support to them due to work commitments, the relocated elders may feel isolated, neglected, and trapped in the new urban environment, with adverse health outcomes (Chi et al. 1999, DaCanhota and Piterman 2001). In addition, as they become more dependent on family members for care, a caregiver burden may result, with their carers caught in a dilemma: feeling obliged to care, but at the same time wanting to be released from the caring load (Yan et al. 2002). As such, the caregiver burden has been shown to be a significant factor in elder mistreatment (Wang et al. 2006). Elsewhere, in non-Chinese populations, models of support services have been developed to address caregiver burden. An example is the Family Caregiver Support model (Nerenberg 2008). Building upon the strengths of family members to change and develop solutions, the model aims to help resolve stresses for families with ailing elders. For elder Chinese and their caregivers, however, seeking help from outside the family may not come naturally. Indeed, they may think that caring for their elders is a family matter and the resultant burden or stress should not be shared with out-siders. Thus, initiatives designed to care for ailing elders and their caregivers in Chinese societies should recognize the cultural norms and values that influence perceived obligations in Chinese families. Specifically, the focus should be on the whole family rather than on individual members, while stressing that the caregiver burden is not a cause for shame but a well-recognized phenomenon. In response to the need to support caregivers of older people, educational and training strategies targeting domestic care-givers of the elderly have been developed by the National Institute of Health in Taiwan (Wang et al. 2006). Similarly, in a poor and deprived district in Hong Kong, where 13.9 percent of the 523,300 residents are 65 or over, a project that builds on well-established community networks has just begun and is designed to provide respite care for incapacitated elders after office hours and during weekends, thus allowing their caregivers to pursue activities of their choice such as social functions or recreational activities (a private community with Yuk, Director of the HKSKH Lady MacLehose Centre, 16 February 2012). Not only does the project bring together joint efforts of human service professionals and volunteers, it also conveys an important message that families are part of the community and that caregiver burden can be better managed with the help of professionals and volunteers.

Under-reporting of elder mistreatment in Chinese societies

Under-reporting of elder mistreatment is not confined to the Chinese. Globally, it has long been recognized that elder mistreatment is probably greatly under-reported (O'Brien et al. 1999). This may be partly because older adults may be too embarrassed to disclose the existence of mistreatment. Others may fail to report mistreatment out of fear, as the abuser may threaten further violence, termination of support, or other reprisals (Fulmer et al. 2011). In Chinese societies, similar reluctance also exists, but the problem may be further complicated by the traditional belief that family matters should remain within the family and not be shared with outsiders, in the interest of preserving family harmony and honor (Lu and Shin 1997, Dong 2005). Such a belief may also be shared by healthcare and social service professionals in Chinese societies, thus inhibiting them from making enquiries into the possibility of elder mistreatment. Furthermore, recent studies conducted in Taiwan have shown that psychological elder mistreatment is a growing but hidden problem (Wang et al. 2006). Identifying psychological elder mistreatment is challenging due to the lack of clear evidence (Washington Adult Protective Services 2004), thus compounding the problem of under-reporting.

To tackle the problem of under-reporting, the assessment of elder mistreatment in Chinese societies should be done systematically, using culturally relevant instruments. For example, the psychological elder abuse scale (Wang 2005) was developed for assessing levels of psychological abuse in Chinese elders. In addition, those who conduct the assessment should be culturally competent in order to recognize what may be considered as mistreatment by Chinese elders, as discussed earlier. Since assessors may vary in their capacity to identify elder mistreatment, it is important that they receive appropriate training to ensure competence and consistency. Community-wide public education programs should also be launched to help those in the community to recognize elders at risk and respond accordingly. Furthermore, crisis hotlines and shelters for victims of elder mistreatment should also be established. This would enable older victims to exercise their right to self-determination by deciding if and when they want to disclose the mistreatment and seek help.

Research

Despite increasing recognition that elder mistreatment is a global problem, there are relatively few research studies on Chinese elder mistreatment. In the following paragraphs, existing evidence relating to prevalence, impact, risk factors, and interventions of elder mistreatment in Chinese societies will be presented.

The prevalence of elder mistreatment in Chinese societies is comparable to that in Western countries such as the United States (NRC 2003, Lauman et al. 2008), Canada (Podnieks 1990, Pittaway and Westhues 1993, Yaffe et al. 2007), and the United Kingdom (Bennet and Kingston 1993, Biggs et al. 2009). In a study of 276 elder Chinese in Hong Kong (Yan and Tang 2004), 27.5 percent of the respondents reported experiencing at least one abusive behavior by their family caregivers during the surveyed year. Verbal abuse (e.g. being subjected to spite, insult, or swearing), with a prevalence rate of 26.8 percent, was the most common form of mistreatment compared to physical abuse (2.5 percent) (e.g. being pushed or shoved) and violation of personal rights (5.1 percent) (e.g. being forced to enter a nursing home, or not being allowed visits by relatives or friends). Overall mistreatment and verbal mistreatment were best predicted by the participants' advanced age, poor visual and memory abilities, the presence of chronic illness, and dependence on the caregivers. In a more recent study into the prevalence and risk factors of elder abuse by family caregivers among older Chinese with dementia in Hong Kong (Yan and Kwok 2011), 18 percent of the 122 family caregivers reported having verbally or physically abused their care recipients during the previous month. Family caregivers who reported more abusive behaviors were those who spent more days co-residing with the care recipients, lacked assistance from a domestic helper, and/or were experiencing a higher level of caregiver burden. The findings showed that verbal and physical mistreatment were prevalent among older Chinese with dementia, and a higher level of caregiver stress was correspondingly associated with a higher level of verbal mistreatment.

In a group of randomly selected elderly Taiwanese (N = 195) who were capable of verbal communication and partially dependent on a caregiver, 22.6 percent scored 10 or above on the psychological elder abuse scale (PEAS), suggesting that they had experienced psychological abuse in the surveyed period (Wang 2006). Also, lower cognitive and physical functioning was strongly related to psychological abuse (Wang 2006). In addition, caregivers of elder Chinese were the focus of three studies conducted in Taiwan. In one of the studies that explored the state and correlated factors of psychological abuse behaviors among caregivers in long-term care facilities in Taiwan, 16.1 percent of the 114 caregiver participants had a score of greater than 40 on the caregiver psychological elder abuse behavior scale (CPEAB), indicating a tendency toward psychological abuse behaviors. Caregivers who displayed a greater tendency toward more abusive behaviors were those who were younger in age, less educated, lacking in geriatric training, and carrying a greater burden (Wang 2005). In another study involving caregivers of elders living in their own home (Wang et al. 2006), only 6 out of the 92 caregivers reported that they had not engaged in any psychologically abusive behavior toward their elder care recipients in the previous six months. Also, female caregivers, caregivers with higher levels of education, and caregivers with heavy burdens demonstrated more severe psychologically abusive behavior. In the third study (Wang et al. 2009), of the 183 caregivers recruited from seven long-term care facilities in Taiwan, those who worked fewer hours, received fewer years of education, lacked social resources, and had more work stress reported higher levels of psychological abuse behaviors when caring for the elderly.

In the PRC, 141 women and 270 men aged 60 years or older attending an urban medical center were recruited to a cross-sectional study investigating elder mistreatment (Dong et al. 2007a). The findings revealed that elder mistreatment was reported by 35 percent of the participants, while female gender, lower education, and lower income were demographic risk factors associated with elder abuse and neglect (Dong et al. 2007a). Other studies conducted in the PRC found that loneliness was positively associated with the risk of elder mistreatment (Dong et al. 2007b); perceived social support, but not instrumental social support, was associated with increased odds of elder mistreatment (Dong and Simon 2010). Furthermore, depression was associated with an increased risk of elder mistreatment in both men and women, even though the increased risk may be modified by greater overall social support, which appeared to have a stronger effect for men than for women (Dong et al. 2010).

There are few studies on the impact of elder mistreatment in Chinese societies. Among the few existing studies, the findings are similar to those reported in Western literature. For example, Yan and Tang (2001) reported that elderly Chinese abused by their caregivers reported significantly more psychological distress. Also, verbal abuse was the most salient predictor of psychological distress among Chinese elders. In Zhang and Yu's (1997) study excessive financial requests and verbal abuse by other family members were found to be significant correlates of elderly people's depressive symptoms.

Notwithstanding the emerging research related to elder mistreatment in Chinese societies, caution must be exercised when comparing the findings as there are variations in definition, sampling technique, method of data collection, and measurement among the studies. Also, few of the studies have elaborated on the cultural sensitivity of the measuring tools used. Exceptions are the PEAS, developed by Wang and her colleagues in Taiwan, focusing on psychological abuse experienced by Chinese elders (Wang et al. 2007), and the 13 questions developed by Dong and researchers in the PRC for identification of physical abuse, psychological abuse, caregiver neglect, financial exploitation, sexual abuse, and abandonment (Dong et al. 2007a).

Conclusion

With rapid social and economic changes in Chinese societies and the erosion of traditional family values, the vulnerability of older people as victims of elder mistreatment has become more apparent. This changing trend has implications for practice, policy, and research. In terms of practice response, existing services and support for older people and their carers should be reviewed and expanded as needed. Crisis hotlines and shelters specially designed for victims of elder mistreatment should be established. Educating the public about healthy aging, family relationships, and elder mistreatment should be strengthened so as to raise public awareness of this often invisible problem. Also, in order to ensure prompt reporting and timely intervention, training should be provided to health and social care professionals, focusing on early detection, identification, crisis management, and intervention regarding elder mistreatment. In relation to policy, existing policy on prevention and intervention regarding elder mistreatment should be reviewed and revised as appropriate. Resources should be allocated not only to expand the existing services but also to ensure that a multidisciplinary approach be adopted to address the needs of older people and their carers. Policy makers should also make public their zero tolerance of elder mistreatment and their intention to bring in sanctions to stop this violation of the rights of older people. Much needs to be done in the research arena in light of the paucity of studies on elder mistreatment in Chinese societies. There is a need to redefine elder mistreatment using the Chinese lens. Similarly, instruments used to identify elder mistreatment among Chinese elders must be validated for cultural sensitivity. The efficacy of elder mistreatment prevention and intervention programs should be tested using robust research designs such as randomized controlled trials. Finally, cross-cultural and cross-national similarities and differences in relation to elder mistreatment should be critically examined in order to advance understanding about this complex phenomenon. Through the concerted efforts of carers, service providers, policy-makers, and researchers, aging can be a healthy process and enjoyed by older people in Chinese societies without the fear of mistreatment.

References

Bennet, G. and Kingston, P. (1993) Elder abuse: Concepts, theories and interventions. London: Chapman and Hall.

Biggs, S., Manthorpe, J. and Tinker, A. (2009) 'Mistreatment of older people in the United Kingdom: Findings from the first national prevalence study'. Journal of Elder Abuse and Neglect, 21: 1–14.

Census and Statistic Department (2011) Statistics and you. Online. Available at <http://www.statistics.gov.hk/publication/free_reference/B8XX0003.pdf> (accessed 10 October 2012).

Chan, A.C.M and Lim, M.Y. (2004) 'Changes of filial piety in Chinese societies'. International Scope Review, 6: 1–16.

Chan, H. and Lee, R. (1995) 'Hong Kong families: At the crossroad of modernism and traditionalism'. Journal of Comparative Family Studies, 26: 83–99.

Chang, Y.C. and Li, J.C.A. (2011) Trends and educational differentials in marriage formation among Taiwanese women. Online. Available at <http://www.rand.org/content/dam/rand/pubs/working_papers/2011/RAND_WR891.pdf> (accessed 21 April 2012)

Chen, Y.C., (2001) 'Chinese values, health and nursing', Journal of Advance Nursing, 36: 270–73.

Chi, I., Chou, K.L., Boey, K.W. (1999) 'Determinants of depressive symptoms among elderly Chinese living alone'. Clinical Gerontologist, 20(4): 15–27.

Chow, N.W.S. (2001) 'The practice of filial piety among the Chinese in Hong Kong' in I. Chi, N.L. Chappel and J. Lubben (eds) Elderly Chinese in Pacific Rim countries: Social support and integration. Hong Kong: Hong Kong University Press.

DaCanhota, C. and Piterman, L. (2001) 'Depressive disorders in elderly Chinese patients in Macau: A comparison of general practitioners consultations with a depressive screening scale'. Australian and New Zealand Journal of Psychiatry, 35: 336–44.

Dong, X. (2005) 'Medical implications of elder abuse and neglect'. Clinical Geriatric Medicine, 21(2): 293–313.

——and Simon, M. (2010) 'Gender variations in the levels of social support and risk of elder mistreatment in a Chinese community population'. Journal of Applied Gerontology, 29(6): 720–39.

——, Simon, M. and Gorbien, M. (2007a) 'Elder abuse and neglect in an urban Chinese population'. Journal of Elder Abuse and Neglect, 19 (3/4): 79–96.

——, Simon, M., Gorbien, M., Percak, J. and Golden, R. (2007b) 'Loneliness in older Chinese adults: A risk factor for elder mistreatment'. Journal of the American Geriatrics Society, 55: 1831–5.

——, Beck, T. and Simon, M. (2010) 'The associations of gender, depression and elder mistreatment in a community-dwelling Chinese population: The modifying effect of social support'. Archives of Gerontology and Geriatrics, 50: 202–8.

Du, P. and Guo, Z. (2000) 'Population ageing in China', in D. Phillips (ed.) Ageing in the Asia Pacific region. London: Routledge.

Fulmer, T., Sengstock, M.C., Blankenship, J., et al. (2011) 'Elder mistreatment', in J. Humphreys and J.C. Campbell (eds) Family Violence and Nursing Practice. New York: Springer Publishing Company.

Harbaugh, C.W. and West, C.A. (1993) 'Ageing trends: China'. Journal of Cross Cultural Gerontology, 8: 271–80.

Ho, D. (1996) 'Filial piety and its psychological consequences', in M.H. Bond (ed.) Handbook of Chinese psychology. Hong Kong: Oxford University Press.

Hong Kong Christian Service (2002) Elder abuse research and protocol. Hong Kong: Hong Kong Christian Service.

Hsu, H.C., Lew-Ting, C.Y. and Wu, S.C. (2001) 'Age, period, and cohort effects on the attitude toward supporting parents in Taiwan'. The Gerontologist, 41: 742–50.

Jones, G.W. (1993) 'Consequences of rapid fertility decline for old age security', in L. Leete and I. Alam (eds) The revolution in Asian fertility: Dimensions, causes, and implications. Oxford: Clarendon Press.

Joseph, A.E. and Phillips, P.R. (1999) 'Ageing in rural China: Impacts of increasing diversity in family and community resources'. Journal of Cross Cultural Gerontology. 14: 153–68.

Kinsella, K. (2000) 'Demographic dimensions of global aging'. Journal of Family Issues. 21: 541–58.

Kwan, A.Y., Cheung, J.C. and Ng, S.H. (2003) 'Revisit of filial piety concept among the young, the adult, and the old in Beijing, Guangzhou, Hong Kong, Nanjing, Shanghai, Xiamen, and Xian'. Unpublished report, City University of Hong Kong, Department of Applied Social Studies.

Laumann, E.O., Leitsch, S.A. and Waite, L.J. (2008) 'Elder mistreatment in the United States'. The Journals of Gerontology, Series B, Psychological Sciences and Social Sciences, 63(4): S248–54.

Lu, L. and Shin, J.B. (1997) 'Sources of happiness: A qualitative approach'. Journal of Social Psychology, 137: 181–7.

Nerenberg, L. (2008) Elder abuse prevention: Emerging trends and promising strategies. New York: Springer.

NRC (2003) Elder mistreatment: Abuse, neglect, and exploitation in aging America. National Research Council. Washington, DC: The National Academies Press.

O'Brien, J.G., Thibault, J.M., Turner, L.C. and Laird-Fick, H.S. (1999) 'Self-neglect: An overview and self-neglect: challenges for helping professionals'. Journal of Elder Abuse and Neglect, 2: 1–19.

Pittaway, E. and Westhues, A. (1993) 'The prevalence of elder abuse and neglect of older adults who access health and social services in London, Ontario, Canada'. Journal of Elder Abuse and Neglect, 5: 77–93.

Podnieks, E. (1990) National survey on abuse of the elderly in Canada: The Ryerson Study. Toronto: Ryerson Polytechnical Institute.

Shen, J. and Dai, E. (2006) Population growth, fertility decline, and ageing in Hong Kong: The perceived and real demographic effects of migration. Online. Available at <http://www.cuhk.edu.hk/shkdi/OP/OP14.pdf> (accessed 21 March 2010).

Tam, S. and Neysmith, S. (2006) 'Disrespect and isolation: Elder abuse in Chinese communities'. Canadian Journal on Aging, 25: 141–51.

Teo, P., Graham, E., Yeoh, B.S.A. and Levy, S. (2003) 'Values, change and inter-generational ties between two generations of women in Singapore'. Ageing and Society, 23: 327–47.

Tsui, A. and Hsu, E. (2011) 'Taipei citizens live longer than others in Taiwan: MOI'. Taiwan News. Online. Available at <http://www.taiwannews.com.tw/etn/news_content.php?id=1740266> (accessed 23 January 2012).

Wang, J.J. (2005) 'Psychological abuse behavior exhibited by caregivers in the care of the elderly and correlated factors in long-term care facilities in Taiwan'. Journal of Nursing Research, 13, 4: 271–9.

——(2006) 'Psychological abuse and its characteristic correlates among elderly Taiwanese'. Archives of Gerontology and Geriatrics, 42: 307–18.

Wang, J.J., Lin, J.N. and Lee, F.P. (2006) 'Psychologically abusive behavior by those caring for the elderly in a domestic context'. Geriatric Nursing, 27, 5: 284–91.

Wang, J.J., Lin, M.F., Tseng, H.F. and Chang, W.Y. (2009) 'Caregiver factors contributing to psychological elder abuse behavior in long-term care facilities: A structural equation model approach'. International Psychogeriatrics, 21, 2: 314–21.

Wang, J.J., Tseng, H.F. and Chen, K.M. (2007) 'Development and testing of screening indicators for psychological abuse of older people'. Archives of Psychiatric Nursing. 21, 1: 40–47.

Washington Adult Protective Services (2004) Reports of abuse, neglect, self neglect, financial exploitation, or abandonment. Online. Available at <www.elderabusecenter.org/pdf/whatnew/litreview040707.pdf> (accessed 15 January 2011).

Yaffe, M.J., Weiss, D., Wolfson, C. and Lithwick, M. (2007) 'Detection and prevalence of abuse of older males: Perspectives from family practice'. Journal of Elder Abuse and Neglect, 19, 1/2: 47–60.

Yan, E. (2012) 'Research on elder mistreatment in Chinese society', in K.L Chan (ed.) Preventing Family Violence: A Multidisciplinary Approach. Hong Kong: Hong Kong University Press.

——and Kwok, T. (2011) 'Abuse of older Chinese with dementia by family caregivers: An inquiry into the role of caregiver burden'. International Journal of Geriatric Psychiatry, 26: 527–35.

——and Tang, C.S.K. (2001) 'Prevalence and psychological impact of Chinese elder abuse'. Journal of Interpersonal Violence, 16: 1158–74.

——and Tang, C.S.K. (2004) 'Elder abuse by caregivers: a study of prevalence and risk factors in Hong Kong Chinese families'. Journal of Family Violence, 19, 5: 269–77.

——, Tang, C.S.K. and Yeung, D. (2002) 'No safe haven: A review on elder abuse in Chinese families'. Trauma, Violence, and Abuse, 3, 3: 167–80.

Yang, K.S. (1997) 'Theories and research in Chinese personality: An indigenous approach', in H.S.R. Kao and D. Sinha (eds) Asian perspectives on psychology. Thousand Oaks, CA: Sage.

Zeng, Y. (1991) Family dynamics in China: A life table analysis. Madison, WI: University of Wisconsin Press.

——and Wang, Z.L. (2003) 'Dynamics of family and elderly living arrangements in China: New lessons learned from the 2000 census', The China Review, 3, 2: 95–119.

——and Yu, L.C. (1997) 'Family and cultural correlates of depression among Chinese elderly'. International Journal of Social Psychiatry, 42: 199–213.

5 Ireland

Amanda Phelan

Introduction

Up until the last decade, elder abuse in Ireland received scant attention. However, since the publication by the Working Group on Elder Abuse of the Irish elder abuse policy document, Protecting our Future (WGEA 2002), a more focused response has been apparent. Recommendations of the report have resulted in the establishment of dedicated services for elder abuse, a reorientation of legislation, a national research centre and improvement in the regulation of residential care for older people. An essential element of the policy has been the emphasis on a multi-dimensional and integrated approach between all relevant stakeholders. This chapter will firstly contextualise older people in Ireland and review the developments in relation to elder abuse in Ireland.

Older people in Ireland

Changing demographics can affect the incidence of elder abuse (Schiamberg et al. 2011). In Ireland, the population of older people has been comparatively low in a European context due to a history of emigration over the past two centuries. Since the Great Famine of 1845–52, many young Irish people emigrated to countries such as America, Australia and the United Kingdom in search of new opportunities. Other impacting factors on Irish current older person demographics include a relatively high birth rate and life expectancy changes (Fahey et al. 2007). Life expectancy has risen from 58 years for both men and women in the period 1925–27 to 76.8 years for men and 81.6 years for women in 2011 (CSO 2011). In a recent 2011 Irish census, there were 4,588,252 people in Ireland. Of this figure, 535,393 people were over 65 years of age, an increase of 14.4 per cent on the previous 2006 census (CSO 2012). The growth in the proportion of people in Ireland over 65 years of age is projected to further increase with estimates that older people will constitute 15.4 per cent of the Irish population by 2021 with over 100 per cent increase in those over 85 years of age in the same timeframe (Morgenroth 2008, Layte 2009).

All older people in Ireland are covered by free medical care, which also covers the cost of most medicines, from the age of 70 years. This has caused significant political debate in recent years as successive governments have attempted to impose a means-based eligibility rather than universal eligibility (Fealy and McNamara 2009, Phelan 2012).

Policy

Elder abuse received little attention in the period up to the late 1990s in Ireland (Horkan 1995). In 1998, the lack of formal service responses was highlighted in an Irish exploratory study on the topic (O'Loughlin and Duggan 1998). Subsequently, a WGEA was established to articulate a comprehensive national policy on elder abuse. The Group extended Action on Elder Abuse's (1995) definition of abuse to incorporate the dimension of a rights based approach. Elder abuse was defined as:

> A single or repeated act or lack of appropriate action occurring within any relationship where there is an expectation of trust which causes harm or distress to an older person or violates their human and civil rights.
>
> (WGEA 2002: 25)

Recommendations from the WGEA were focused on an integrated, contexualised person-centred approach to addressing elder abuse in Ireland. This approach emphasised a linkage between elder abuse and wider social policy and included areas such as public awareness, advocacy for and empowerment of older people, education of various professionals, legislation, public awareness, issues pertaining to mental capacity, legislative protection, the establishment of a national research centre and a dedicated service to respond to allegations of elder abuse. Recognising that elder abuse often has a criminal dimension, the role of the Garda Siochana (Irish police) was made explicit in cases where an offence had occurred.

Irish policy (WGEA 2002) identified elder abuse as manifesting itself in psychological, physical, sexual and financial abuse, neglect and discriminatory abuse. Abuse by strangers and self-neglect were specifically identified as outside the remit of the terms of reference of WGEA (2002). However, in 2009, the Health Service Executive (HSE) extended their referral criteria to include extreme cases of self-neglect. This subsequently led to the development of a formal HSE policy to address self-neglect in 2012 (HSE 2012a).

The implementation of WGEA (2002) was overseen by the Elder Abuse National Implementation Group (EANIG). In terms of assessing the implementation process, the WGEA (2002) recommendations included a formal national review of progress in policies, procedures, service responses and legislative changes. In 2009, PA Consulting carried out this review and noted that much progress had occurred in the health sector in relation to responding to elder abuse. However, the review acknowledged further directions for policy improvement in terms of increased agency collaboration to potentialise the protection of older people. Furthermore, it was observed that additional integration of elder abuse policy within a wider health and social context was needed (PA Consulting 2009). Issues such as increased legislative protection, continued public awareness campaigns, caregiver regulation and professional education were also identified as areas for improvement. Ensuring that such interconnections were realised has been bolstered by the establishment in 2008 of a ministerial position with a portfolio that includes a specific responsibility for older people.[1] This has resulted in a determined emphasis on policy in relation to older people. Moreover, recognising that the protection of older people transcends a specific elder abuse focus, other policy developments have occurred in relation to a dementia-specific policy, a caregivers' strategy, a healthy ageing strategy and a review of the rights of older people in Ireland, all of which are fundamental to underpinning a safe and equitable environment for Irish older people.

Service response

In Ireland, the HSE is responsible for the delivery of public health services and is comprised of four regional areas. Within the HSE, there is a dedicated Assistant National Director with specific responsibility for services for older people. In response to WGEA (2002), a formal, dedicated service was established to respond to elder abuse in 2007 and was situated within the HSE. The service is led by a national elder abuse steering committee and there are four regional HSE steering groups. While the national steering group take an overall strategic approach to standard planning, implementation and evaluation, the regional groups operationalise these approaches at a local level. Each regional area also has a dedicated officer for the protection of older people and there are 32 senior caseworkers nationally who receive elder abuse referrals, coordinate case management and lead on multi-disciplinary responses to elder abuse cases as well as raising awareness and delivering training on elder abuse (PA Consulting 2009). Since the service's establishment, the national elder abuse steering group has published annual statistics. Year on year there has been an increase in case referrals from 927 in 2007 (HSE 2009) to 2,302 in 2011 (HSE 2012b). Of the 2011 figures, 1,867 of referred cases cited an alleged perpetrator, 429 were cases of self-neglect and the remaining 6 were described as organizational abuse (HSE 2012b). Females were over-represented in referrals (63 per cent), as were older people over 80 years of age. Although many referrals related to only one type of abuse (68 per cent), 24 per cent detailed two types of abuse with 8 per cent having more than two types of abuse. The most common form of abuse in referrals was psychological abuse (29 per cent), followed by financial abuse (19 per cent), self-neglect (18 per cent), neglect (17 per cent), physical abuse (10 per cent), sexual abuse (2 per cent), discriminatory abuse (1 per cent) and other (4 per cent). Most case referrals related to abuse in the older person's own home environment (81 per cent), while the remainder related to settings such as nursing homes and the homes of relatives. The most common perpetrators were family members, predominantly a son or daughter (44 per cent). Of the total number of case referrals (n = 2,302), 637 (34 per cent) older people were identified as having some form of health issue, for example physical ill health, dementia or mental health challenges (HSE 2012b). These referrals are generally underestimations compared to prevalence studies (Naughton et al. 2010, Amstadter et al. 2011, Lifespan of Greater Rochester et al. 2011), thus, under-referral is a constant concern.

In the context of service responses, the HSE also established four working groups who lead on particular strategic priorities. These are a) the media and public awareness group, b) the policies, procedures, protocols and guidelines group, c) the staff awareness and curriculum group and d) the financial abuse of older people group. In relation to the media and public awareness group, public awareness campaigns have been used in the local and national media to enhance understandings of elder abuse and its unacceptability in Irish society. Evaluations have also occurred to identify the impact of the 2010 'Open your Eyes' media campaign using a focus group methodology. Findings reveal the effectiveness of improving public awareness on both the issue of elder abuse and the context within which it occurs (HSE 2012b). Other successes have been demonstrated in the effectiveness of the HSE DVD training material and information leaflets as well as the annual World Elder Abuse Awareness Day conference (in collaboration with the International Network for the Prevention of Elder Abuse and the National Centre for the Protection of Older People).

The policy and procedures group have made significant advances in terms of protocols for making a will in residential and day services, the transfer of elder abuse cases between local health offices, the prevention of elder abuse: best practice guidelines for non-governmental organisations and a review of the HSE's own policy on responding to allegations of elder abuse. The HSE staff awareness and curricula group have reviewed the curriculum content for relevant disciplines in relation to elder abuse and lobbied for its inclusion in academic programmes which did not cover this material. In addition, training has occurred for professionals in financial institutions, An Garda Siochana and the legal sector (HSE 2012b).

The final working group focused on financial abuse of older people. Financial abuse was specifically identified as an issue in the Irish policy on elder abuse (WGEA 2002) and financial abuse was the most frequent type of abuse to be identified in the Irish prevalence study (Naughton et al. 2010). The HSE National Financial Abuse of Older Persons Working Group is comprised of membership from differing government departments, the Irish League of Credit Unions, An Garda Siochana, the Law Reform Commission, the National Consumer Agency, the Irish Banking Federation, the Department of Social and Family Affairs, An Post and the Office of the Financial Regulator. Work to date has included a review of the Financial Regulator's

Consumer Protection Code and recommendations were made to the Financial Regulator on how abuse could be minimised for vulnerable customers such as older people.

The National Centre for the Protection of Older People

One of the recommendations of WGEA 2002 was the establishment of a dedicated research centre to focus on elder abuse in Ireland. In 2008, the National Centre for the Protection of Older People (NCPOP) (www.ncpop.ie) was established in University College Dublin (UCD). Led by the UCD School of Nursing, Midwifery and Health Systems, this Centre represents a collaboration between UCD School of Applied Social Science, the UCD School of Public Health and Population Science, UCD School of Medicine and Medical Science and the UCD Geary Institute. The Centre's dominant focus is to conduct Irish-based research, review international literature in relation to elder abuse issues and deliver regular seminars focused on NCPOP study findings or relevant presentations from invited guest speakers.

Projects completed by the NCPOP include specific literature reviews and studies on elder abuse and its context in Ireland. Literature reviews focused on issues such as legislation in relation to elder abuse (Lyons 2009a), public perceptions of older people and ageing (Lyons 2009b), public perceptions of elder abuse (Lafferty 2009), a critical review of elder abuse screening tools (Phelan and Treacy 2011) and the financial abuse of older people (Fealy et al. 2012).

A number of studies have generated insights into elder abuse in Ireland. The Irish prevalence study used a random route-finding technique in 150 Irish electoral divisions to interview 2,021 older people face to face in their homes (Naughton et al. 2010). Participants were stratified into three age groups: 65–69 years, 70–79 years and 80 plus years. Data were collected based on socio-demographics, health status, social support, the experience of abuse and neglect, the impact of and response to abuse, and the perpetrator characteristics. Findings revealed a prevalence of elder abuse of 2.2 per cent by people in a position of trust in the previous twelve months. When these figures are extrapolated to the general population, an estimated 10,201 older people were subject to abuse in the community. However, if the perpetrator variable included those in the wider community (i.e. those not classicly termed in a position of trust), the prevalence figure rose to 2.9 per cent. Abuse by perpetrators in a position of trust since the age of 65 years was found to be 4.0 per cent, while such abuse in the wider community increased figures to 5.5 per cent (Naughton et al. 2010). When the prevalence figures are compared with the HSE referrals, there is a gap between the incidence of elder abuse and cases which come to the attention of the formal services. This corresponds with the iceberg theory of elder abuse (DHSS 1998), which suggests that many elder abuse cases do not come to the attention of official services and under-reporting has been identified in the literature as an issue of concern (DHSS 1998, Lachs and Pillemer 2004, WHO 2008, O'Brien 2010).

Two NCPOP studies focused on newspaper analysis to identify issues related to elder abuse (Fealy and McNamara 2009, Phelan 2009). The first study considered how ageing was constructed in selected national newspapers following the Irish government's threatened withdrawal of universal free medical cards to older people over 70 years of age (Fealy and McNamara 2009). This threatened withdrawal resulted in a march by over 10,000 older people on the Irish Parliament and, ultimately, the rescinding of the government's proposals. The second study examined newspaper discourses following an expose of poor practices in an Irish nursing home (Phelan 2009). Findings from both studies revealed that older people were constructed in vulnerable positions. Moreover, the reportage of newspapers was rarely neutral and editorial commentary varied within the context of tabloid and broadsheet. Both studies also advocated caution on the use of language, in particular language that perpetuated stereotypes of older people and polarised positions of government and older people (Phelan 2009, Fealy and McNamara 2009).

In a study which reviewed senior caseworkers' management of elder abuse cases, an in-depth interview approach was taken with a sample of 18 participants (O'Donnell et al. 2012). Elder abuse was considered by the participants as a complex issue which involved a careful balance between the older person's self-autonomy and the degree of risk, vulnerability and capacity due to the abuse. Each case was described as unique and could challenge the senior caseworker (O'Donnell et al. 2012). The management of cases demanded an ethical approach, which involved navigating family conflict and addressing normalised, challenging family behaviours. An essential element of case management was inter-disciplinary and inter-agency collaboration, although negotiation of roles and understandings in such alliances could be difficult. Senior caseworkers also described the complexity of aligning case management to available resources, particularly in an environment of finite resources. In particular, limited legislation pertaining to the regulation of solicitors and care professionals and in relation to underpinning their own role was identified as challenging. Senior caseworkers also articulated concern regarding their isolated working practice, the lack of clinical supervision and the need for standardised work practices within the service (O'Donnell et al. 2012). Similar findings were also observed in a study of Irish community nursing services and the management of elder abuse (Phelan 2010).

Another study was undertaken on the experiences, coping strategies and support needs of older Irish people who have been abused (Lafferty et al. 2012). In-depth interviews occurred with nine community-dwelling older people, who had received support services from senior caseworkers. The participants reported experiences which mirrored all types of elder abuse. The abuse impacted on the physical and emotional health of the older person as well as impacting on their social circumstances. Various strategies were employed by the participants to cope with the abuse, such as avoiding the issue, confronting the perpetrator, finding a place of sanctuary and rationalising the abuse. Some of the participants described how they drew on personal strengths to cope with the abuse. In terms of seeking help, most participants received help through third party intervention, such as other family members or friends, as well as from both statutory and voluntary bodies (Lafferty et al. 2012). However, the participants reported that issues such as non-recognition of the abuse, a fear of sourcing assistance and difficulties in accessing limited services could provide significant barriers to seeking help (Lafferty et al. 2012).

Further research in progress in the NCPOP includes a survey of staff–resident interactions and conflicts in residential care settings for older people, piloting of the Elder Abuse Suspicion Index (Yaffe et al. 2008) and the Older Adult Financial Exploitation Measure (Conrad et al. 2010), an evaluation of the HSE training for elder abuse, carer stress in relation to elder abuse and the empowerment of older people as a preventative and ameliorative mechanism in elder abuse. Further literature reviews will focus on elder abuse in the context of older people and dementia, abuse in residential care settings: best practice and elder abuse services and interventions.

Elder abuse in the public eye

All forms of media have the ability to influence societal perspectives in the context of politics, culture and social life (Bell 1998, Kitzinger 2000). One of the major catalysts in raising Irish public awareness of elder abuse was Raidió Teilifís Éireann's broadcast of two television programmes using undercover filming of poor practices. The first programme, Prime Time Investigates: Home Truths (RTÉ 2005), caused huge public alarm and generated much subsequent coveragage in newspapers, radio and other media forms. The Home Truths programme was significant due to the enormous public outcry it caused and the intensive debate it sparked in the Oireachtas (Irish Parliament) on how older people in residential care were protected from abuse. Although this nursing home was subsequently closed down, two formal inquiries were commissioned (O'Neill 2006, DOHC 2009) and identified issues pertaining to staff competency in relation to working with older people, a lack of individualised care planning, a lack of impact assessment of major bed capacity expansion in the nursing home and the inadequacies of the existing inspection process by the HSE in 2005. Significantly, this broadcast provided a powerful catalyst to the establishment of the Health Information and Quality Authority (HIQA) which is an independent body responsible for regulation and standards of residential care facilities in Ireland.

The second television broadcast employed a similar approach of undercover film footage to highlight deficiencies in the provision care support services to older people in their own homes in Ireland. Prime Time Investigates: The Homecare Scandal programme was broadcast on 13 December 2010

(RTÉ 2010). Although the HSE has a service to provide home care, it also funds private care agencies to deliver care through 'home care packages'. In Ireland, the private home care enterprise expanded hugely with numbers rising from approximately 10 companies in 2000 to approximately 150 in 2010. Concerns raised by this broadcast (RTÉ 2010) included the relative ease of registering as a company in Ireland to provide homecare, a lack of appropriate training of the caregivers, particularly in relation to dementia, a failure to deliver the negotiated duration of care, a lack of standardised police vetting or ensuring suitable references of caregivers and a lack of appropriate responses to complaints by the private care agencies. Although the HSE provided funding for private care, in many instances there was a disconnect between the formal HSE services and the private care provision in the context of supervision of care and communication of care planning. The programme also demonstrated the vulnerability of the caregiver being employed by the care agency as, in some cases, the European Union Working Time Directives (EP and ECM 2003) were disregarded and underpayment or non-payment of employees was evident. Although the government of the day indicated that regulation in the home environment was not required, recent recommendations from the Irish Law Reform Commission (2011) have lobbied for the regulation of formal care services in the community.

The public scrutiny of private areas, such as the older person's home or residential care facilities for older people, has revealed major concerns in regard to standards of care in Ireland. Older people in these environments may not realise that the care delivery is substandard and the power differentials between the older person and formal caregivers can imbue a perceived help-lessness which exacerbates the possibility of abuse perpetration, either on an individual level or in the context of the organisation and delivery of care. Both broadcast programmes identified the need to tighten regulation of care service delivery in settings for older people. This is particularly important in the context of older people in receipt of such care and are therefore more vulnerable due to a dependency which requires such care (McDonald et al. 2012).

Legislation

The general literature on older people's specific legal needs is scant (Basu and Duffy 2010). Although the Irish Constitution (Bunreacht na Éireann) specifically states a responsibility to safeguard the 'aged' (Article 4, Section 2, Government of Ireland 1937), there is no explicit legislation specifically for older people, nor is the reporting of elder abuse mandatory. However, generic legislation can be used to pursue elder abuse allegations. For instance, the Domestic Violence Act (Government of Ireland 1996a) can be used to protect an abused person. This legislation also stipulates that action can be taken on behalf of a person if fear or trauma prevents the person from taking action. In this context, consent for action from the abused person is not necessary although consultation is.

In 2003, the Irish Law Reform Commission recognised the need for improved legislative protection for older people made recommendations to address deficits in a consultation paper. A further consultation paper acknowledged that many of the issues raised in the 2003 consultation paper also pertained to all vulnerable adults (Law Reform Commission 2005, 2006). One issue of particular concern related to mental capacity. While the Power of Attorney Act (Government of Ireland 1996b) allows a person to nominate a legal representative for specific decision making, the person must have full mental capacity. On the opposite end of the legal spectrum, the archaic Lunacy Regulation Act (Government of Ireland 1871) allows a person without capacity to be made a ward of the Courts. Moreover, the Law Reform Commission observed the limitations of the current restricted medical model of assessing mental capacity and recommended that mental capacity assessment should be established through a functional model which was considered to promote a rights based approach (Rickard-Clarke 2005). These changes, outlined in the Scheme of Mental Capacity (DJE 2008), are due for debate by the Oirteachas (Dáil Éireann, or House of Deputies, and Seanad Éireann, or Senate) and will then enter the Irish Statute Book.

Other legislative proposals which impact on protecting older people include those for ensuring standards in long-term care facilities (Government of Ireland 2010). Although such legislative improvements enhance the protection of older people, gaps remain. In relation to the laws of agency (Government of Ireland 2009), additional refinements are necessary to deter financial abuse, particularly with regard to the collection of the state pension (Rickard-Clarke 2011). The rights of older people in Ireland have also been reviewed by the Seanad Éireann (Houses of the Oireachtas 2012) and particular impetus has been given to improve legislation and policies for older people to ensure equality and equity as Irish citizens. Furthermore, legislation needs to address pragmatic issues which assist in the protection of older people, in particular areas such as the legal advice on the repercussions of actions in relation to areas of will making or property/financial transfer (Pearson 2011, Rickard-Clarke 2011).

Health Information and Quality Authority (HIQA)

HIQA was established in 2007 and represents an amalgamation of the Social Services Inspectorate (SSI) and the Irish Health Services Accreditation Board (IHSAB). HIQA is responsible for setting and monitoring standards in residential care facilities for children, older people and people with disabilities in Ireland. HIQA can also carry out investigations when concerns regarding care are identified and offer recommendations to the Minister for Health.

Ireland has a mixture of public, private and voluntary residential care facilities for older people. In 2009, HIQA published its first care standards in relation to residential care for older people. This document outlined 32 standards which are subdivided into six sections: rights, protection, health and social care needs, quality of life, staffing, the care environment and governance and management. Recognising the particular needs of older people with dementia, criteria for dementia-specific residential care units for older people were articulated. HIQA standards focus on 'a road map of continuous improvement to support the continued development of person-centred care' (HIQA 2009: 4). These standards changed the landscape of regulation in nursing homes in Ireland as inspections occurred in all residential care facilities, rather than just private and voluntary facilities, which had previously been the case. Significantly, proactive steps have been taken in holding residential care facilities to account if appropriate standards are not achieved, with the ultimate sanction being deregulation as a nursing home. In promoting a transparent inspection and quality service, HIQA also provides public access to its inspection reports which can assist older people and their relatives in a choice of residential care facilities via its web site (www.hiqa.ie).

In relation to elder abuse, section two of HIQA's (2009) care standards stipulates that each residential facility has a policy to prevent, detect and respond to elder abuse. This includes guidelines to facilitate protective disclosure of information, regular staff training on the issue and protection of the residents' assets. The protective disclosure of information in the HIQA standards concurs with the Health Act (Government of Ireland 2007). However, Transparency International Ireland (2010) argues that a generic approach to disclosures in the public interest is essential as the 'sectoral' approach promoted by the Health Act (Government of Ireland 2007) is problematic. Concerns are particularly focused on the statement that 'a person who makes a disclosure who knows or reasonably ought to know is false is guilty of an offence' [my italics] (Government of Ireland 2007) as this provides 'for the most severe of the penalties upon the lowest level of (objective) culpability' (Transparency International-Ireland 2010: 26). Thus, continued debate on enhancing and making disclosure comprehensive will promote the identification of abuse, especially in residential care.

Conclusion

Elder abuse is a complex issue. There is an increased awareness by both the public and statutory bodies on the duty of care to protect older people and to enhance their lives as equal citizens of Irish society. In Ireland, elder abuse received relatively little interest in any domain until the publication of WGEA (2002). This seminal document has been the catalyst of major legislative, practice and research responses in the context of Irish society's awareness of the topic and its prevention and intervention in elder abuse cases. The ethos of WGEA (2002) has been the immersion of elder abuse in the context of broader health, legislative and social care. This concurs with the necessity that a society's response to elder abuse needs to be comprehensive, cohesive and multi-dimensional (Mixson 2010, Nerenberg 2010), and empowerment of the older person is central to any developments (Pearson 2011). Despite the major steps taken in Ireland to understand and ameliorate elder abuse, an on-going focus needs to be sustained to ensure the protection of older Irish people. This involves a comprehensive approach which is flexible enough to allow continuous evaluation of the Irish context and the implementation of plans for emerging issues of concern.

Note

1 Minister of State, Department of Health and Department of Justice, Equality and Defence with responsibility for disability, equality, mental health and older people.

References

Action on Elder Abuse (1995) 'Action on elder abuse bulletin1' Online. Available at <http://www.elderabuse.org.uk/> (accessed 30 March 2006).

Amstadter, S.B., Zajac, K., Strachan, M., Hernandez, M.A., Kilpatrick, D.G. and Acierno, R. (2011) 'Prevalence and correlates of elder mistreatment in South Carolina: The South Carolina mistreatment study', Journal of Interpersonal Violence, 26, 15: 2947–72.

Basu, S. and Duffy, J. (2010) 'Providing legal information and advice to older people: As much a question of accessibility as affordability', European Journal of Law and Technology, 1,3: 1–32.

Bell, A. (1998) 'The discourse structure in news stories', in A. Bell and P. Garrett (eds) Approaches to Media Discourse, London: Blackwell.

Conrad, K.J., Iris, M., Ridings, J.W., Langley, K. and Wilber, K.H. (2010) 'Self-report measure of financial exploitation of older adults', Gerontologist, 50, 6: 758–73.

CSO (2011) 'Women and men in Ireland 2011'. Central Statistics Office. Online. Available at <http://www.cso.ie/newsevents/pr_womenandmen2010.htm> (accessed 20 April 2012).

——(2012) Profile 2: Older and younger, Dublin: Stationery Office.

DHHS (1998) The National Elder Abuse Incidence Study: Final Report, New York: The Administration for Children and Families and The Administration on Aging by The National Center of Elder Abuse at The American Public Human Services Association in Collaboration with Westat, Inc.

DJE (2008) Scheme of mental capacity, Dublin: Department of Justice and Equality.

DOHC (2009) The Commission of Investigation (The Leas Cross Nursing Home): Final Report. Department of Health and Children. Dublin: Stationery Office.

EP and ECM (2003) Directive 2003/88/EC of the European Parliament and of the Council concerning certain aspects of the organisation of working time. European Parliament and European Council of Ministers. Online. Available at <http://eurlex.europa.eu/LexUriServ/LexUriServ.do?uri=OJ:L:2003:299:0009:0019:EN:PDF> (accessed 17 February 2011).

Fahey, T., Maitre, B., Nolan, B. and Whelan, B.T. (2007) A social portrait of older people in Ireland. Dublin: Stationery Office.

Fealy, G. and McNamara, M. (2009) Age and age identity in Irish newspapers. Dublin: University College Dublin National Centre for the Protection of Older People.

Fealy, G., Donnelly, N., Bergin, A., Treacy, M.P., Phelan, A. (2012) Financial abuse of older people: A review. Dublin: University College Dublin National Centre for the Protection of Older People.

Government of Ireland (1871) Lunacy Regulation Act (Ireland). Dublin: Stationery Office.

——(1937) Bureacht na hÉireann. Dublin: Stationery Office.

——(1996a) Domestic Violence Act. Dublin: Stationery Office.

——(1996b) Power of Attorney Act. Dublin: Stationery Office.

——(2007) Health Act. Dublin: Stationery Office.

——(2009) Social Welfare (Consolidated claims, payments and controls) (Amendment) (No. 6) (Nominated persons) Regulations. Dublin: Stationery Office.

——(2010) Health Act 2007 – Care and Welfare of Residents in Designated Centres for Older People –(Amendment) Regulations 2010. Dublin: Stationery Office.

HIQA (2009) National quality standards for residential care settings for older people in Ireland. Dublin: Health Information and Quality Authority.

Horkan, E.M. (1995) 'Elder abuse in the Republic of Ireland', in J.I. Kosberg and J.L. Garcia (eds) Elder abuse: International and cross-culture perspective. Binghamton NY: Haworth Press.

Houses of the Oireachtas (2012) Seanad public consultation committee report on the rights of older people, Dublin: Seanad.

HSE (2009) HSE elder abuse: Service developments 2008: Open your eyes. Dublin: Health Service Executive.

——(2012a) HSE policy and procedures for responding to allegations of extreme self-neglect. Dublin: Health Service Executive.

——(2012b) Open your eyes: There's no excuse for elder abuse. Dublin: Health Service Executive.

Kitzinger, J. (2000) 'Media templates: Patterns of association and the (re)construction of meaning over time', Media, Culture and Society, 22, 1: 61–84.

Lachs, M. S. and Pillemer, K. (2004) 'Elder abuse', The Lancet, 364: 1263–72.

Lafferty, A. (2009) Public perceptions of elder abuse: A literature review. Dublin: University College Dublin National Centre for the Protection of Older People.

——, Treacy, M.P., Fealy, G., Drennan, J., Lyons, I. (2012) Older people's experiences of mistreatment and abuse. Dublin: University College Dublin National Centre for the Protection of Older People.

Law Reform Commission (2003) Consultation paper on law and the elderly. (LRC CP23–2003). Dublin: Law Reform Commission.

——(2005) Consultation paper on vulnerable adults and the law: capacity (May) (LRC CP37–2005). Dublin: Law Reform Commission.

——(2006) Report on Vulnerable Adults and the Law (LRC 83–2006). Dublin: Law Reform Commission.

——(2011) Legal aspects of professional home care (LRC 115–2011). Dublin: Law Reform Commission.

Layte, R. (2009) Coping with population change in Ireland: The implications for healthcare. Dublin: Economic and Social Research Institute Research Bulletin.

Lifespan of Greater Rochester et al., (2011) Under the radar: New York State elder abuse prevalence study. Lifespan of Greater Rochester, Inc., Weill Cornell Medical Center of Cornell University, and the New York City Department for the Aging. New York: New York Department of Ageing.

Lyons, I. (2009a) Elder Abuse and Legislation in Ireland. Dublin: University College Dublin National Centre for the Protection of Older People.

——(2009b) Public perceptions of older people and ageing. Dublin: University College Dublin National Centre for the Protection of Older People.

McDonald, L., Beaulieu, M., Harbison, J., Hirst, S., Lowenstein, A., Podnieks, E. and Wahl, J. (2012) 'Institutional abuse of older adults: What we know, what we need to know', Journal of Elder Abuse and Neglect, 24, 2: 138–60.

Mixson, P.M. (2010) 'Public policy, elder abuse, and adult protective services: The struggle for coherence', Journal of Elder Abuse and Neglect, 22, 1/2: 16–36.

Morgenroth, E. (2008) The impact of demographic change on demand for and delivery of health services in Ireland 2006–2021, Report 2: Demographic projections for the period until 2021. Dublin: Economic and Social Research Institute.

Naughton, C., Drennan, J., Treacy, M.P., Lafferty, A., Lyons, I., Phelan, A., O'Loughlin, A. and Delaney, L. (2010) Abuse and neglect of older people in Ireland: Report on the national study of elder abuse and neglect (Report Summary). Dublin: University College Dublin National Centre for the Protection of Older People.

Nerenberg, L. (2010) 'Promoting practice-based policy' Journal of Elder Abuse and Neglect, 22, 3: 335–9.

O'Brien, J. (2010) 'A physician's perspective: Elder abuse and neglect over 25 years', Journal of Elder Abuse and Neglect, 22, 1/2: 94–104.

O'Donnell, D., Treacy, M.P., Fealy, G., Lyons, I., Phelan, A., Lafferty, A., Drennan, J., Quin, S., O'Loughlin, A. (2012) Managing elder abuse in Ireland: Senior caseworkers' experiences. Dublin: University College Dublin National Centre for the Protection of Older People.

O'Loughlin, A. and Duggan, J. (1998) Abuse, neglect and mistreatment of older people: An exploratory study. Dublin: National Council of Ageing and Older People.

O'Neill, D. (2006) The nursing home review. Dublin: Health Service Executive.

PA Consulting (2009) Review of the recommendations of Protecting Our Future: Report of the WGEA. Dublin: Department of Health and Children.

Pearson, K.C. (2011) 'Legal implications of ambivalence in caregiver relationships seminar: The legal and policy challenges of financial elder abuse'. Dublin: University College Dublin National Centre for the Protection of Older People Seminars (22 February).

Phelan, A. (2009) 'Examining newspaper reports of care in an Irish nursing home:A discursive analysis'. Dublin: University College Dublin National Centre for the Protection of Older People.

——(2010) 'Discursive constructions of elder abuse: Community nurses' accounts', unpublished thesis, University College Dublin.

——(2012) 'Older people and citizenship', in D. Petty and C. McFarland (eds) Citizenship-practices, types and challenges. New York: Nova.

——and Treacy, M.P. (2011) A review of elder abuse screening tools. Dublin: University College Dublin National Centre for the Protection of Older People.

Rickard-Clarke, P. (2005) Guardianship: A new structure for vulnerable adults – Law Reform Commission's recommendations. Dublin: Law Reform Commission.

——(2011) Financial abuse: The legal and regulatory gaps seminar: The legal and policy challenges of financial elder abuse. University College Dublin: National Centre for the Protection of Older People Seminars (22 February).

RTÉ (2005) Prime Time Investigates: Home Truths. Raidió Teilifís Éireann. Online. Available at <http://www.rte.ie/news/av/2005/0621/leascross_av2048320.html> (accessed 10 January 2010).

——(2010) Prime Time Investigates: The Homecare Scandal. Raidió Teilifís Éireann. Online. Available at <http://www.rte.ie/news/av/2010/1213/primetimeinvestigates.html> (accessed 15 January 2011).

Schiamberg, L.B., Barboza, G.G., Oehmke, J., Zhang, Z., Giffore, R.J., Weatherill, R.P., Von Heydrick, L. and Post, L.A. (2011) 'Elder abuse in nursing homes: An ecological perspective', Journal of Elder Abuse and Neglect, 23, 2: 190–211.

Transparency International Ireland (2010) 'An alternative to silence: Whistleblowing protection in Ireland'. Online. Available at <http://www.transparency.ie/Files/2010_Alternative_to_Silence_Ireland_v1.pdf> (accessed 12 March 2012).

WGEA (2002) Protecting our future. Working Group on Elder Abuse. Dublin: Stationery Office.

WHO (2008) A global response to elder abuse and neglect: Building primary health care capacity to deal with the problem worldwide – Main report. World Health Organisation. Geneva: WHO.

Yaffe, M.J., Wolfson, C., Litwick, M. and Weiss, D. (2008) 'Development and validation of a tool to improve physician identification of elder abuse: The Elder Abuse Suspicion Index (EASI) ©', Journal of Elder Abuse and Neglect, 20, 3: 276–300.

6 Israel

Ariela Lowenstein and Israel (Issi) Doron

Introduction

In most developed nations, declines in fertility, improved health and dramatic increases in life expectancy have generated growing numbers and proportions of older people. Such social change challenges existing social priorities concerning the individual, family and social lives. The aging of the population is a global phenomenon, even if its pace varies in different countries (Kinsella 2000). Aging affects all age groups and there are critical interdependencies between family generations along different stages of the individual and familial life course (Hagestad 2003). This phenomenon of global aging poses challenges to families, organizations and states (Lowenstein 2005). Greater longevity also causes a secondary aging process – an increase in the number of disabled elderly who might need more care and support. Older dependency rates rise substantially and increasingly there will be fewer adults to care for a growing number of older persons. This adds burdens to families and welfare states, which are the two major pillars of support in old age, particularly in the face of constraints in welfare state spending (Daatland and Lowenstein 2005, Silverstein et al. 2006). The situation becomes even more complicated in view of changing family structures that impact on intergenerational family relations and the willingness and ability of families to support their aging family members. Additionally, the increase in labor force participation of women, who are still the traditional caregivers, puts further constraints on families abilities to care for frail older family members.

The post-modern approach to the study of families in changing social realities challenges us to rethink concepts of social solidarity, obligation, and mutuality between generations. In particular, the physical, mental and financial vulnerability and dependency of many seniors, compared to younger adults, continue to give rise to concerns over the risk of abuse and neglect that older populations may face. An increasing stress on family members caring for older adults may result in rising levels of abuse and neglect.

The unique character of Israeli society, especially its Jewish and Muslim traditional familial values, contributed to the fact that until the late 1980s and early 1990s very little attention has been paid to elder abuse and neglect.

Public opinion as well as the political and scientific view was that Israel was unique in its positive attitudes toward the aged, and that the phenomenon of elder abuse or neglect did not exist. This "idealistic" picture of Israel as an "elder-abuse-free society" was shattered in the 1990s by academic research. In the wake of studies conducted by Lowenstein and Ron (1995, 2000b), Sharon and Zoabi (1997) and others, awareness has been raised among researchers, practitioners and policy-makers to the phenomenon of family violence in general, and elder abuse and neglect in particular. Thus, elder abuse has become more of a major concern as it has major consequences for the well-being and physical health of the older population. The family itself was found to be a major source of elder abuse, which often arises out of the tension in response to the burdens in caring for the elderly and their well-being is also a major concern (Myres-JDC-Brookdale Institute 2011).

Since the revelation of the phenomenon about two decades ago, Israel has been characterized by swift transitions and dynamic changes regarding elder abuse and neglect. Research, policies, legislation, and social interventions have flourished, especially during the past decade. The phenomenon has moved to the forefront of public and political awareness.

The major aim of this chapter is to review and discuss the advances in research, legislation, policies and practice which are geared to meet the needs of abused and neglected elderly and their families in Israel. Accordingly, the chapter presents the following:

- a short overview of demographic factors and trends, reflecting population attributes and needs;
- a brief outline of the current welfare system, describing policies for older people and basic service structures. It will provide a background for policy development in the area of elder abuse and neglect;
- developments in practice experiences, as affected by policy and legislation.

Israeli society

The State of Israel was established in 1948. It is still a young and evolving democracy with an exceptional mix of modern and traditional values. On one hand, it is a modern country with high standards of education, technology, and health. On the other, a strong traditional and family-oriented culture mixes the Jewish majority's traditions and religious values with those of the country's Muslim, Christian, and Druze minorities (groups that constitute about 20 percent of Israel's population) (Brodsky et al. 2010).

Israeli society is a multi-cultural, pluralistic society that includes a variety of national, religious, and ethnic groups; diverse communities such as the kibbutz; new immigrants vs. long-term residents and native-born citizens, Jews and Arabs. The population's diversity and the aged among them impact needs, expectations, and patterns of elders support. Thus, Israel can serve as a natural laboratory for understanding effects of culture and ethnicity on elder care, as well as on elder abuse and neglect. Israel is also an urbanized welfare state. Its welfare policies and legislation are shaped by a mixture of governmental and market forces, all of which impact elder abuse and neglect.

In Israel, as in the modern world generally, society is undergoing a process of population aging. In 1948, when the State was established, the Jewish population was relatively young: some 28,500 of its citizens – less than 4 percent of the population – were over 65 years of age. Data from the 2010 census show that the aged (65+) comprise 10 percent of the total population – close to 760,000. While the overall population grew by about 3.5 times growth during this period, the older population grew by some 7 times more. Another indication of the aging of Israel is the increase in the number of the "old-old" – the 75 years and older group. Whereas the 65 years and older group doubled between 1970 and 1990, the number of those aged 75 years and older tripled, and the sector that grew the fastest was the 80 years and older. There are differences between the Jewish and the non-Jewish older populations. Within the Jewish sector, the percentage is now 12 percent while among non-Jews the elders comprise only 4.2 percent due to higher fertility rates (Brodsky 2010). But the proportion of the aged in the Arab population is increasing more rapidly than in the Jewish community.

The aging of Israeli society is primarily the result of increased life expectancy. In 1965 life expectancy was 70.5 years for males and 73.2 years for females. By 2010 it had risen and reached 79.3 years for men and 83.8 for women. Aging is also related to the composition and aging of cohorts from previous immigration waves. These waves, especially from the former Soviet Union during the 1990s, brought a high percentage of older people (16 percent). Close to 19 percent of older Jews are disabled in activities of daily living (ADL, measured with the Katz scale). The percentage is higher among new immigrants (close to 17 percent) and even higher among non-Jews (nearing 30 percent). It is congruent with data from the United States (US) indicating that socio-cultural factors are related to the incidence of chronic disease among elders. This segment of the population needs closer care and assistance, which is still provided mostly by family members and in some cases can cause abuse and neglect (Brodsky et al. 2010).

The aging of Israeli society can also be viewed from the angle of the Elder Support Ratio: the number of people above 65 to every 100 people of working age. In the 1960s the Elder Support Ratio in Israel was about 10:100. By 2003 it had almost doubled, to 19:100. The Israeli population is expected to continue to age, and it is forecasted that by 2025 the proportion of old people will reach 14 percent. In addition, there will be a further increase in life expectancy. Almost twice as many older men (81 percent) compared to older women are married and the majority of elders live with a spouse; only 24 percent live alone. Among aged new immigrants, 70 percent live with their children because of housing and financial difficulties, especially during the first years of immigration (Katz and Lowenstein, 1999).

Most aged people have an informal support network, with spouses being the main source, followed by children (Habib and Tamir 1994). There is a strong emphasis on the role of the family in caring for its elders, as reflected, for example, by the relatively low rate of institutionalization (4.4 percent). We can anticipate that changes in the composition of the older population will result in continued increase of the "high-risk" groups: those 75 years and older, women, holocaust survivors and new immigrants. These projections mean that needs for long-term care will rise and that more resources will have to be allocated to develop community services and support family caregivers. In this new millennium, Israel faces the dual challenge of meeting current needs more adequately while keeping pace with anticipated needs.

Criminal code definition

As will also be detailed later in this chapter, under the Israeli Criminal Code (Article 368c) any person who physically, mentally, or sexually abuses a "helpless adult" – either by active behavior or by omission and neglect – can be punished with up to seven years in prison (nine years if that person is legally responsible for that helpless adult). The law defines "helpless adult" as any adult who, due to age, sickness, physical or mental disability or cognitive impairment, or any other reason, cannot take care of his or her basic needs, health or safety (Article 368a).

The Israeli criminal code does not include financial abuse within the chapter that covers the protection of helpless adults (however, in other parts of the criminal code there are specific articles which constitute fraud or financial exploitation as a criminal offence – but this is done within a general context and not specifically in the context of the protection of helpless adults). The criminal code itself does not define what is meant by "abuse" but it has been established in Israeli case law that "abusive" behavior is behavior that has elements of cruelty, humiliation, or terror. This is usually associated with an on-going or prolonged behavior, although "abuse" can also occur in a one-time scenario. In this context, the helplessness and the unique characteristics of the victim are relevant for the construction of the "abusive" nature of the actions. Nevertheless, there is still uncertainty under Israeli law as to the exact borderlines of the term "abuse" as case law on this topic is still scarce.

Policy

Up to the end of the 1980s there was no real awareness of elder abuse and neglect in Israel, as mentioned. Thus, the problem was discussed only in general terms, without reference to its social context or special characteristics (Shnit 1976). Toward the end of the 1980s empirical research on the topic began, in part as a result of an interdisciplinary US–Israeli conference on elder abuse that took place in Israel. The conference also addressed the broader issue of victimization of the older population (Wolf and Bergman 1989, Lehman 1989, Lowenstein 1989). Additionally, the 1989 Law of Protection of the Helpless gave the impetus needed to deal with the issue. The study by Lowenstein (1989) was the first empirical study on the topic of elder abuse and neglect in Israel. Research has increased during the 1990s (Green 1997, Kerem 1995, Lowenstein and Ron 1995, 1999, 2000a, 2000b; Ronen and Neikrog 1993, Zoabi 1994), a trend that has continued to the present (e.g. Alon 2004, Band-Winterstein et al. 2010) Ben Natan et al. 2010, Buchbinder and Winterstein 2003, Cohen et al. 2006, Cohen et al. 2007, Iecovich et al. 2004, Iecovich 2005, Katzman and Litwin 2002, Rabi 2006, Zoabi 2000.

As outlined by Kosberg et al. (2006), unlike the US, early work on elder abuse in Israel also included empirical work on maltreatment in institutions. All the earlier studies, however, similarly to the US, were based on lay or professional perceptions of the problem, and the likely existence of elder abuse was extrapolated from findings about the caregiving burden of the family. Studies were limited mostly to small samples living in a particular locale.

A significant point of reference was the publication of the Lowenstein and Ron (1995) study. For the first time in Israel a systematic study of the phenomenon, although restricted to the Haifa area, revealed the incidence of elder abuse, identified typologies of victims and perpetrators, and established an etiology of abuse. This research spawned several other studies investigating specific aspects, such as spousal abuse (Lowenstein and Ron 1999, Ron and Lowenstein 1999). The results of the earlier survey were later expanded (Lowenstein and Ron 2000a). Other studies corroborated the findings that most elder abuse occurs within domestic settings, mainly by family caregivers (e.g. Katzman and Litwin 2002, Iecovich et al. 2004).

The next point of reference and progress in this field was made in 2002, when public discourse peaked with the publication of the 'Report on the means required to prevent and deal with elder abuse and neglect' (Eshel 2004). Commonly referred to as the Eshel Report, the document presented conclusions drawn by a committee that included representatives from all strata of Israeli society.

It seems that since the publication of that report, a significant change has occurred in Israel regarding elder abuse and neglect. The major development and point of reference in scientific research took place in 2005, when the first National Survey of Elder Abuse and Neglect in Israel, funded by Eshel was published (Eisikovits et al. 2005, Lowenstein et al. 2009). The study findings were presented to the President of Israel in a highly publicized meeting, received wide press coverage, and were later discussed in a meeting of the Parliamentary Committee of Labor, Social Affairs, and Health (Protocol No. 364, 28 February 2005). A workshop organized to present the results and to highlight activities in the field attracted some 200 professionals from all over the country. The findings of this national survey provided, for the first time, a broad scientific picture (and a harsh one) of the state of elder abuse and neglect in Israeli society. One has to bear in mind, though, that the high figures of abuse and neglect found among community-dwelling elders, both Jews and Arabs – about 18 percent – relative to other studies, especially European surveys, were related to a broad definition as well as using a multitude of survey instruments.

Since the publication of these findings there have been several developments in Israel in policy, legislation and practice which will be outlined below. In 2006, for the first time, a national conference was held in Tel-Aviv with the participation of government ministers and senior officials to mark the International Elder Abuse Awareness Day. This conference placed the issue clearly on the public agenda.

Legislation

Although general awareness of elder abuse began to surface in Israel only in the late 1980s, the country's welfare authorities and legal establishment had had to deal with cases of abuse and violence directed at older people long before. Thus, over the years Israel has enacted various laws to cope with such abuse and this has resulted in four "legislative generations." Understanding this process of development, as described by Doron et al. (2005), makes it easier to understand the current state of Israeli law.

The first statutory generation: paternalism and social intervention

The first generation of laws relating to older people at risk of mistreatment was enacted, for the most part, during the 1950s and 1960s. At that time, the Israeli state was attempting to move away from British mandatory law, which it had adopted when the state was created, and was working to create a body of independent and original legislation. During this period many laws were passed that granted relatively wide-ranging powers to the country's welfare authorities, including the authority to intervene in the lives of vulnerable persons, such as children, the retarded, and the insane (as they were named at the time). Two main laws enacted at that time are relevant for the aged: the Law of Legal Competence and Guardianship 1962, and The Law for the Defense of Protected Persons 1966. Both these laws are still being used to deal with the issue of elder abuse and neglect.

The Law of Legal Competence and Guardianship 1962 was the first Israeli law to address the subject of legal competence. It deals with a broad range of legal competence issues, providing legal mechanisms that can be used to help individuals who are no longer competent in the eyes of the law. The most important of these is laid out in Clause 33, which states that the court can appoint a guardian for an adult who is mentally ill or deficient, or otherwise unable to care for him or herself. Because it was created as part of the movement to compile a general civil code of Israeli law, this law does not specifically refer either to older people or to the issue of elder abuse and neglect. In reality, however, it has been applied mainly to older people unable to look after their own affairs (Doron 2004). In many cases, the appointment of a guardian has rescued the older people concerned from exploitation, neglect, or abuse, and ensured that they received appropriate care and concern. As a result, Israel's welfare authorities still view this law as one of their principal "working tools."

A second central piece of legislation of the first generation was the Law for the Defense of Protected Persons, 1966. This was the first law to explicitly mention older people in the context of abuse or neglect. In it, a "protected person" was defined as "a minor below the age of 14, or a person who, because of injury, mental defectiveness, or old age is unable to deal with his vital needs." In many respects, this section is reminiscent of the authority bestowed by adult protection legislation in North America (Kerem 1995): it grants welfare officials the authority to follow the procedures required to protect older persons. This legislation directs the courts to act as a mechanism for supervision and control. In reality, however, the ability of the courts to act in this capacity is limited because they must act on the basis of the professional opinions submitted by welfare officials. Because of the wide-ranging powers granted by this law, methods of intervention and types of action can vary greatly, and welfare officials have a wide range of discretionary powers in all matters relating to the choice of a court order. Moreover, it should be noted that empirical research has found that in many elder-guardianship proceedings, insufficient weight is given to the autonomy and liberty of older individuals and legal measures are frequently overly paternalistic (Doron 2004).

The second statutory generation: criminal law and mandatory reporting

For almost twenty-five years after the first-generation legislation was passed, there was no change in Israeli law in relation to elder abuse and neglect. This reflected the fact that the public and the scientific community were not generally aware of the problem, and that the welfare community had already reached an ideo-logical consensus about what constituted suitable methods of intervention in cases of neglect and injury of older people. This state of affairs changed only with the emergence of a new legislative generation at the end of the 1980s.

Although it was not intended specifically to address the issue of elder abuse and neglect, Amendment 26 to the Penal Code, 1989, lent itself to this use because it was designed to address the needs of "the helpless" (Kadman 1992). The preamble to the law stated that "injury to one who is unable to defend him/herself, such as children, the old, and the disabled – hereinafter 'the helpless' – justifies special consideration on the part of the legislator" (Proposal for [Amendment to] Penal Law 1989).

Amendment 26 has two principal aspects. The first is its explicit assertion that abusing "helpless persons," physically, mentally, or sexually, whether by omission or commission, is a criminal offence subject to severe punishment. This was the first time that the broad range of harmful behavior typical of elder abuse had been identified clearly and unambiguously in criminal law.

The second major aspect of Amendment 26 reflects the fact that the legislators had become aware that elder abuse and neglect occurred behind closed doors and was an issue that people were either afraid or unwilling to report. To expose this social problem and allow the legal authorities to act, the law required individuals to report any case, or suspected case, of abuse to a welfare officer or to the police. This obligation applied to all members of the public, but particular emphasis was placed on the fact that professional care workers were specifically mandated to report any abuse or neglect of older persons.

In real life, however, empirical data in Israel suggests that there is a wide gap between "the law on the books" and the reality. As reported by Alon (2004), data collected by the Chief Welfare Officer from Services for the Elderly of the Ministry of Labor and Social Affairs indicates that in 2000 and 2001, only 360 reports per year were made to the police – a very low rate compared to the rates of abuse and neglect described in the previous parts of this chapter. Moreover, as Alon (2004) reports, social workers in Israel prefer to use therapeutic tools rather than legal tools when encountering cases of elder abuse and neglect.

The third statutory generation: protection, therapy, and domestic violence

Whereas the transition from the first to the second generation of legislation was a slow process, the transition to the third statutory generation occurred relatively quickly. Three years after Amendment 26, a completely new law was enacted: the Law for the Prevention of Violence in the Family, 1991. This legislation was enacted as a result of a report produced by a committee on violence in the family headed by the Assistant Attorney General (Karp Commission Report 1989). Once again, as in the case of the second generation, the legislation was not targeted at older people as such, and their needs were "packaged" with those of women being abused in a family context.

The aim of the new law was to provide temporary relief to victims of sexual, physical, and mental abuse within the family unit, its chief innovation being the elimination of the approach that views welfare officers or the police as the solution to the problem of intra-family violence. The legislative innovation of the third generation was the adoption of a legal instrument that rested on civil law and could be set in operation quickly and independently by the victim or by a relative. The assistance provided by this legislation is mainly defensive and practical, and includes such practices as physically removing the aggressor(s) from contact with the victim, and prohibiting them from approaching the victim in any manner, entering her or his apartment, or even simply staying in a defined vicinity ("protective order"). The 1991 law also allows the court to recommend treatment and to compel the aggressor to undergo such treatment, stating that:

> When a protective injunction is given, the court is entitled, at the time of the imposition of the injunction or at a later date, to direct the person to bind him/herself to undergo treatment by an agent nominated by the court.

At least in the first years of its operation, the rate of usage of protective orders was low and questions were raised as to the legal efficiency of the law (Makies 1995).

Emergence of the fourth generation: empowerment

In certain respects, both second- and third-generation laws are still in the process of development and assimilation, which makes it difficult to identify with certainty what constitutes the next generation of Israeli law. Nevertheless, it is possible to identify some legislative developments that reflect new statutory approaches unlike those of previous generations.

The new legislative developments are characterized by the use they make of the findings of research conducted on elder abuse and neglect in the 1990s. They also demonstrate that Israel is committed to implementing the Madrid International Plan of Action on Ageing (United Nations 2002), to which it is a signatory. Both the research considered by the legislation and the Madrid plan of action indicate how important awareness, knowledge, professional training, and empowerment are in dealing with the abuse of older persons (Biggs et al. 1995, Podnieks and Baillie 1995, United Nations 2002).

Although it does not involve primary legislation, the series of internal directives issued by the Director-General of the Ministry of Health in 2003, offers an example of this legislative development. All the directives dealt with the identification of victims of violence within the family (Director-General's Circular 2003a). One of the circulars focuses on several specific issues and states that one of its aims is "to increase awareness of the phenomenon of elder abuse and neglect" (Clause 2) and "to broaden and deepen identification of and care for the aging population, from the moment that suspicion is aroused" (Clause 2.3). The document also states that a team should be formed in every medical institution to identify and report cases of elder abuse and neglect, that specialized education and training should be developed and that the team should consist of social work, medical, and nursing professionals (Director-General's Circular 2003b).

It is interesting to note two recent developments in Israeli law. The first was when a Pensioner Party had representation in the Israeli Parliament (the Knesset, in the period 2006–9). As part of its political agenda, it enacted a new section to Israel's criminal code, adding a new and specific criminal offence of "Assault of an Elderly" (368f), which mandates the courts to include mandatory imprisonment punishment, unless there are unique circumstances that justify otherwise. This was a symbolic move to show the public's revolt at the phenomenon of elder abuse.

The second interesting development was the unique case of extreme neglect of an older woman by her grandchild, who brought her to his house promising to care for her, but in fact, exploited her financially while neglecting her physically. While the court convicted him of criminal neglect, he was acquitted on the charge of abuse of a helpless adult, based on doubts that were raised about the actual "abusive nature" of his behavior. This decision stirred public debate and criticism on the court's narrow construction of the term "abuse" in the context of the inter-relationships between the grandchild and his helpless grandmother.

A recent development is the establishment of an inter-ministerial committee which works on recommendations for introducing changes in the existing legislation regarding guidelines for professionals with respect to the definition of a "helpless person" and for obligation to report. This initiative has not resulted in any new legislation, but should in the future reduce the ambiguity that currently exists around the legal construction of the term "helpless persons."

Practice responses

The main impetus in dealing with elder abuse came from advocacy by Eshel and the relevant ministries. The national committee established by Eshel to investigate needs in the field of elder abuse submitted a report in August 2002. Following the report, Eshel continued its work by:

- developing pilot programs for community service models of interventions;
- introducing new regulations and protocols for general hospitals, long-term care institutions, and community health organizations;
- establishing a "help line" for victims of elder abuse;
- developing case materials for professionals in the field and educational systems;
- developing training programs for professional staff and volunteers working in the service system; and
- developing knowledge and information on elder abuse in Israel.

Establishing special units for prevention and intervention

The Ministry of Welfare, the National Insurance Institute, and Eshel started operating a pilot program for abuse prevention and intervention in several municipalities (two of them rural councils). A unique aspect of the project is the collaboration between the Center for the Prevention of Domestic Violence and the Welfare Department for the Elderly at each local welfare office. The units include a social worker (coordinator), a para-professional, an advising geriatric physician and a lawyer/legal expert. Currently such special units operate in 14 local authorities, especially in the larger municipalities.

The units employ various models of individual and team work, establishing multi-disciplinary teams (involving, for example, the police, the legal system, and voluntary organizations) and working with hospitals and homes for the aged. In addition, they are engaged in raising public awareness in general and among various professionals regarding elder abuse and neglect. They are also recruiting partners and professionals in the community for advancing actions on elder abuse at the community level. Some of the municipalities activate various support groups, for example for older abused women and for family caregivers to prevent abuse. An evaluation research of the work of these units revealed that a very large number of older victims were identified and treated. In about one fourth of the cases the abuse was completely eradicated. In two-thirds of the cases a major improvement was witnessed.

Another major activity is the establishment of a mobile multi-disciplinary team aimed at assisting in diagnosis and recommendations for interventions. The team includes a senior welfare officer for the court, a legal expert, a geriatric physician specializing in psychiatry, and the director of a center for prevention of domestic violence. The team operates within the social services framework of the Tel Aviv municipality.

A special model for intervention was developed for rural councils in view of the large incidence of cases of economic exploitation and abuse related to the status of the "inheriting son." This is a unique project, stemming from legal regulations that allow only one son to inherit the family agricultural holdings, which often leads to acts of abuse, exploitation, and neglect of older parents (Danon v. Eshed 1999).

Coping with elder abuse in the health system

In November 2003, the Director General of the Ministry of Health issued a detailed procedure for identifying and reporting elder abuse and neglect in the health care system (community clinics, hospitals, and long-term care institutions). The procedure requires establishing a special committee headed by a social worker. The committee is responsible for receiving reports, reporting to a welfare officer for the court or to the police, and informing the Ministry of Health about cases of elder abuse. Patients subjected to abuse and neglect are referred for continued treatment. In addition, the committee is responsible for training the organization's staff in this area.

Specifically, this joint program of Eshel and the Ministry of Health includes responsibility for:

- allocating a budget for a national coordinator and three district coordinators;
- developing and implementing training programs for professionals in health care organizations in order to implement and deploy the regulations

and the Ministry of Health procedure (forming committees, enhancing the process of identifying and reporting elder abuse and neglect).

In the next three years, the program will be deployed throughout the country.

Help line for victims of elder abuse and for family members

The help line enables older victims of abuse to call anonymously and obtain advice and practical information through a special telephone help line service. The service is operated by Eran, an organization employing 1,000 volunteers which maintains a crisis hot line. Eshel trained 300 of these volunteers to deal specifically with issues of elder abuse and neglect, and the service is publicized by them.

Case materials for professionals

A manual has been prepared for professionals to be used in training programs and during supervision (Ines-Kenig et al. 2007). The manual includes topics concerning elder abuse and case material. The case material is based on the work of an interdisciplinary team in Tel-Aviv that advises municipal social workers on specific cases. The manual has been tested and will have been disseminated. In addition, several movies were produced as learning tools.

Education and training

Education and training are important components of effective responses to elder abuse. Training has been and remains integrated into all aspects of the programs developed both for social workers and professionals in the health system. For example, 150 social workers and 'officers for the court' were trained recently to identify and intervene in cases of elder abuse. Special workshops and supervision is provided on a regular basis.

On the academic level, in the Department of Aging Studies (which grants an MA degree in Gerontology) at the University of Haifa, a special course on elder abuse will be offered.

Conferences

Conferences have been held in various cities around the country, some for professionals of various disciplines, and others for senior citizens:

- The Center for Research and Study of Aging at the University of Haifa, in cooperation with Eshel and the National Insurance Institute, organized a large workshop after publication of the results of the national survey.
- Maccabi Health Services (one of the largest HMOs) and Eshel held a seminar on the topic of elder abuse for family physicians and nurses.

- At the conference of the Israel Gerontological Society several special sessions on the topic of elder abuse and neglect were organized.
- At the Non-profit Associations conference a special session on the topic of elder abuse was introduced.
- The Ministry of Health and Eshel held two seminars for professionals from health care organizations (hospitals and long term care institutions).

Training manuals and materials

A manual to assist professionals in identifying elder abuse and neglect and a book on elder abuse intervention and prevention was published (Berg-Warman 2009). In addition, guidelines were developed for professionals within the health system.

Tools to identify elder abuse and neglect

Two major tools have been developed – one for the evaluation and identification of the risk of being abused or neglected was developed and tested by a team from Haifa University and two hospitals one in Haifa and the other in Jerusalem. The tool was tested, evaluated and is being introduced for use by various professionals through different simulation methods (Cohen et al. 2006, 2007).

The other was the Elder Abuse Suspicion Index (EASI) developed by Professor Mark Yaffe in Canada (Yaffe et al. 2009), which was to be used mainly by family physicians. The tool has been translated into Hebrew (using the back translation method) and validated by being introduced to several focus groups of interdisciplinary teams and groups of physicians. Data were collected by 15 physicians in northern Israel on a small sample of 75 of their clients. The rate of abuse identified was rather low at this point. The work will continue with other professionals (Halperin and Lowenstein 2012).

A national forum for inter-organizational coordination

The Ministry of Social Affairs (www.molsa.gov.il) has initiated a forum where professionals from various disciplines and different organizations are represented. The forum is dedicated to the discussion of fundamental issues and the formulation of procedures for inter-organizational coordination for coping with the phenomenon. The forum includes a wide representation of the relevant ministries, Eshel, major NGOs working with the elderly, representatives of the heads of the special units from several municipalities, the police, the prosecutor's office, and academia.

As part of advocacy efforts, other voluntary organizations which operate to meet the needs of the older population in general have also begun to work in the areas of elder abuse and neglect. Most of them focus on legal interventions and elders rights. The non-profit organization Yad-Riva was established in

1984 to provide legal aid for older persons. Their services include social aid and emotional support provided by social workers who volunteer to accompany needy older persons to court and provide support for them.

Ken Lazaken ("Yes for the Elderly") is another voluntary organization managed by professionals from the geriatric, social work, legal, nursing, and occupational therapy fields. Its aim is to fight against infringement of elders' rights and dignity, to identify elders' needs, and to provide appropriate answers to those needs. A complaint officer and a defense attorney handle elders' rights issues. As part of its activities, the organization is forming a lobby for the older population to promote legislation on elders' rights, including elder abuse and neglect.

'Law in the Service of Elderly' (LSE 2006) is an organization established in 2002 that operates to promote the rights of the older population in Israel through advocacy and legal activities. It aims to establish a legal resource center in Israel on elders' rights, to change and create legislation in this field, to educate and advocate on behalf of the older population, to publish popular and professional legal materials in the field of elders' rights, and to cooperate with national and international organizations with similar goals.

The General Federation of Trade Unions in Israel is a social movement that unionizes seniors and pensioners across the country. Their main goal is to protect the rights and benefits of pensioners and help them achieve adequate pensions, healthcare, and quality of life. The activity is provided voluntarily by pensioners (The New Histadrut, Internet Web page). Recently they enlisted the President of Israel to work toward creating a National Council on issues of Elder Abuse and Neglect.

Knowledge development and dissemination of research

Though comprehensive empirical data is still sparse, some basic characteristics of elder abuse and neglect in Israel have been identified. Lowenstein and Ron (2000b) interviewed professionals working with older persons in the Haifa area who indicated that during the preceding year 280 older persons in their care reported having been exposed to abuse (0.5 percent of the city's aged population at the time). Almost half of the interviewees described how older persons were suffering from lack of proper care; while a third were subjected to emotional abuse. Twenty five percent of those who reported that they had been abused were subjected to physical abuse, and 17.2 percent were exploited financially.

Katzman and Litwin (2002) investigated four categories of abuse and the characteristics of the abused in a care unit in a town near Tel-Aviv. They found that about 65 percent of the 163 old people who were in care in 2001 were subjected to psychological abuse, about 60 percent were exploited financially, and 47 percent were abused physically. Zoabi (1994, 2000) investigated elder abuse in the Arab community in Israel. His respondents, 128 professionals working with the aged, reported 434 cases of abuse, about 2.5 percent of those in care. Around 66 percent of the victims suffered from emotional abuse, 11 percent from financial exploitation, a similar proportion from neglect, and 3.5 percent from physical abuse.

Alon (2004) explored the degree to which social workers, working with the aged in welfare departments in Israel, planned to use relevant legislation to intervene in cases of elder abuse or neglect. Four hundred forty nine workers were interviewed. Social workers' preferences were examined by asking participants to rate their intentions of using treatment, legal intervention, or both in six hypothetical situations depicting elder abuse and neglect. The study showed that all respondents were aware of the problem of mistreatment and had in their care older people who had been subject to abuse and neglect. Findings also showed significant preference for using treatment interventions in all situations depicting abuse and neglect.

Iecovich (2005) compared abuse among new immigrants and the general Israeli population looking at 120 "identified" cases and found that new immigrants were more exposed to abuse and neglect than veteran elders. Iecovich et al. (2004) studied abuse in an "identified" sample of 120 elderly. Their data indicate that unmarried women who were more frail and disabled and who lived with others were at greater risk of all types of abuse and neglect. Conflictual family relations were the most prevalent cause.

The most recent comprehensive information available on elder abuse and neglect in Israel is contained in the 2005 National Survey on Elder Abuse and Neglect in Israel. In general, this survey, first of its kind in Israel, aimed to examine the incidence, prevalence, and severity of various forms of abuse and neglect; to examine the nature of abuse from the perspectives of the victims; to examine the correlates and predictors of abuse and neglect; and to develop profiles of elders at risk. Data were gathered by personal interviews in the homes of a representative random urban sample of 1,045 Jewish and Arab elders living in the community. The findings revealed that 18.4 percent of Israel's older population were exposed to at least one type of abuse (physical, emotional, sexual, limitation of freedom, and financial exploitation) or neglect during the 3 to 12 months preceding the study; the rates were similar among Jews and Arabs (Eisikovits et al. 2005, Lowenstein et al. 2009). Relatively high were verbal abuse (close to 4 percent) and economic exploitation (about 6 percent). Moreover, 18 percent reported neglect in answer to primary needs such as nutrition, medical services, and personal hygiene. Women were victims of physical abuse more than men, and old Arab women were the most vulnerable. Physical and sexual violence, verbal abuse, and limitation of freedom occurred mostly among partners, and financial exploitation mostly by adult children. When the perpetrators were partners, they had more chronic health problems, physical disabilities, dementia, and emotional problems. When they were adult children, they usually lived with the victims, were unemployed, had various mental health and substance abuse problems, and were often in the process of separation or divorce (the complete report can be found at www.eshelinfo.org.il).

Surveys on neglect in Israel are scant, partial, and address specific aspects of the phenomenon based on data from local samples that are usually not representative of the older population on a national scale. Most studies focused on abuse, with neglect as an additional rather than the primary focus (Zoabi 1994, Lowenstein and Ron 2000b, Katzman and Litwin 2002). Studies that focused specifically on neglect explored it among particular populations such as Arabs (Sharon and Zoabi 1997) and in specific settings such as hospitals (Cohen et al. 2006), and reported frequencies ranging from 1.25 percent to 6 percent. An attempt has also been made to develop different screening tools (Cohen et al. 2007).

The reported sense of neglect may also be the result of changes in family values in Israeli society. As Israel moved from a collectivistic to a more individualistic society, solidarity among family members (although still higher than in other Western countries) is increasingly associated also with conflict and feelings of ambivalence between generations (Lowenstein 2007).

Recently a qualitative study on elder self-neglect was conducted in Israel (Band-Winterstein et al. 2012). The study was based on a sample of 16 self-neglecting elders while data collection was performed through in-depth semi-structured interviews, followed by content analysis. The key finding of this study suggested that elder self-neglect is not necessarily an issue of old age, but is related to the person's life history. Self-neglect, as a way of life, accompanied the participants into old age, but it was not originated there. Regarding elder abuse in residential settings the data is scarce. The research literature shows that many cases of elder maltreatment in long-term care facilities, although required by Israeli law, are not reported to the authorities. The full prevalence of the phenomenon is unknown (Gibbs and Mosqueda 2004, Lindbloom et al. 2007).

The purpose of a relatively recent large study on the topic was to examine and analyze maltreatment in nursing homes in Israel. Data was collected quantitatively from 510 staff members in 24 nursing homes (out of the 300 operating in Israel), mostly from nurses and some from physicians and directors of the homes. The findings indicate that slightly more than half of the staff sampled reported abusing elderly residents over the past year involving one or more types of maltreatment, where about two-thirds of the cases were incidents of neglect. In addition, 70 percent reported that they had been present at incidents in which another staff member abused an elderly resident. The findings show that staff attributes, i.e., the degree of emotional burnout and residents' traits, i.e. their cognitive status impact physical and mental abuse, while institutional features – staff turnover rate and their level of emotional fatigue, which is higher in some for-profit facilities, impact physical and mental neglect (e.g. Ben Natan et al. 2010; Ben Natan and Lowenstein 2010). The study's findings were corroborated in a cross-sectional study of quality in nursing homes, by the Ministry of Health where assessment teams were used. The Ministry for Health study found that for-profit nursing homes provide poorer care than non-profit nursing homes, possibly due to a conflict between the demands of patient care and the desire to maximize profits in for-profit institutions (Clarfield et al. 2009).

Discussion and summary

This chapter attempted to identify and discuss the developments in research, legislation, as well as within the service system, regarding elder abuse and neglect in Israel. The manner in which these three areas have dealt with the issue has advanced significantly over the last decade. The compilation of scientific findings, and especially national estimates of the incidence and prevalence of abuse and neglect, affected both legislation and service developments and placed the issue on the public and professional agendas. But numerous challenges are still facing Israeli society in its attempt to address elder abuse and neglect. These challenges are scientific, institutional/organizational, legal and political.

Changes in values and political beliefs regarding elder abuse and neglect can also be traced through the evolution of the different legislative generations as they moved from paternalistic and invasive legislation, through the use of criminal legislation and the provision for treatment, to the provision of empowering laws that provide information and places choices in the hands of the victims. These legal changes indicate a significantly increased awareness in public and academic activity with regard to elder abuse and neglect. These developments, however, also raise several challenges.

The scientific challenge

Despite the findings of the national survey and other recent studies and the legislative developments that have taken place, the extent of elder abuse and neglect in Israel is still not fully known. In part, this lacuna stems from an overall lack of knowledge about violence in the country, how often violence occurs or what characteristics and components contribute to such events, as no central organization plots this phenomenon systematically. By the same token, some dimensions and characteristics of elder abuse, such as institutional abuse, are sparse.

More specifically, there are spheres or aspects of elder abuse and neglect that are still in need of empirical data, for example, abuse and neglect in institutional settings (sheltered housing, assisted living, and nursing homes) elder abuse and neglect within specific minority groups (the Druze, Ethiopians, immigrants from the former Soviet Union); and elder abuse by formal caregivers in home-care and community-care settings. Further data is needed also to understand the "unresearched" groups by conducting focused studies on particular sub-samples to cover their subgroup dynamics.

The existing knowledge gaps are not confined to Israel, and exist in other societies as well. But because of the country's unique cultural and religious nature, elder abuse and neglect in Israel may differ from that found in other

Western societies. Thus, more specific comparative cross-cultural and cross-national research is needed to explore potential differences and similarities.

The institutional/organizational challenge

The formal and organizational authority to combat and deal with elder abuse and neglect is vested in different governmental and professional agencies. In practice, this has often resulted in fragmented and uncoordinated legal and service responses to elder abuse and neglect. Thus, the legal reality stands in stark contrast to the collaborative and multidisciplinary approach that is actually required to successfully address elder abuse and neglect (Quinn and Tomita 1997, Quinn and Heisler 2002). The issue is multifaceted and complex. Therefore, services and interventions should strive to be multi-professional and use interdisciplinary approaches. This was clearly reflected in the creation of the special units in the local municipalities and in the developments in the health care system.

Future advancements in this field must support further multidisciplinary collaboration and coordination, especially between the health and welfare systems, but also involving the police, the legal systems and the courts, on both local and national levels. This will require developing clear guidelines, protocols, and methods of multi-organizational and interdisciplinary interventions. Creation of the national forum where representatives from all ministries and agencies are involved is an important step in this direction.

The legal challenge

Despite the rich and multi-generational legislative developments that have occurred in the field of elder abuse and neglect in Israel, certain issues still require attention and action because they are either not covered by existing laws or are covered only partially (Salpeter 2002). These issues include financial abuse and exploitation, abuse in an institutional context, and the need for certain legal instruments for planning to combat elder abuse and neglect. Further development of specific legislation is needed to ensure that the range of abusive and neglectful actions or omissions used to harm older people is completely covered by Israeli law.

Another legal challenge is the need to abandon the existing paternalistic and ageist legal approach. For example, the legal terms embedded in the laws of the first statutory generation express outdated and ageist social concepts. Use of the broad categories these laws contain (such as "mental diseases" or "defectiveness") to justify paternalistic interventions in the affairs of older individuals is no longer justifiable. Nor is there any place for approaches that grant broad authority for intervention without providing a clear and specific definition of legal incapacity and strong measures for procedural justice.

Experience has shown that these laws can themselves be used to mistreat older individuals. The most obvious example is the way in which the Law of

Legal Competence and Guardianship can be applied. Empirical research and the State Comptroller's report have both shown that this law is sometimes used to unnecessarily and excessively restrict older people's rights to autonomy (State Controller 2003, Doron 2004).

The political challenge

One noteworthy aspect of developments in Israel regarding elder abuse and neglect is that the voice of the older population is not heard enough. Indeed, many activities, legislative initiatives, and social interventions having to do with this phenomenon have been implemented with very limited input from the representatives of older people or their advocacy organizations. Strikingly, this has occurred despite the fact that many professional organizations, human rights organizations, and organizations representing the rights of children and women were involved in the legislative process.

The older population has suffered in part because the various policy solutions considered above were developed to address the abuse of children, women, or simply "helpless people," rather than being specifically designed to meet the needs of older people. Models developed to help children in distress (such as those of the second generation of legislative development) or to aid women experiencing family violence (such as those developed during the third generation of legislation) were applied automatically to older people without conducting any form of independent assessment. Thus, legislative development has ignored the special characteristics of abuse against older persons and has contributed to the stigmatization of older people as helpless (Phillips 1989, Wolf 1989, Biggs et al. 1995).

Israel is not the only country that failed to ensure that the voice of older people was heard when legislative reaction to abuse was formulated. International research has shown that the exclusion of older people from discussions about their interests is not uncommon (WHO/INPEA 2002). Other countries have also copied the statutory provisions enacted for older people from those intended to promote the rights of children or women (Saphiro 1992). Recognizing this, Israel must assure that older people can voice their own needs in any future legal and service developments.

The financial challenge

A financial analysis of many of the policies pertaining to elder abuse and neglect in Israel shows that many of them do not require specially allocated resources to deal with the issue. For example, from a legal perspective, application of many of the relevant laws, particularly those of the first three generations of laws, relies on existing, general financial and institutional systems and comprehensive budgets. Or, to use another example, welfare officials who deal in general with older people receive their budgets from the Ministry of Welfare and from local authorities and do not receive extra budgets for dealing with elder abuse and neglect. Such responsibilities to deal specifically with elder abuse and neglect should be undertaken over and above their other legal responsibilities in working with older people – unlike welfare officials dealing with children or women at risk, who receive extra funding for these legal responsibilities.

It is not by accident that only the fourth generation laws, which are still in their early stages of development, require resource allocation to help fight elder abuse. The laws that call for education, professional training, and efforts to promote the detection of abuse and to raise public awareness all state that social resources must be allocated to help achieve these objectives. The unwillingness to allocate financial resources to benefit older people may stem from the fact that they are still not a politically strong social group. Although any funds allocated to help the aged would have to come at the expense of other, politically stronger groups (Pearson and Richardson 1993), it must be recognized that progress in the struggle against elder abuse can be made only if the law also provides for necessary resources and new services.

Conclusion

Israel has made considerable progress in its attempts to confront elder abuse and neglect. Dramatic changes and progress had been made in the scientific, legal, and policy-organizational spheres, with new service developments, especially during the past decade. Many innovative initiatives, new laws, and social programs have been created to deal with issues of neglect and abuse. For example, legislative development in the field has reached a point where the question is not whether there is a law that allows the state to intervene on behalf of an abused older person, but which of the many existing laws is most appropriate for the case in question.

Israel can be characterized today as being at a crossroads (Doron et al. 2005). Having reached a relatively mature stage, it must recognize that it has not yet faced all the challenges involved in dealing with elder abuse and neglect, and has to make a clearer decision about these issues for the future. First, there is broad recognition that the dimensions of the phenomenon are much larger than had previously been understood, and that often these problems are not identified by the service system. Thus, there is a significant need to enhance awareness of service providers and their willingness to come to terms with this challenge. Second, the risks of elder abuse are much greater when the elderly person becomes disabled or develops dementia. Thus, with the growing numbers of elderly people who face these difficulties the potential extent of elder abuse has increased significantly. Third, the extension of life expectancy and the fact that the period of caring by the family has been so prolonged increases both the burden on the family and the risk of abuse by the family or by non-family carers. Thus, the elderly experiencing these problems need advice and consultation, including legal advice and emotional support and counseling. This is also true of their families.

Awareness of the different family dynamics within different subcultures in countries of immigration such as the US, Canada, and Israel also varies and is reflected in the concept of "cultural relativity." Cultural relativity is a complex issue that must consider family norms, tolerance of behaviors regarded as abusive by family members and professionals, expectations for care, and who should provide it. For example, data generally shows that women are the traditional caregivers of older family members. But in certain cultures, as in Japan or in the Arab sector of Israeli society, the eldest son is expected to become the caregiver. Accordingly, ethnic and cultural norms should be considered when developing programs in the field and cultural diversity should be more researched (Kosberg et al. 2006).

In sum, three main policy issues emerge while legislative and service efforts in the area of elder abuse and neglect are being considered. First, to what degree should the criminal–legal approach be dominant? If this is an appropriate direction, then more resources should be allocated for implementing the existing laws. Such resources should provide for more training and knowledge dissemination within the police and court systems, and introduce more coordinated and collaborative work between these systems and the health and social service professionals. Such an attempt has been made by the inter-ministerial national forum. Second, what types of professional interventions should be developed and implemented? An example was presented above of special units created by local authorities to improve working models in this area. Third, what should be the division of responsibility between the health and welfare systems, on one hand, and the police and the legal system, on the other? Again, the emphasis should be on more coordinated work and joint projects, wherever possible. This is beginning to be the norm, as more and more professionals in these systems are trained jointly and learn to collaborate for the benefit of abused older persons.

References

Alon, S. (2004) 'The intent of social workers caring for older people to operate legal or therapeutic interventions in cases of elder abuse', unpublished thesis, University of Haifa.

Band-Winterstein, T., Lowenstein, A. and Eisikovits, Z. (2010) 'Abuse and neglect of the elderly in his family', in I. Brick, and A. Lowenstein (eds) The Elderly and the Family Jerusalem: Eshel (Hebrew).

Band-Winterstein, T., Doron, I., and Naim, S. (2012) 'The meaning of self-neglect'. Journal of Aging Studies,26, 2: 109–18.

Ben Natan, M. and Lowenstein, A. (2010) 'Study of factors that affect abuse of older people in nursing homes'. Nursing Management, 17, 8: 20–24.

Ben Natan, M., Lowenstein, A. and Eisikovits, Z. (2010) 'Psycho-social factors affecting elders' maltreatment in long-term care facilities', International Nursing Review, 57, 1: 113–20.

Berg-Warman, A. (2009) Evaluation of a project to prevent and treat elder abuse and neglect in the urban sector. Jerusalem: Myers-JDC Brookdale Institute.

Biggs, S., Phillipson, C. and Kingston, P. (1995) Elder Abuse in Perspective. Buckingham: Open University Press.

Brodsky, J., Shnoor, Y. and Be'er, S. (2010) The elderly in Israel: Statistical abstracts 2009. Jerusalem: Eshel.

Buchbinder, E., and Winterstein, T. (2003) '"Like a wounded bird": Older battered women's life experience with intimate violence', Journal of Elder Abuse and Neglect, 15, 2: 23–44.

Clarfield, A.M., Ginsberg, G., Rasooly, I., Levi, S., Gindin, J., Dwolatzky, T. (2009) 'For-profit and not-for-profit nursing homes in Israel: Do they differ with respect to quality of care?' Archive Gerontology and Geriatrics, 48, 2: 167–72.

Cohen, M., Halevi-Levin, S., Gagin, R., Friedman, G. (2006) 'Development of a screening tool for identifying elderly people at risk of abuse by their caregivers', Journal of Aging and Health, 18: 660–85.

Cohen, M., Halevi-Levin, S., Gagin, R., and Friedman, G. (2007) 'Elder abuse: Disparities between elders' disclosure of abuse, evident signs of abuse and high risk of abuse', Journal of the American Geriatric Society, 55, 8: 1224–30.

Daatland, O.S., and Lowenstein, A. (2005) 'Intergenerational solidarity and the family–welfare state balance', European Journal of Ageing, 2, 3: 174–82.

Danon v. Eshed (1999) Family Court Ruling, Tsfat, 23220/1999.

Director-General's Circular (2003a) Information transfer between medical institutions regarding minors and helpless persons who are victims of domestic violence. Jerusalem: Ministry of Health (Hebrew).

——(2003b) Permanent commissions domestic violence and sexual abuse of minors and helpless persons. Jerusalem: Ministry of Health (Hebrew).

Doron, I. (2004) 'Ageing in the shadow of law: Elder guardianship in Israel', Journal of Aging and Social Policy, 16, 4: 59–77.

——, Alon, S. and Nissim, O. (2005). 'Time for policy: Legislative response to elder abuse and neglect in Israel', Journal of Elder Abuse and Neglect, 16, 4: 63–82.

Eisikovits, Z., Winterstein, T. and Lowenstein, A. (2005) The national survey on elder abuse and neglect in Israel. Haifa: Center for Research and Study of Aging, University of Haifa and Eshel.

Eshel (2004) Report of the committee on the means required to prevent and deal with elder abuse and neglect. (Eshel = The Association for the Planning and Development of Services for the Aged in Israel.) Jerusalem: JDC-Eshel.

Gibbs, L. and Mosqueda, L. (2004) 'Confronting elder mistreatment in long-term care', Annals in Long-Term Care, 12, 4: 30–35.

Green, N. (1997) 'Attitudes and social reactions of home care workers towards domestic elder abuse', unpublished thesis, University of Haifa.

Habib, J. and Tamir, J. (1994) 'Jewish aged in Israel: Sociodemographic and socio-economic status', in Z. Harel, D.E. Biegel, and D. Guttmann (eds.) Jewish aged in the United States and Israel. New York: Springer.

Hagestad, G.O. (2003) 'Interdependent lives and relationships in changing times: A lifecourse view of families and aging', in R. Settersten (ed.) Invitation to the life course: Toward new understandings of later life. Amityville, NY: Baywood.

Halperin, D. and Lowenstein, A. (2012) 'Validating the EASI tool for identification of elder abuse by physicians'. A paper presented at the bi-annual scientific meetings of the Israeli Gerontological Society, Tel-Aviv, February.

Iecovich, E. (2005). 'Elder abuse and neglect: A comparison between the general elderly population and elderly new immigrants'. Family Relations, 51: 436–47.

——, Lankri, M. and Drori, D. (2004) 'Elder abuse and neglect: A pilot incidence study in Israel', Journal of Elder Abuse and Neglect, 16,3, 45–63.

Ines-Kenig, O., Alon, S., and Ben-David, V. (2007) Manual for professionals. Jerusalem: Eshel (Hebrew).

Kadman, I. (1992) 'The law for prevention of abuse of minors and helpless persons: A turning point in the Israeli society's approach towards child abuse', Social Security, 38: 135–46 (Hebrew).

Karp Commission Report (1989) Investigation policies, indictments, and court proceedings in family violence crimes. Jerusalem: Government Press (Hebrew).

Katz, R. and Lowenstein, A. (1999) 'Adjustment of elderly Soviet immigrant parents and their adult children residing in shared households: An intergenerational comparison'. Family Relations, 48: 43–50.

Katzman, B. and Litwin, H. (2002) Protecting the elderly and preventing violence against them. Jerusalem: The National Insurance Institute (Hebrew).

Kerem, B. (1995) Protection of the elderly. Jerusalem: Eshel (Hebrew).

Kinsella, K. (2000) 'Demographic dimensions of global aging', Journal of Family Issues, 21, 5: 541–58.

Kosberg, J., Lowenstein, A., Garcia, J, and Biggs, S. (2006) 'Study of elder abuse within diverse cultures', Journal of Elder Abuse and Neglect, 15, 3/4, 71–90.

Lehman, H. (1989) 'Fraud and abuse of the elderly', in R. S Wolf and S. Bergman (eds) Stress, conflict, and abuse of the elderly, Jerusalem: JDC-Brookdale Monograph series.

Lindbloom, E.J., Brandt, J, Hough, L.D. and Meadows, S.E. (2007) 'Elder mistreatment in nursing home: A systematic review'. Journal of American Medical Directors Association, 8, 9, 610–16.

Lowenstein, A. (1989) 'The elderly victim and the welfare services', in R.S. Wolf and S. Bergman (eds) Stress, conflict and abuse of the elderly. Jerusalem: Brookdale Series, pp. 99–110.

——(1999) 'Elder abuse in residential settings in Israel'. Journal of Elder Abuse and Neglect, (Special Issue), 10, 1/2: 133–52. Reprinted in F. Glendenning and P. Kingston (eds) (1999) Elder abuse and neglect in residential settings. New York: Haworth Press.

——(2005) 'Global aging and the challenges to families', in M. Johnson, V.L. Bengtson, P.G. Coleman, T. Kirkwood (eds) Cambridge Handbook on Age and Aging. Cambridge: Cambridge University Press.

——(2007) 'Solidarity-conflict and ambivalence: Testing two conceptual frameworks and their impact on quality of life for older family members', Journal of Gerontology Social Sciences 62, 2: S100–107.

——and Ron, P. (1995) Elder abuse by family members who care for them. Haifa: The Center for Research and Study of Aging (Hebrew).

——and Ron, P. (1999) 'Tension and conflicts factors in spousal abuse in second marriages of the widowed elderly', Journal of Elder Abuse and Neglect, 11, 1, 23–45.

——and Ron, P. (2000a) 'Adult children of elderly parents who remarry: Etiology of domestic abuse', The Journal of Adult Protection, 2, 4, 22–32.

——and Ron, P. (2000b) 'Elder abuse in a domestic context in Israel: Victims' typology and abuse etiology', Society and Welfare, 20, 2: 175–92 (Hebrew).

——, Eisikovits, Z., Band-Winterstein, T. and Enosh, G. (2009) 'Is elder abuse and neglect a social phenomenon? Data from the first national prevalence survey in Israel', Journal of Elder Abuse and Neglect, 21, 3: 253–60.

LSE (2006) 'Law in the service of the elderly' Online. Available at <http://www.elderlaw.org.il> (accessed 3 January 2012).

Makies, R. (1995) 'The law of prevention of domestic violence', in F. Radai, C. Shalev and M. Leiben-Kobi (eds) The status of women in law and society. Tel-Aviv: Shoken (Hebrew).

Myres-JDC-Brookdale Institute (2011) Overview of social needs in Israel. Jerusalem: Myres-JDC-Brookdale Institute.

Pearson, M. and Richardson, S. (1993) 'Insidious abuse? Who is responsible for societal neglect?', in P. Decalmer and F. Glendenning (eds) The Mistreatment of Elderly People London: Sage.

Phillips, L. (1989) 'Issues involved in identifying and intervening in elder abuse', in R. Filinson and S.R. Ingman (eds) Elder abuse: Practice and policy. New York: Human Sciences Press.

Podnieks, E. and Baillie, E. (1995) 'Education as the key to the prevention of elder abuse and neglect', in M.J. MacLean (ed.) Abuse and neglect of older Canadians: Strategies for change. Toronto: Thompson Educational Publishing.

Proposal for [Amendment to] Penal Law (1989) Law proposal no. 1947, 146, 2 August.

Quinn, M.J. and Heisler, C.J. (2002) 'The legal response to elder abuse and neglect', Journal of Elder Abuse and Neglect, 14, 1: 61–77.

Quinn, M.J. and Tomita, S.K. (1997) Elder abuse and neglect: Causes, diagnosis, and intervention strategies, (2nd edn). New York: Springer Publishing Company.

Rabi, K. (2006) 'Israeli perspectives on elder abuse', Educational Gerontology, 32: 49–62.

Ron, P. and Lowenstein, A. (1999) 'Loneliness and unmet needs of intimacy and sexuality: Their effect on the phenomenon of spousal abuse in second marriages of the widowed elderly', Journal of Divorce and Remarriage, 31, 3/4: 69–90.

Ronen, M. and Neikrog, S. (1993) 'The perception of elder abuse in Israel' Society and Welfare, 14, 1: 17–30 (Hebrew).

Salpeter, R. (2002) 'Holes in the protective legislation of the elderly in Israel', Dorot, 60: 26–8 (Hebrew).

Saphiro, J. (1992) 'The elderly are not children', US News and World Report, 13 January.

Sharon, N. and Zoabi, S. (1997) 'Elder abuse in a land of tradition: The case of Israel's Arabs', Journal of Elder Abuse and Neglect, 8, 4: 43–58.

Shnit, D. (1976) 'Protection of the elderly in Israeli law', Gerontology, 7: 6–19 (Hebrew).

Silverstein, M., Cong, Z., and Li, S. (2006) 'Intergenerational transfers and living arrangements of older people in rural China: Consequences for psychological well-being', Journal of Gerontology: Social Sciences, 61B, 5: S256-S266.

State Controller (2003) 'State Controller's Report'. Jerusalem: Government Press

United Nations (2002) Madrid Political Declaration and International Plan of Action on Ageing. New York: United Nations

WHO/INPEA (2002) Missing voices, views of older persons on elder abuse. Geneva: World Health Organization.

Wolf, R.S. (1989) Helping elderly victims: The reality of elder abuse. New York: Columbia University Press.

——and Bergman, S. (eds) (1989) Stress, conflict and abuse of the elderly. Jerusalem: Brookdale Series.

Yaffe, M.J., Wolfson, C., and Lithwick, M. (2009) 'Professions show different enquiry strategies for elder abuse detection: Implications for training and interprofessional care', Journal of Interprofessional Care, 23, 6: 646–54.

Zoabi, S. (1994) 'Elder abuse in the Arab sector: Myth or reality?', unpublished thesis, Hebrew University (Hebrew).

——(2000) 'Structural and interactional characters of older Israeli Arabs suffering from abuse', unpublished thesis, Hebrew University (Hebrew).

7 Kenya

Isabella Aboderin and Nesta Hatendi

Introduction

In contrast to other world regions, issues of elder abuse have thus far remained peripheral to public, policy and social scientific debates in, or on sub-Saharan Africa (SSA). Nonetheless, recognition of and concern about the challenge of elder abuse in SSA has grown over the past decade, driven largely by advocacy efforts of non-governmental (NGO) and community-based organisations (CBO) working on issues of older persons in the region. Two international organisations that have played key roles in this regard are HelpAge International, a global network focusing on the issues of older persons, and the International Network for the Prevention of Elder Abuse (INPEA), which appointed its first Africa Regional Representative in 2003 and, by 2009, had established 13 African country chapters (Aboderin and Ajomale 2009).

At an academic level, a budding interest in the abuse of older persons as a subject of inquiry in SSA is exemplified by a small number of general overviews (Mba 2007) as well as a first discussion of the contexts, types, causes and human rights implications of elder abuse published in 2004 (Ferreira 2004). The growing interest of elder abuse in SSA for international debates is illustrated by the inclusion of African perspectives in recent global examinations of the issue – this volume included (e.g. Ajomale and Aboderin 2008).

The mounting concern about elder abuse in SSA countries centres on strong perceptions (thus far unsubstantiated by robust trend data) that the incidence of maltreatment of, and violence against, older persons is rising in African communities. The perceived increase is broadly viewed as a function of pervasive economic strain and rapid social change, including urbanisation, in SSA countries, compounded in some communities by conflict, natural disasters and the HIV epidemic, and interacting with persistent aspects of traditional culture and gender discrimination.

Against a backdrop of typically minimal formal social old age security or care provision, the interplay of these factors is believed to exacerbate older persons' vulnerability to poverty and abuse by undermining societal as well as family care and protection mechanisms for older persons. Within this context, and drawing on conceptual work developed for Latin America (Moser and Clark 2001), Ferreira (2004) identified five key types of violence against older persons in SSA:

- 'economic violence' by family or household members aimed at seizing an older persons' assets, such as pension income or ownership of the house. Upon failure to relinquish the assets when pressured, perpetrators may seize control of them collectively through violent means (Keikelame and Ferreira 2000, HelpAge International 2002);
- witchcraft accusations and consequent mistreatment, even killing, of older persons. Based on explicit, traditional spiritual beliefs in witchcraft, such abuse is viewed as being typically directed at widows;
- domestic violence against older persons, occurring in the context of strained relations or disharmony within households or families;
- 'community violence', including criminal violence (assault, robbery, rape or vandalism) and gang warfare, which affect older persons through generalised feelings of fear and insecurity as well as obstructed access to basic services and social participation; and
- political violence, linked to civil wars and armed conflict, leaving older persons displaced or left behind, separated from family.

Separately, Ajomale and Aboderin (2008), based on insights from Nigeria, identified two possible additional dimensions of elder abuse in SSA:

- state-perpetrated 'elder abuse', including de facto age-discrimination in the provision of basic services such as health care or agricultural support, as well as harsh pension eligibility verification exercises and regular, extended defaulting in the payment of pensions; and
- abusive cultural practices, including in particular harmful traditional widowhood rites and customs.

Policy developments

Signifying a 'success' of advocacy and academic efforts thus far, issues of abuse and discrimination against older persons have received increasing direct, formal recognition in mainstream African human rights debates and instruments. At the regional level, stimulated by clauses in the African Union Policy Framework and Plan of Action on Ageing calling for strengthening of legal instruments to protect older persons' rights within family and society, provisions on elder abuse are now incorporated in the 'Protocol on the Rights of Older Persons in Africa' currently being finalised by the African Commission on Human and People's Rights (AU/HAI 2003). By the same token, a recent regional meeting of the Network of African National Human Rights Institutions (NANHRI) focused on advancing advocacy and practice on the rights of older persons broadly, and elder abuse specifically (NANHRI 2011).

Echoing the growing acknowledgement of the issue in regional rights fora and frameworks, a number of individual SSA countries have developed national-level policy or legal responses on elder abuse. The pioneering and thus far unique Older Persons Act (2006) of South Africa explicitly prohibits and provides a framework for reporting of and litigation against abuse of older persons (South African Government 2006). Other countries, such as Kenya, Ghana, Tanzania, Mozambique, Uganda, Cameroon, while lacking a comparable legal base, have developed and ratified national policies on ageing, which typically recognise and contain provisions on elder abuse (Aboderin 2011).

Despite the advances at general policy level, however, formal programmatic and practice responses to the mistreatment of older persons are scant and, where they exist, as in South Africa, lack coherence and effectiveness (Mathiso 2011). The reasons for the gaps have not been formally investigated. However, two factors emerge prominently:

- a strong and pervasive normative discourse and associated assumptions about the strength of traditional African values of respect for its elders, which preclude any possibility of elder abuse and hamper national or regional debates on the matter (Ajomale and Aboderin 2008); and
- the lack of systematic, culturally grounded classificatory and explanatory frameworks for identifying and understanding the spectrum of conditions, practices or outcomes that constitute mistreatment and abuse of older persons in individual sub-Saharan African country contexts. The rudimentary typology proposed by Ferreira (2004), has not so far been developed further into such frameworks. At the same time, currently used international definitions, such as that proposed by the World Health Organization or INPEA, while useful as a starting point, lack the necessary context-specificity to capture key features of elder abuse in SSA settings. Neither definition, for example, encompasses culturally biased, collectively perpetrated dimensions of abuse such as witchcraft accusations and widowhood practices, or state-perpetrated abuse and mistreatment, which often do not occur within 'relationships' of trust.

The absence of grounded classificatory frameworks of elder abuse in SSA societies means there is as yet little basis for generating evidence on the scope and determinants of the problem, and thus for promoting and developing systematic and appropriate legal and service responses to mitigate it. Against this background, the subsequent sections describe current perspectives on and understandings of the incidence of elder abuse in Kenya and discuss the status of policy, legal, practice and research responses on the issue.

Elder abuse in Kenya

Country and demographic contexts

Kenya, one of sub-Saharan Africa's largest economies, is located on the east coast of the African continent. Kenya's population is estimated to be close to 43 million and to comprise 42 ethno-linguistic groups. A large majority of Kenyans (78 per cent) live in rural areas. Christianity is the dominant religion in the country, with 10 per cent of the population being Muslim and an additional 10 per cent holding traditional beliefs (UNPD 2011, CIA 2011). Kenya's economy depends mainly on service and agricultural sectors, has shown considerable growth in recent years and has good growth forecasts. Nonetheless, Kenya remains a low income country. It is classified as a low human development country, ranked 128th out of 169 countries with comparable data, and is beset by pervasive poverty and grave inequality in the distribution of welfare in the population (UNDP 2011).

Close to half of the population are estimated to live below the national poverty line, and 1 in 5 are estimated to live below the absolute $1.25 a day threshold (World Bank 2012). Kenya, like other SSA countries has a large younger population, with the share of older persons aged 60 and above currently only 4.2 per cent. However, this figure is projected to more than quadruple to 20 per cent by the end of the century. In the same time span the absolute number of older persons will rise almost 19-fold from currently 1.7 million to 32 million (UNPD 2011).

Status and foci of the debate

Within this context, official concern about issues of ageing has intensified in recent years, including a recognition of the incidence of abuse of older persons. This is exemplified in the 2009 report of the Kenya National Commission on Human Rights *Growing old in Kenya: Making it a positive experience* (KNCHR 2009) and its subsequent official briefing on 'Kenya's enforcement of the rights of older persons' (KNCHR 2011: 2), which highlight the occurrence of 'Neglect and other forms of physical and/or mental abuse' and, specifically, notes that 'older persons in some of the regions have been targeted and subjected to torture and extra judicial executions on allegation of practising witchcraft'. As illustrated by the above quote, the major concrete focus in considerations of abuse of older persons in Kenya is the incidence of accusations of witchcraft – that is of engaging in the practice of causing harm to others by supernatural means (Sleap 2011) – which is levelled at older persons and can result in their subsequent banishment and ostracisation, or even torture, maiming, lynching or killing. Other potential forms of elder abuse have received little, if any, attention. The almost exclusive focus on witchcraft-related abuse of older persons is fuelled by explicit reporting in the national media and ensuing public debate especially of extreme cases, such as those documented in several communities in Kilifi, Kisii and Nyamira counties of Kenya. In May 2008, for example, Kenyan daily newspapers, reported the death of 11 older persons, mostly women, who were burned to death in a witch-hunt near the town of Kisii. The killings shocked the nation. Witness reports indicated that more than 100 mostly young people gathered machetes and knives and stormed the village of Kegogi after midnight, broke into the houses of suspected witches and killed them. A few days before the incident, a group of schoolchildren had reportedly found a book containing minutes of a 'witches meeting', which listed community members who were due to die and witches who would be responsible (BBC 2008). In 2009, similar killings of 5 elderly persons were reported (Odhiambo 2009).

In total, HelpAge International estimates based on local records suggest that 42 older people were killed in Kisii District in 2008 and 23 in Coast, Rift Valley and Nyanza provinces in 2009 (HelpAge International 2009). More recently, in January 2012, the Kenyan Press reported the lynching of 22 older people, in a spate of separate attacks (News 24 Kenya 2012). The reports underscore that allegations of witchcraft and sorcery against older people can emanate from their own children, grandchildren, friends and neighbours as well as the wider communities in which they live. They are based on entrenched cultural beliefs in the existence and potency of witchcraft. Thus, accusations of witchcraft are typically levelled in relation to a particular ill or misfortune, including illnesses or death that befalls a family or community and is ascribed to the older person. In the 2009 killings, for example, one older victim was accused of bewitching a boy who later turned out to be epileptic and to have fits (Odhiambo 2009). In some communities labels of 'witch' or 'wizard' appear to be attached to older persons more loosely based solely on physical attributes such as wrinkles, red eyes and grey hair (Masha 2011).

Crucially, community beliefs in witchcraft remain reflected in the Kenyan legal code in the form of a Witchcraft Act from the colonial era (1925), which has not been repealed to date. The Act, Chapter 67 in the Laws of Kenya, Section 3, states that:

> any person, professing a knowledge of so-called witchcraft or the use of charms, who advises any person applying to him how to bewitch or injure persons, animals or other property, or who supplies any person with any article purporting to be a means of witchcraft, shall be guilty of an offence and liable to imprisonment for a term not exceeding ten years.

Similarly, Section 4 of the Act provides that:

> any person who, of his pretended knowledge of so-called witchcraft, with intent to injure, uses or assists to use or causes to be put into

operation such means or processes as may be calculated to cause fear, annoyance or injury in mind person or property to any person shall be guilty of an offence and liable to the same punishment as is provided in section 3 (Kenya Law Reports 2012: Chapter 67, sections 3 and 4).

A key feature of the public debate on witchcraft-related violence against older persons in Kenya is the absence of an explicit link to the concept of and discourse on elder abuse. Instead, discussions are framed narrowly only in relation to questions about the persistence of traditional beliefs in witchcraft. Partly as a consequence, no systematic examination of the meaning and causes of witchcraft-related maltreatment as a form of elder abuse has been undertaken in Kenya. In the absence of such inquiry, various speculative explanations as to what drives witchcraft accusations against older persons have been put forward by community leaders, law enforcement agents and district and local government officials. All point to underlying resource constraints, in particular land scarcity, within contexts of broad illiteracy or poor education in rural communities. One view considers witchcraft accusations as a means by which adult children avoid supporting their older parents who may no longer be able to contribute to the economic welfare of the family and are therefore perceived as burdens. Another view posits such accusations as a way of settling scores, including domestic disputes, forcing the accused to leave the homestead and resulting in relatives sub-dividing the older persons' land among themselves.

Definitions of elder abuse as understood through policy, practice, informal understandings or older people themselves

Given the absence of broad public awareness of, and debate on, the concept of elder abuse in Kenya, no policy or legal document thus far provides, refers to or highlights the need for an effective definition of elder abuse. Rather, official references to the abuse of older persons – such as in Kenya's recently ratified (2009) National Policy on Ageing and Older Persons and the statements of the Kenya National Commission on Human Rights – only speak loosely of neglect, physical or mental abuse and violence as part of calls for the development of national responses to the phenomenon (Kenya Government 2009, KNCHR 2009).

Policy responses

As indicated by the policy calls, Kenya so far lacks a direct formal response to the incidence of elder abuse. However, the National Policy on Older Persons and Ageing (NPOPA), which builds on Kenya's recognition of various international rights and policy frameworks, including the UN Principles for Older Persons (1991), the Madrid International Plan of Action on Ageing (MIPAA) (UN 2002) and the African Union Plan of Action and Policy

Framework on Ageing (AU/HAI 2003), provides a basis for the forging of such a response. Indeed, the NPOPA explicitly calls for the development of 'a comprehensive national strategy involving all stakeholders to stop exploitation, abuse and violence against older persons, especially targeting older women. This should include a supportive legal framework, public education and training/capacity building' (Kenyan Government 2009: 41).

Parallel appeals for such government action to protect vulnerable older persons have been issues as part of civil society and media campaigns such as 'Age Demands Action' (ADA), organised by HelpAge International and its affiliate HelpAge Kenya.

In the absence of a systematic government strategy, responses to cases of witchcraft accusations and related violence against older persons have remained improvised – with local authorities and role players taking ad hoc decisions on how cases are handled.

Police inquiries thus tend to be protracted, especially where witchcraft accusations involve tightly knit family structures, and fear of reprisals and expulsion from communities hamper investigations. Community responses vary depending on the perspectives and engagement of local leaders or the presence of civil society organisations dedicated to providing protection to those accused. An example of the latter were community interventions provided by HelpAge Kenya, with support from UN Women in Kisii Central and Nyamira Districts of Nyanza province in 2009. The measures included an awareness campaign on elder abuse involving all stakeholders and including older persons as well as tailored communication with younger people to address negative perceptions and often media-propagated images of older persons as burdens and victims (HelpAge International 2009, HelpAge Kenya 2009).

A second example of a community response, encouraged by local law enforcement officers, is the employment of traditional rituals, such as Mijikenda rituals, administered by traditional healers to persons accused of witchcraft. Arguably an action of abuse in themselves, such 'trial by ordeal' measures appear to be viewed locally as an acceptable means of establishing guilt or innocence of a charge of witchcraft, given the perceived inability of official court procedures based on formal requirements of 'proof' to do so (Masha 2012).

A final example, in the Vitengeni division of Ganze district, involved action by a local chief who liaised with a local rescue and rehabilitation centre (Kaya Godoma), to admit older women and men who had been accused of witchcraft by younger local people and who had fled their homes in fear of their lives (Masha 2011). Besides offering shelter, the centre obtained the services of a traditional healer to administer tests to the accused, which would be accepted by the community, to prove their innocence. Originally set up by the Ganze District Cultural Association as a mechanism for preserving traditional values and customs, the Centre is presently a safe haven for a considerable number of older people fighting abuse caused by witchcraft and sorcery accusations – as illustrated in the case study reported in the media below. By 2012, the camp held 46 older women and men who had escaped persecution in this regard (Masha 2012). In addition, young people were recruited to carry out civil education and campaigns to combat local beliefs tied to an identification of witches specifically by physical attributes. While no robust trend data exists, indications are that the campaign has succeeded in reducing the incidence of witchcraft accusations against older persons (HelpAge Kenya 2009).

Case study: response through a local rescue and rehabilitation centre

At 76, Mzee Ponda Changa was forced to leave his home at Kabaoni Village in Kilifi District to avoid being killed by his son, who had accused him of being a witch. Changa says he left home eight months ago and is now staying in Malanga, Ganze district, where he found a refuge following attempts on his life. 'My son has attempted to kill me several times. He once beat me seriously outside a chief's office in Takaungu on claims that I bewitched his sister. I decided to flee to save my life,' said Changa … 'My son plans to sell off the land, which I am totally opposed.' He says police refused to assist him when he reported the matter, saying the officers have been demanding money from him which he does not have. 'I have lodged my case to the area chief and Kilifi Police Station but nothing has come of it,' says Changa (Masha 2011).

Legislation

Thus far, Kenya possesses no dedicated legislation on the issue of elder abuse broadly, and on witchcraft-related accusations and mistreatment of older persons specifically. As indicated above, however, calls for the development of such a legal framework are made explicitly in the National Policy on Older Persons and Ageing. In the interim, certain aspects of existing generic legislation in Kenya may lend themselves to addressing cases of abuse of older persons. The Witchcraft Act (1925) itself, while impeding a categorical prohibition of witchcraft accusations, does contain clauses regulating how such charges should be handled. The stipulations in effect prescribe a formalised process and proscribe informal accusations and 'mob violence'. Thus, Article 6 of the Act states that

> Any person who accuses or threatens to accuse any person with being a witch or with practising witchcraft shall be guilty of an offence and liable to a fine not exceeding five hundred shillings or to imprisonment for a term not exceeding five years: Provided that this section shall not apply to any person who makes an accusation to a District Commissioner, a police officer, a chief or any other person in authority.

At a more general level, a potentially powerful legal basis for addressing instances of elder abuse in Kenya is provided by the country's new constitution, which was ratified in 2010 (National Council for Law Reporting 2010). The Bill of Rights incorporated in Article 57 of the constitution specifically provides for the protection of the rights of the older members of society, including the right to be free from abuse:

The State shall take measures to ensure the rights of older persons–

(a) to fully participate in the affairs of society;
(b) to pursue their personal development;
(c) to live in dignity and respect and be free from abuse; and
(d) to receive reasonable care and assistance from their family and the State.

Unfortunately, however, while the Bill of Rights includes in-depth provisions on the rights of children, young people and people with disabilities across key dimensions such as access to education, healthcare or employment, education among others, it provides no such elaboration on the specific rights of older persons.

The gap compounds the major hurdles to successful litigation of witchcraft related abuse of older persons that are posed by the lack of clear definitions of the 'crime', entrenched beliefs in witchcraft, witness intimidation and reluctance to testify. As a result of the obstacles, perpetrators of witchcraft accusations and mistreatment are, for the most part, not brought to justice (US Dept of State 2010).

Practice responses

In the absence of a systematic official framework for addressing cases of elder abuse in Kenya, responses by practitioners, as indicated above, remain ad hoc and uncoordinated and shaped by subjective perspectives and approaches of individual role players or community-based organisations in affected localities.

Research

As indicated above, virtually no focused inquiry into the nature, scope and drivers of elder abuse in Kenya has been undertaken. At the same time, the accuracy of available official figures on human rights violations, based on data collected locally by law enforcement agencies, remains circumscribed. A notable exception to the dearth of research on elder abuse in Kenya is a small-scale, qualitative study conducted by HelpAge International and its affiliate HelpAge Kenya in the Kisii District, which aimed to explore the frequency and, through case studies, the basis of witchcraft accusations against older persons (HelpAge International 2009). Study findings suggested a link between witchcraft accusations against older persons and a shortage of uncultivated land, crop failure, poor milk production by cows, school drop outs, polygamy, loss of wealth and alcoholism in families, as well as physical vulnerability and poverty of the older person under charge. In many of the case studies researched, family members or close neighbours played a key role as accusers of older relatives. A key recurring motive was found to be the intended acquisition or inheritance of land from the older person.

Conclusion

At the outset of this chapter we argued that the absence of a systematic, culturally appropriate framework to define, classify and explain what constitutes elder abuse of older persons in individual sub-Saharan African countries is a major factor impeding coherent national responses to such abuse. The case study from Kenya has underscored the impacts that the absence of such a framework have. Its lack not only hinders the furnishing of a specialised policy and legal architecture and subsequent formal strategies to manage and prevent forms of elder abuse that have received attention, in this case witchcraft accusations against and subsequent mistreatment of older adults. It also precludes an acknowledgment and measurement of, and subsequent advocacy for service responses to, the spectrum of other forms of elder abuse that are likely to exist in the country.

In concluding this chapter, we wish to underscore, therefore, the fundamental importance of and urgent need for incisive research and conceptual efforts to develop a classificatory framework for elder abuse in Kenya as in other SSA states. The effectiveness of such a framework will be strengthened if it builds on parameters of existing international definitions and the initial typology developed by Ferreira (2004). In addition, the framework crucially must be grounded in an understanding of the perspectives of key stakeholders – in particular older 'victims' and younger perpetrators themselves and how these relate to broader, meso- and macro-level factors (Ajomale and Aboderin 2008). An explicit comparative perspective in research on the above, seeking to identify and understand similarities and differences with other world regions, will not only deepen an understanding of the drivers of elder abuse locally, local determinants issues, but will also serve to advance the scientific debate on elder abuse globally.

In parallel to an endeavour to forge a classificatory and explanatory framework for elder abuse in Kenya, there is a need for research to evaluate and action to expand existing community-based interventions on witchcraft-related elder abuse. This should include the establishment and publicisation of robust mechanisms to encourage and protect those who report elder abuses related to witchcraft, as well as an extension of rescue centres and civic education campaigns driven by young people, as described above. Rehabilitation processes to support older persons who want to return need to be fostered concurrently. In addition to concrete practice responses, efforts are required at broader, national level advocacy and awareness raising. These ought to include media training on issues of ageing and the portrayal of older persons broadly, and on concepts and discourses on elder abuse, specifically.

Development of the above responses may usefully draw on experiences and lessons learnt in other African and/or developing world countries. By the same token generated insights, frameworks and interventions may –especially if brokered through regional-level platforms for South–South exchange – serve as starting points and models for advancing responses to elder abuse in other African countries.

References

Aboderin, I. (2011) 'Understanding our ageing world assessment of national level implementation of the Madrid International Plan of Action on Ageing (MIPAA) in the Africa region'. Consultancy Report submitted to HelpAge International/UNFPA

——and Ajomale, O. (2009) 'Understanding and addressing elder abuse in sub-Saharan Africa: Status and challenges'. Paper presented at the INPEA World Elder Abuse Awareness Day Conference, 5 July, Paris.

African Union and HelpAge International (2003) Policy Framework and Plan of Action on Ageing. Nairobi: HAI Africa Regional Development Centre.

Ajomale, O. and Aboderin, I. (2008) 'Elder abuse in sub-Saharan Africa: Perspectives from Nigeria'. Paper presented at the 4th World Ageing and Generations Congress, 28–30 August, St Gallen, Switzerland.

BBC (2008) 'Witches burnt to death in Kenya'. BBC News online, 21 May, available at <http://news.bbc.co.uk/2/hi/africa/7413268.stm> (accessed 17 March 2012).

CIA (2011) 'World fact book'. Online. Available at <https://www.cia.gov/library/publications/the-world-factbook/geos/ke.html> (accessed 19 March 2012).

Ferreira, M. (2004) 'Elder abuse in Africa: What policy and legal provisions are there to address the violence?', Journal of Elder Abuse and Neglect, 16, 2: 17–32.

HelpAge International (2002) State of the world's older people 2002. London: HelpAge International.

——(2009) 'International Statement on Recent Killings Related to Witchcraft Accusations in Kenya'. Online. Available at <http://www.globalaging.org/elderrights/world/2009/Witchcraft.htm> (accessed 19 March 2012).

HelpAge Kenya (2009) 'World Elder Abuse Awareness Day (WEAAD) Report'. Online. Available at <http://www.inpea.net/images/WEAAD2009_Report_HAK.pdf> (accessed 19 March 2012).

Keikelame, M.J. and Ferreira, M. (2000). Mpathekombi, ya bantu abadala: Elder abuse in black townships on the Cape Flats. Cape Town: HSRC/UCT Centre for Gerontology, University of Cape Town.

Kenya Law Reports (2012) 'Laws of Kenya'. Online. Available at <http://www.kenyalaw.org/kenyalaw/klr_home/> (accessed 21 April 2012).

Kenyan Government (2009) National Policy on Older Persons and Ageing. Nairobi: Government of Kenya.

KNCHR (2009) Growing old in Kenya: Making it a positive experience. Nairobi: Kenya National Commission on Human Rights.

——(2011) 'Brief on Kenya's enforcement of the rights of older persons'. 4 April, Nairobi: Kenya National Commission on Human Rights.

Masha, J. (2011). 'Dad, just go to hell!'. The Standard, 10 July. Online. Available at <http://www.standardmedia.co.ke/mag/InsidePage.php?id=2000038677andcid=349and> (accessed 16 March 2012).

——(2012) 'Six escape lynching on suspicion of witchcraft'. The Standard. 13 March, p. 10a.

Mathiso, S. (2011) 'Realising the rights of older persons in South Africa' Economic and Social Rights in South Africa Review, 12: 3–5.

Mba, C.J. (2007) 'Elder abuse in parts of Africa and the way forward', Gerontechnology, 6: 230–35.

Miruka, K. (2011) 'Plotting to kill parents', The Standard, 31 August.

Moser, C. and Clark, F. (2001) Victims, perpetrators or actors? Gender, armed conflict and political violence. London: Zed Books.

NANHRI (2011) 8th Biennial Conference of the Network of African National Human Rights Institutions: Advancing the Human Rights of Older Persons and Persons with Disabilities – the Role of African National Human Rights Institutions Nairobi: Network of African National Human Rights Institutions.

National Council for Law Reporting (2010) 'The Constitution of Kenya 2010'. Online. Available at <http://www.kenyalaw.org/kenyalaw/klr_app/frames.php> (accessed 16 March 2012)

News 24 Kenya (2012) 'Kenya cops probe 22 witch killings'. News 24 Kenya, 12 January. Online. Available at <Kenya.news24.co,/National/News/Kenya-copes-probe-22-witch-killings-20120112> (accessed 12 April 2012).

Odhiambo, J. (2009) 'Horror of Kenya's 'witch' lynchings'. BBC News, 26 June. Online. Available at <http://news.bbc.co.uk/2/hi/8119201.stm> (accessed 16 March 2012).

Sleap, B. (2011) Using the law to tackle accusations of witchcraft: HelpAge International's position. London: HelpAge International.

South African Government (2006) 'Older Persons Act 2006' Government Gazette, 497, 29346, 2 November. Online. Available at <http://www.info.gov.za/view/DownloadFileAction?id=67839> (accessed 17 March 2012).

UN (2002) United Nations Madrid: International Plan of Action on Ageing. New York: United Nations.

UNDP (2011) Human Development Report 2011. Equity and Sustainability: A Better Future for All. New York: United Nations Development Programme.

UNPD (2011) World Population Prospects: The 2010 Revision. UN Population Division. Online. Available at <http://esa.un.org/unpp/> (accessed 17 March 2012).

US Dept of State (2010) Human Rights Report: Kenya. Online. Available at <http://www.state.gov/j/drl/rls/hrrpt/2010/index.htm> (accessed 14 March 2012).

World Bank (2012) Poverty and Equity Data. Online. Available at <http://poverty data.worldbank.org/poverty/home> (accessed 19 March 2012).

8 Latin America

Lia Daichman and Liliana Giraldo

Introduction

Since first identified more than forty years ago as a social and health problem, elder abuse, like other forms of violence, has been recognized as a public health and human rights issue and a criminal justice concern. Elder abuse has become a worldwide phenomenon and the discrimination and mistreatment of older persons and its nature as a hidden problem is no longer something unusual. Consequently elder abuse is acknowledged as an issue in most Latin American countries.

The concept of elder abuse, as such, is now emerging markedly influenced by the rapidity of socio-economical change, weakening of the extended family, rising of elderly populations and growing concern for human rights, equality and justice. It crosses legal, ethical and health care domains within society's major institutions, making it a complex issue with moral, socio-cultural, political, and personal ramifications. However, today, concern about elder abuse has driven a worldwide effort to increase awareness of the problem and encourage development of prevention and intervention programs. Such foci are predicated on the belief that elders are entitled to live out their advancing years in peace, dignity, good health, and security.

Daichman et al. (2002) suggested that structural inequalities in both the developed and developing countries have resulted in low wages, high unemployment, poor health services, gender discrimination and a lack of educational opportunities. In particular this has contributed to the vulnerability of older persons. For elders in the developing world the risk of communicable diseases still exists and environmental hazards present yet another threat. Increasingly, older people in Latin America will be subject to the long-term, incurable and often disabling diseases associated with old age in the developed countries.

Neglect and abuse are culturally defined phenomena which reflect distinctions between acceptable and unacceptable interpersonal behaviors. These distinctions denote moral values, standards and conduct. The perceptions of unacceptable behaviors, cultural norms and moral standards can vary within complex societies. Therefore it is necessary to examine elder abuse and neglect from different perspectives in order to understand the meaning of these phenomena. It is also essential that the societal descriptions, norms and laws are sensitive to the various groups they are intended to serve (Hudson 1998).

There are abundant myths and stereotypes associated with older people which, combined with the lack of knowledge about the violence phenomena generally, and elder abuse specifically, hinder recognition of the abuse. While the developed countries have emphasized individual and family attributes as predictors of elder mistreatment, the developing nations have given more weight to societal and cultural factors.

Societal factors are currently considered important as risk factors for elder abuse all over the world; cultural norms and traditions such as ageism, sexism and a culture of violence are also now recognized as playing an important underlying role. Developing nations have given more weight to societal and cultural factors such as the inheritance systems and land rights, social construction of gender, rural–urban migration, and a loss of tradition rituals and arbitration roles of elders within the family through the modernization process (Wolf et al. 2003).

The Latin American region

The Latin American region includes Central America, South America and the Caribbean, with over thirty countries and nearly 603 million people (UN 2011):

- Central American countries: Belize, Costa Rica, El Salvador, Guatemala, Honduras, Mexico, Nicaragua, and Panama;
- Caribbean countries: Cuba, Dominica, Dominican Republic, Grenada, Haiti, Jamaica, Puerto Rico, Trinidad and Tobago and some other islands; and
- South American countries: Argentina, Bolivia, Brazil, Chile, Colombia, Ecuador, Guyana, Paraguay, Peru, Surinam, Uruguay and Venezuela.

The demographic revolution, never experienced before, in all regions of the world, is a global phenomenon and one of the main achievements of the twentieth century. By 2050 there are likely to be 2 billion older people, representing 22 percent of the global population. The longevity rate increase could be well considered a success, making the twenty-first century the ageing century.

Since 1950, life expectancy at birth increased globally by 21 years, from 46.6 years in 1950–55 to 67.6 years in 2005–10. On average, the gain in life expectancy at birth was 24.6 years in the less developed regions and 11.1 years in the more developed regions (UN 2009). Trends in the ageing process demonstrate that females tend to live longer than males and that there are more older females living alone than older males. These changes could result in deep implications for elders' human rights and might also put urgent pressure on facing up to discrimination, especially to older females, in a more comprehensive and systematic way (UN 2010).

The demographic panorama of Latin America and the Caribbean is changing and is expected to accelerate over the coming years. Population ageing makes it imperative to provide for their needs, which are growing steadily. In Latin America and the Caribbean, more than 57 million inhabitants are aged 60 or over and by 2050 the overall number of older persons will have reached 180 million, thus comprising more than a quarter of the population. Another figure provided by ECLAC (2010) is that by around 2040 the population of Latin America and the Caribbean will experience a shift unprecedented in the region's history: there will be more older people than children. This situation will come earlier for some countries than others (UN 2011).

A key indicator is related to the ageing index, which refers to changes in the rate at which the population of older adults grows in comparison with the younger population. In Latin America there are differences among countries depending on where they are on the demographic transition. Countries might be grouped by the 2010 ageing index: the first group consists of Argentina, Brazil, Chile, Cuba and Uruguay, which have the highest aging index, with Cuba having the oldest population in the region. In 2010, the number of older Cubans was almost the same as the number under 15 years of age. The second group shows moderate increases in the ratio of older persons: Colombia, Costa Rica, Ecuador, Mexico and Panama. Costa Rica and Mexico are noteworthy in that from 2025 they will deviate from the group, with ageing indices of 88 and 68, respectively (UN 2012).

The ageing index follows a more consistent path in the third group, at least for the first half of the century. These are countries in full demographic transition: in El Salvador, Paraguay, Dominican Republic, Venezuela and Peru the process accelerates in 2055. The fourth group, Bolivia, Guatemala, Nicaragua, Haiti and Honduras, clearly shows that the country with the youngest population in the region is Guatemala. Its ageing index in 2010 was 15 older persons per 100 persons under 15 (UN 2012).

In general, Latin America had around 36 older persons per 100 persons under 15 in 2010. The Latin American region is characterized as being one of the most urbanized areas globally, where about 78 percent of the population lives in urban settings. This is a particular feature in countries such as Uruguay, Argentina, Colombia, Chile and Venezuela, where urban inhabitants make up about 90 percent of the population. Fertility has fallen precipitously over the past decades, thanks to the changing demographics of the ageing population, and is now near the 2.1 replacement rate in most major countries. Consequently, by 2050 there will be as many people turning 60 each year in Latin America as being born. In the developed regions, the population aged 60 and over is increasing at the fastest pace ever (growing at 2.4 percent annually before 2050 and 0.7 percent annually from 2050 to 2100). It is expected to increase by more than 50 percent over the next four decades, rising from 274 million in 2011 to 418 million in 2050 and to 433 million in 2100 (UN 2011).

Compared with the developed world, the population of the less-developed regions is ageing much more rapidly. Over the next three decades, the population aged 60 years or over in the developing world is projected to increase at rates far surpassing 3 percent per year and numbers are expected to rise from 510 million in 2011 to 1.6 billion in 2050 and to 2.4 billion in 2100 (UN 2009).

Gender

The older female population has undergone a unique internal ageing process, as evinced by the 2010 data which show that one in every three older women in Latin America was 75 or older (UN 2011). Although in most countries life expectancy is higher for women than for men, the same is not always true of the quality of life since they tend to spend more years with functional limitations as a result of inequities experienced through their lives. Most elderly women are often not in very good health and quite vulnerable as they are particularly poor and more likely than men to be on their own. They have more chance of being widowed, having received a lower standard of education and experiencing a poor nutritional state. Restricted access to health services and to the labour market in earlier life often left them with very few resources in their old age (Daichman 2004). Gender-related issues vary between different societies and cultures. Past and present evidence shows that in many societies women have a lower status than men, leading them not only to a poorer diet but also to less access to education, risk of sexual violence, physical abuse and exclusion from decision-making (Ageways and HelpAge International 2002).

Ageing affects men and women in different ways as they have different roles throughout their lives, leading them also to different experiences and needs into their old age. Many of these differences are related to unequal power relationships. Women are also disproportionably represented among the very old and the most disadvantaged as they constitute the "inevitable caregivers."[1]

Older women are not a homogeneous group. They have a great diversity of experience, knowledge, skills and abilities. Women's socio-economic situation depends on a wide range of demographic, political, environmental, cultural, labour, personal and family issues. Their contributions to society in public and private life, as community leaders, as entrepreneurs, caregivers, advisors and mediators, among many other roles are invaluable, but yet are not generally recognized. Policies and programs that do not address gender issues, the ones relating to the way that society treats people according to whether they are male or females, are bound to promote inequality.

Older women are very often exposed to situations of multiple risks. Despite the fact that 17 countries in the region have adopted laws on domestic violence, in six of them, there is no protection for older persons, and even when the abuse is recorded in those of advanced age, the guarantees of protection are insufficient (OEA 2011). Laws and policies on gender equality are often not specific with respect to age and therefore, not sufficient to ensure effective protection for this vulnerable group.

In Latin America, researchers are beginning to relate to and examine issues on ageing, gender, discrimination and elder abuse and neglect, but data is lacking. Some fairly recent results show a clear trend which indicates that older women are more likely to be abused than older men and those men and, in particular husbands and sons, make up as one of the largest category of abusers (Giraldo 2010).

Many females face neglect and bad practices when they are considered passive in their productive and reproductive roles and perceived as a burden; in addition to that, widowhood and divorces exacerbate discrimination. The lack or limited access to health services for common geriatric diseases prevents older women's enjoyment of their real capacity and their own human rights. The full development and advancement of women can only be achieved if attention is focused on the life cycle course and recognizing different stages of this journey, for example, childhood, adolescence, adulthood and old age, and how this impacts on their rights as they are getting older.

Age and sex discrimination continue to be tolerated in many countries and accepted at an individual, institutional and political level and very few Latin American countries have a proper legislation on this respect. Gender stereotypes, traditional practices and customs may damage all domains of older females' lives, especially in the context of family life, community roles, media images, attitudes of employers, health workers and other service providers. Negative perceptions can, therefore result in psychological, verbal and financial abuse. Older women are discriminated by the lack of opportunity "to participate in politics and in the process of decision making" (UN 2010: 4).

The lack of identity "indocumentadas", as well as lack of transportation can deny women access to the things they are entitled to have, including the right to vote. Older women, especially widows are particularly vulnerable to financial exploitation and abuse; mainly when their legal capacity is denied and control is by lawyers or other family members without the older woman's consent. Thus, they are easily robbed and might lose all they have (UN 2010).

Specific areas of concern

Mistreatment of older people in both public and private spheres is a concerning aspect for Latin Americans. This was identified as a growing problem in the Latin American region and one that requires countries to adapt to the new context of the demographic and epidemiological situation through specific protection measures. Both older men and older women suffer from discrimination, but they do experience it in different ways. The impact of gender inequalities are exacerbated in old age and based on deeply rooted cultural and social norms. Examples include the result of the inequitable distribution of resources, abuse and neglect and limited access to basic services. Specific forms of discrimination may differ in situations where equal opportunities and choices about education, labour, health, family and private life have been "more limited or stimulated at an earlier stage" (Daichman 2012).

Access to justice is another area in which older persons may also be at a disadvantage; given that very often proceedings lasting several years can mean that these individuals never have their claims processed, particularly in cases of economic and inheritance abuse (OEA 2011). ECLAC (2010) has also analyzed the situation of aging in prisons. Without distinguishing between the levels of country's development, it has been affirmed that older persons in prisons do not receive the care they properly need.

In Latin America and the Caribbean, 50 percent of older people do not have sufficient resources to meet their daily needs, while a minimal proportion of the region's countries have health promotion goals in place for the over 60 years of age population. The PAHO review notes the existence of thousands of older persons living in a situation of discrimination, impotence, and neglect (PAHO 2011). The incidence of poverty among older people is just as high and is a pressing problem on the well-being of older persons as opposed to the rest of the population. This may increase risk as abuse tends to be associated with infirmity, lack of support networks, limited schooling, and a productive life marked by informality or intermittent employment (UN 2011).

In some areas, the lack of access to communication links, adequate housing, social services, loneliness and isolation presents problems for some older people, while those living in rural areas or slums, suffer from a severe lack of basic resources for survival, social security, access to health systems and information on opportunities to access and exercise their rights. Furthermore, older females, members of minority groups, ethnic or indigenous, or those who are displaced or out of their homelands experience a higher degree of discrimination.

Prevalence and research of elder abuse and discrimination in the Latin America region

Prevalence studies have been restricted mostly to some developed nations. In developing countries there is practically no systematic collection of statistics or prevalence studies. However, crime and social service records, journalistic reports and small scale studies provide evidence that abuse, neglect, discrimination and financial exploitation of older people appear to be widely prevalent (Daichman 2005). Thus, the magnitude of the problem of abuse of older adults in the region is still uncertain. However, some countries have made efforts to draw attention to the phenomenon through prevalence studies as well as taking into account elder's and health professional's views and perceptions, using different methodologies in terms of definitions, types of abuse, tools, sample sizes, target population, health centers, day care centers, long term institutions and within the community. The comparison with international studies is also difficult because of different cultural and social characteristics of the studied populations, and the methodologies used to carry them out.

Investigations in the Latin America region reveal a prevalence of abuse of older adults ranging from 3 percent to 30 percent, for example: 3.6 percent in Cuba (Docampo et al. 2009), 14.7 percent in Argentina (Gil 2002), 16.2 percent in Mexico (Giraldo 2006), 17.3 percent in Paraguay (Riveros 2006), 21 percent in Brazil (Lopes et al. 2006), and 24.8 and 30 percent in Chile (Quiroga et al. 2001, WHO 2008). There are similarities between studies' results despite methodological and conceptual differences which emphasize the following matches:

- A significant percentage of the adult population suffers from one or more types of abuse at the same time.
- Most of the elderly population does not report, because they may or do not know how, or are frightened to do so.
- The most common type of abuse is psychological abuse and is not exclusive to older people with physical dependence or other mental health problems.
- Abuse occurs in all socioeconomic status, educational levels, religion, gender and age.

Abusive situations may be committed by males and/or females with different kinds of relationship with the older adult. This contravenes the stereotypical view that males can be the main physical aggressor.

Perpetrators

Although research studies in Latin America have used different methodologies, to examine the mistreatment of older people, there is a consensus that the main perpetrators are frequently sons and daughters, followed by the spouse or partner, other relatives and friends, and then informal caregivers who provide their care (Viviano 2005, Giraldo 2006, Martina et al. 2010). Although the definitions of abuse and methodological approaches used vary in Latin American studies, the following section presents an overview of this phenomenon within the region. Findings highlight that a uniform definition of elder abuse and neglect for all cultures and ethnicities is limited without paying attention to cultural and subjective aspects of a given situation. A generic understanding is, therefore, problematic and can neglect important contextual issues. Moreover, professionals' understanding and sensitivity towards aspects of culture and ethnicity is essential when making a judgment about a given case, including appropriate intervention. However, acknowledging such limitations, these studies have made visible the problem of mistreatment of older persons and given similar prevalence rates between some countries of the region, although these results differ from some found in developed countries.

Types of abuse

Research in Latin America reported psychological abuse as the most frequent in the older population, followed by physical, financial, sexual abuse and neglect. Common manifestations of psychological abuse include insults, disqualification (meaning disregard, disrespect, to disqualify someone), humiliation, rejection and threats (Giraldo 2006, Martina et al. 2010).

Elder abuse is usually categorized as:

- Physical abuse: the infliction of pain or injuries, physical coercion and physical/ pharmacological restraint to an older person.
- Psychological/emotional abuse: the infliction of mental anguish or distress in an older person.
- Financial/material abuse: the illegal or improper exploitation and/or misuse of funds, and or economic resources from an older person.
- Sexual abuse: non-consensual contact of any kind with an older person.
- Neglect: the refusal or failure to fulfill a care-taking obligation including/ excluding a conscious and intentional attempt to inflict physical or emotional distress on an older person (WHO and INPEA 2002).

Another type of elder abuse is structural abuse (societal) defined by the INPEA Latin American Experts as the lack of adequate health and social policies, bad practice and non-fulfillment of the existing legislation, presence of social, community and cultural norms which disqualify and give negative images of ageing, causing harm or distress to an older person, and expressed as discrimination, marginality and social exclusion (UN 2003). The majority of elders, who had been interviewed, in addition to those from other age groups, affirm that societal abuse is the most frequent type of abuse, at least in most of the developing countries (WHO and INPEA 2002).

Institutional abuse

Although there are no significant studies on institutional abuse in the Latin American Region, mistreatment of older people has been identified in facilities for continuing care (such as nursing homes, residential care, hospitals and day care facilities) in almost every country where such institutions exist. Various people may be responsible for the abuse: a paid member of the staff, another resident, a voluntary visitor, relatives or friends. It had been suggested that the spectrum of abuse and neglect within institutions spans a considerable range and may be related to any of the following:

- The provision of care – for example, resistance to changes in geriatric medicine, erosion of individuality in the care, inadequate nutrition and deficient nursing care, such as lack of attention to pressure sores.
- Problems with staffing – for example, work related stress and staff burnout, poor physical working conditions, insufficient training and psychological problems among staff.

- Difficulties in staff–resident interactions – for example, poor communication, aggressiveness on the part of residents and cultural differences.
- Environment – for example, a lack of basic privacy, dilapidated facilities, the use of restraints, inadequate sensory stimulation, and a proneness to accidents within the institution (Daichman et al. 2008).

Risk factors

Elder abuse is a public health, social and human rights multidimensional problem, that could be explained and probably understood using the ecological theory, which takes a multi-dimensional perspective. Studies in Latin America have found several, complex risk factors which can encompass the dynamics of the individual or inter-individual relationships, societal causes and causes within the social context. Risk factors for elder abuse may be located in Table 8.1.

Table 8.1 Risk factors for elder abuse

Circumstances	• Female gender • Advanced age • Absence of significant other or peers (i.e. widowed, divorced or separated) • Lack of a social network (isolation)
Health	• Evident and frequent injuries • Physical dependence and/or impairment • Symptoms of depression • Cognitive impairment and mental illness • Deafness, speech problems, difficulties in understanding
Family	• History of family violence • Economic dependence of the victimizer (habitat and/or economic) • Victimizer's addiction to drugs and alcohol
Socio-Cultural	• Social and economic situation in past decades • Changes in the family structure • Migrations • Social Inequalities • Older person's self-perception, myths and stereotypes on old age
Most elders identified other risk factors as (WHO/INPEA 2002)	• Being old • Being ill • Living alone • Isolation • Family history of mistreatment • Lack of a social network • Lack of information about available resources. • Poor contact with peers • Intergenerational conflict • Lack of respect

Cultural specific risk factors for elder abuse in a Brazilian urban area may also include family members who work in drug dealing (WHO 2008). Also living in a "Favela"1 increases the level of vulnerability due to the violent environment, caused mainly by drug trafficking. This situation plus the impediment of free movement might contribute to a higher isolation of older persons and prevent proper action and intervention when there is a suspicion of abuse (WHO 2008).

Few existing data exist in Uruguay; however, the most common type of elder abuse is family abandonment, followed by economic abuse, psychological violence, neglect and physical abuse. As age increases, so does risk particularly after 70 years old and over (Lorenzo 2010).

Elder abuse is an extremely complex phenomenon. Risk Factors cannot explain all types of elder mistreatment, because different types involve different risk factors, which could be related to elder abuse and neglect. Barriers to the conduct research and the implementation of consistent safeguarding policies for older people are explained by the strong silence and taboo nature around the topic. A lack of systematization of official records within public and private institutions and social network support structures with poor clear definitions of the concept of elder mistreatment and neglect might only increase this already problematic situation.

Strategies, policies and practices

The Madrid Plan of Action on Ageing (UN 2002) and its political Declaration has been adopted by all the United Nations Member Countries. This Declaration emphasized the importance of raising awareness of prevention of and intervention in abuse and violence of older persons and has functioned to put the issue into the context of universal human rights. In response, Latin American countries have developed a series of policies, strategies, legislations and activities related to the wellbeing of the ageing population. Moreover, under the Plan, two new areas were identified as requiring urgent action in Latin America, namely the elders and HIV/AIDS, and the abuse of elder people worldwide. However, despite such improvements using a human rights focus, additional efforts are urgently required to prevent the abuse of older people in Latin America.

As regards laws and policies on gender equality, they are also non-specific with respect to age and, therefore, not sufficient to ensure effective protection for this vulnerable group. Official policies, which have a special emphasis on older people, are rather slow to incorporate the theme of elder abuse and discrimination on the basis of gender and ageing. Some examples of policy and legislation related to the rights and protection of older people may be observed in Latin America. Some of these laws are relatively recent while others modify existing legislation to incorporate the context of old age. A review of pertinent legislation is located in Table 8.2.

Despite such advances, most of the policies and legislation in Latin America do not stipulate abuse of older people as a crime. There is an absence of

Table 8.2 Legislation

Country	Law
Argentina	Law 24.417 (1994), Protection Law against Family Violence, enforced to start in Buenos Aires DC, but already in many other provinces.
	The Family Tribunals Courts (Tribunales de Familia) are the Civil Courts with competence respecting this law. It allows the possibility to denounce through the "Centro de Denuncia Inmediata", which means people might do it without legal assistance.
	2007–2008
	The National Ministry of Social Development under resolution 215/07, delegates on the National Direction for Social Polices for the Aged the responsibility of taking over the policies of Prevention on Discrimination and Mistreatment towards the older population.
Bolivia	Article 68, Constitution of the State. Law on Rights and Privilege on Third Age (N1886); Law 3323 on Health Insurance FOR elders. Law against interfamilial and domestic violence–National Plan on AGEING (2010–2015).
Brazil	Law 10.741 (2003), (Estatuto do Idoso), is a law on protective elders rights.
Chile	Law 20.427 (2010) amending the Law 20.066, on domestic violence, and other legislation to include the abuse of older persons in the National Legislation.
Colombia	Law 19.325 (1994) on domestic violence and abuse but does not include mistreatment of the elderly, specifically.
Costa Rica	Law 7586 (1996) Domestic Violence, mentions that "persons sixty years or more" are specific subject of violence. Law 7935 on Older People.
El Salvador	Law 717 (2002) Comprehensive Care for Older Persons.
Guatemala	Decree Law 80–96 (2005) Protection of the Elderly People. Act on the Prevention, Punishment and Eradication of domestic violence.
Mexico	Rights Act of Older People (2002).
	Penal Code section 200 (2011). Reforms to the Federal District Penal Code. Criminalizing violence against the elderly. Alleged perpetrators are charged and prosecuted.
Nicaragua	Law 720 (2010). Senior's rights to live with dignity and security, free of exploitation, physical abuse, psychological or any other action that goes against his person or property.
Peru	Law 28803 (2006), which guarantees the rights of elders and their families and have determined their obligation to provide for them towards their welfare.
	Law 26763 (1997) across the board incorporates the older persons as liable for actions that shape violence.
Republican Dominican	Law 352-98 (1998) on Protection of the Person "aging".

appropriate legislation in many countries and in most cases complaints and allegations are covered by the domestic family violence laws, which are not necessarily sensitive to the needs of older people who may be suffering from abusive situations.

Due to the lack of a comprehensive approach within some Latin American countries, there is a lack of programs to address elder abuse, although there have been several prevention activities, such as the "Train the trainer seminars" (Havana, Buenos Aires, Puebla, etc.). Such programs focus on teaching professionals and primary health care workers, who look after older people in health and social services, to promote the rights and safety of older people. Other specific areas focus on the education of the caring professions in the context of postgraduate lectures on the elder abuse and its management. However, even with such preliminary education, professionals struggle to deliver appropriate responses in cases of elder abuse.

Several Latin American countries, however, have begun to develop programs to prevent and intervene in abusive situations.

• Argentina: "Proteger" (to protect) was established in 1998 in Buenos Aires DC, and is one of the Argentinean government's current programs on the promotion of social welfare and old age and which deals with abusive situations. Professionals and other workers are given six-months training in gerontology, focusing mainly on the prevention of violence, the guarantee of elder rights and intervention in cases of mistreatment and neglect. "Proteger" also runs a free helpline.

Also, the National Ministry of Social Development, under Resolution 215/07, delegates on the National Direction of Elder's Policies (DINAPAM), the responsibility of developing policies on prevention, discrimination and mistreatment towards the elderly population and launching a National Prevention Program on Discrimination and Elder Abuse in collaboration with the International Network for the Prevention of Elder Abuse (INPEA) Argentina and International Longevity Center (ILC) Argentina (Daichman 2009).

• Chile: Since the implementation of Law no. 20,427 of March 2010, which amended earlier laws on domestic violence by specifically including the mistreatment of older people in the national legislation, a national program for all regions in Chile has been launched and due to be implemented in 2012. This will focus on coordinating all necessary actions for prevention of and intervention in abuse of older people as well as fostering an adequate elder's assistance network for the victims.
• Brazil: Although Brazil has adopted the Elderly Act, a law that makes reporting of suspicions or proven cases of elder abuse mandatory, there is a lack of available training and insufficient guidelines for health professionals. This is evidenced by a lack of clarity on appropriate actions and procedures in elder abuse cases which these health professionals come into

contact with in professional practice (WHO 2008). This phenomenon is quite common throughout the region and is not a unique Brazilian reaction.

- Uruguay: In Montevideo there are two centers which focus on addressing elder abuse. The first was established in 2006 and is a result of the initiative of the Inter-Center Collaboration with the Older Adult (CICAM) Foundation, which since 1991 had been working for the Rights of Older Adults. In addition, the civil partnership Care Center for the Elderly (CAAM) started operating in 2010 to look after people whose rights were violated. However, despite such advances, there is a need to establish such programs on a national level in Uruguay (Lorenzo 2010).

In considering the status of addressing elder abuse in the Latin American countries, there are neither enough specific protocols for the prevention and intervention of elder abuse nor sufficient training. Furthermore, education on elder abuse is not standardized within the institutions where health professionals work with older adults.

The creation of a National Institute on Ageing in Uruguay is an important step in the promotion of elder's rights and other countries should follow. During the last few years, certainly, within the Latin America and the Caribbean region, initiatives have begun to emerge for the prevention of discrimination against elders, and greater recognition and defense of their rights.

Conclusion

Elder abuse is an issue which is emerging in the Latin-American region. There are some important issues within this emergence. Structural inequalities mainly in developing countries have resulted in high unemployment, low wages, poor sanitation, gender discrimination and a lack of opportunities for education. This has contributed to an increase in the vulnerability of older people. Consequently, there are still millions of elders in developing countries who had been denied their rights as they experience isolation, poverty, violence, abuse and limited access to health services, education and legal protection. Moreover, the lack of a regular and sufficient economic income can result in older people being forced to work in inadequate and poorly paid jobs in order to provide not only for themselves but for their families. As with any age group, human rights violations can result in serious health problems and consequences. In recognition of such challenges for older people in Latin America, efforts have been made to increase awareness about the magnitude of the problem and promote the development of prevention and intervention programs. However, policies and health and social programs must be constructed cautiously as they can promote or violate older people's human rights, depending on the way they were designed and implemented.

Essentially, the prevention of elder abuse requires integration and involvement of Latin American society's multiple sectors as well as promoting equality through acknowledgement of the gendered nature of abuse.

Caregivers and professionals working with older people, together with the older population and their families, should be able to have a more comprehensive knowledge about discrimination and elder mistreatment. Health workers, especially those in primary care, can play a fundamental role as they are more likely to encounter abusive situations. However, it is essential that they are trained and educated to recognize, diagnose and manage elder abuse cases, and that there would be a responsive, comprehensive and supportive service behind. It is also important that health professionals and older persons are aware of legal assistance available to assist them. This encompasses both knowledge on using the legislation and lobbying on areas which are not covered by existing statutes and laws.

At a societal level, the importance of education and information dissemination, both formal, informal and through the media is central to changing existing negative stereotypes related to old age and promoting positive messages to facilitate the empowerment of elders. Empowerment should enable older people to access appropriate services, to act on their behalf, to exercise their rights and advocate for their own interests. Violation of human rights may only be effectively prevented if a social culture is fostered that promotes intergenerational solidarity and has zero tolerance for any form of violence.

Further research is essential in Latin America to examine elder abuse within a local and cultural environment. Research on the prevention of elder abuse should lead to contextualized prevention policies which are sensitive to the needs of Latin American older people. Such research is imperative to ground coherent policies, planning and practices and would provide reliable data in the region.

Intervention research and intervention programs are also necessary to plan and evaluate coherent policies on violence prevention, age and gender discrimination and to enhance older people's human rights at local, national and regional levels. Responsible agencies and NGO organizations should form partnerships, reducing duplication and resources waste and enhancing trust in collaborative efforts. This will also promote reliable, efficient and effective services for older people in the area.

Finally, countries in the Latin American region need to be proactive as well as reactive to their responses to the abuse of older people. Information is knowledge, knowledge is power and power enables us to respond to this major challenge. Awareness of the problem and actions needed are crucial to achieve recognition of the issue and social and health changes should follow. Latin American elders have become aware of their needs and rights and are ready for the great challenge. Thus, a convention for rights for older persons (UN 2011) is no longer a utopian ideal. The journey has begun in the region to ensure the rights of each older person and for them to enjoy a quality of life which fundamentally promotes their safety.

Ultimately the challenge to all professionals involved in the area is not only to raise awareness and provide education and training on the subject.

We must get into action and prevent elder abuse, which is still by far the best possible intervention. To listen to what has been said already, carefully heard or published about elder abuse, but more than that, strongly believe and act upon it.

Note

1 A favela is the term for a shanty town in Brazil, most often within urban areas. In the late eighteenth century, the first settlements were called African neighborhoods.

References

Ageways and HelpAge International (2002) Violence and abuse. Online. Available at <http://www.helpage.org/resources/helpage-newsletters/?ssearch=Violence+and +abuseandadv=1andtopic=0andregion=0andlanguage=0andtype=0> (accessed 22 December 2011).

Daichman, L. (2004) 'Elder abuse in the Latin American countries', in T. Tatara (ed.) A survey on intercultural differences in the perceptions about future concerns, governmental functioning and elder rights protections in five countries. Tokyo: (Japanese).

——(2005) 'Elder abuse in developing nations', in M. Johnson, V. Bengston, P. Coleman and T. Kirkwood (eds) The Cambridge handbook of age and ageing. Cambridge: Cambridge University Press.

——(2009) 'ILC–Argentina Report', in ILCA (ed.) Global Ageing Report: Threats to Longevity. New York: International Longevity Center Global Alliance.

——(2012) 'Seminar on Discrimination and Ageing'. Paper on Discrimination, old age and gender ILC–Brazil, Rio de Janeiro, Brazil, March.

Daichman, L., Bennett, G. and Wolf, R. (2002) 'Abuse of the elderly', in E. Kruge (ed.) World Report on Violence and Health. Geneva: World Health Organization.

Daichman, L., Aguas, S. and Spencer, C. (2008) 'Elder abuse', in K. Heggenhougen and S. Quah (eds), Enciclopedia Internacional sobre la Salud Pública. San Diego, CA: Academic Press.

Docampo, S.L., Barreto, L.R. and Santana, S.C. (2009) 'Comportamiento de la violencia intrafamiliar en el adulto mayor', Revista Archivo Médico de Camagüey, Online. Available at <http://www.scielo.sld.cu/scielo.php?script=sci_arttextandpid=S1025–02552009000600010andlng=esandnrm=iso>. ISSN1025–0255> (accessed 22 December 2011).

ECLAC (2010) 'Strategy proposal, from the perspective of Latin America and the Caribbean, for advancing towards an international convention on the human rights of older persons'. Committee on Population and Development. Online. Available at <http://www.eclac.org/publicaciones/xml/1/39461/LCL3220_CEP2010_I.pdf> (accessed 30 July 2012).

Gil, G.C. (2002) Violencia, abuso, maltrato y/o trato negligente en la Tercera Edad. El suicidio en America Latina Vs la UE en la Tercera Edad. (E-book) Córdoba, Argentina: Universidad Nacional de Córdoba website Online. Available at <http://www.aniorte. eresmas.com/archivos/violenc_abus_maltrat_3edad.pdf> (accessed 5 December 2011).

Giraldo, L. (2006) Los malos tratos a personas adultas mayores: Una caracterización sociodemográfica en la Ciudad de México. Mexico City: El Colegio de México.

——(2010) 'El maltrato de personas adultas mayores: una mirada desde la perspectiva de género', Debate Feminista, 21, 42: 151–64.

Hudson, M. (1998) 'Elder abuse: Two Native American views', The Gerontologist, 38, 5: 538–48.

Lopes, V., Oliveira, J., and Falbo, G. (2006) 'Maus-tratos contra idosos no município de Camaragibe, Pernambuco (Elder abuse in Camaragibe, Pernambuco)'. Rev. Bras. Saúde Matern. Infant., Recife, 6, 1: S43–8.

Lorenzo, L. (2010) 'Derechos que no caducan'. La Diaria, Uruguay, 31 August.

Martina, M., Nolberto, V., Miljanovich, M., Bardales, O. and Gálvez, D. (2010) 'Violencia hacia el adulto mayor: Centros Emergencia Mujer del Ministerio de la Mujer y Desarrollo Social. Lima-Perú, 2009'. Rev. Perú. Epidemiol, 14, 3: 1–7.

OEA, 2011. 'Report on the situation of older persons in the hemisphere and the effectiveness of binding universal and regional human rights instruments with regard to protection of the human rights of older persons'. Online. Available at <http://www.globalaging.org/agingwatch/situation%20hemisphere.pdf> (accessed 30 July 2012).

PAHO (2011) 'Permanent Council of the Organization of American States: Report on the situation of older persons in the hemisphere and the effectiveness of binding universal and regional human rights instruments with regard to protection of the human rights of older persons'. Working Group on Protection of the Human Rights of Older Persons. Online. Available at <http://www.globalaging.org/aging watch/situation%20hemisphere.pdf> (accessed 10 December 2012).

Quiroga, L.P., Wagemann B.H. and Torres A.G. (2001) 'Caracterización y frecuencia del maltrato a adultos mayores en áreas urbanas'. Cuad Med. Soc. Santiago de Chile, 42, 1/2: 30–35.

Riveros, R.M. (2006) Índices y subíndices de malos tratos en los adultos mayores. Asunción-Paraguay: Facultad de Ciencias Médicas-UNA.

UN (2002) 'Political declaration and Madrid international plan of action on ageing, Second World Assembly on Ageing, Madrid, Spain 8–12 April'. Online. Available at <http://www.social.un.org/index/Portals/0/ageing/documents/Fulltext-E.pdf> (accessed 31 July 2012).

——(2003) 'Report of the regional intergovernmental conference on ageing: Towards a regional strategy for the implementation in Latin America and the Caribbean of the Madrid International Plan of Action on ageing, Santiago, Chile, 19–21 November'. Economic Commission for Latin America and the Caribbean. Online. Available at <http://www.cepal.org/publicaciones/xml/9/15009/lcl2079i.pdf> (accessed 6 January 2012).

——(2009) World Population Ageing 2009. New York: Department of Economic and Social Affairs. Online. Available at <http://www.un.org/esa/population/publications/WPA2009/WPA2009_WorkingPaper.pdf> (accessed 6 January 2012).

——(2010) Convention on the elimination of all forms of discrimination against women: General recommendation No. 27 on older women and protection of their human rights. New York: Department of CEDAW. Online. Available at <http://www2.ohchr.org/english/bodies/cedaw/docs/CEDAW-C-2010-47-GC1.pdf> (accessed 6 January 2012).

——(2011) 'Statistical Yearbook for Latin America and the Caribbean'. Online. Available at <http://www.eclac.cl/publicaciones/xml/7/45607/LCG2513b.pdf> (accessed 28 July 2012).

——(2012) 'Population ageing: Latin America and the Caribbean Demographic Observatory, Year VI, No. 12, October 2011'. Online. Available at <http://www.eclac.cl/publicaciones/xml/2/46772/OD12_WEB.pdf> (accessed 28 July 2012).

Viviano, T. (2005) Violencia familiar en las personas adultas mayores en el Peru: Aportes desde la casuística de los centros emergencia mujer/ programa nacional contra la violencia familiar y sexual. [E-book] Peru: Online. Available at <http:// www.mimdes.gob.pe/files/PROGRAMAS%20NACIONALES/PNCVFS/mimdes_ adultos_mayores_libros.pdf> (accessed 5 December 2011).

WHO (2008) A global response to elder abuse and neglect: Building primary health care capacity to deal with the problem worldwide: main report. [E-book] Geneva: World Health Organization. Online. Available at http://<http://www.who.int/ ageing/publications/ELDER_DocAugust08.pdf> (accessed 22 December 2011).

WHO and INPEA (2002). Missing voices: Views of older persons on elder abuse. Geneva: World Health Organization and International Network for the Prevention of Elder Abuse.

Wolf, R., Bennett, G. and Daichman, L., (2003) 'Abuse of the elderly', in B. Green, M. Friedman, J. Jong, S. Solomon, T. Keane, J. Fairbank, et al. (eds) Trauma intervention in war and peace: Prevention, practice and policy. New York: Kluwer Academic, Ch. 6.

9 Norway

Astrid Sandmoe

Introduction

Norway is a rather affluent and sparsely populated country in the northern hemisphere. Johns and Hydle (1995), two of the first Norwegian researchers to examine elder abuse, recorded that Norwegians in the early 1990s held firm beliefs regarding the welfare state and that older people appeared to have few concerns about support systems when growing old. The situation is likely to be similar today, especially for those in good health. Norwegian older people generally have good health, an adequate income and/or pension and enjoy a good standard of life. However, comprehensive reforms have changed the health and social system, and, based on public discussion, there are some indications that people do not trust the state's ability to meet their health care needs in any situation (Stamsø 2009). The naïve belief that the Norwegian welfare state could prevent most problems including elder abuse, was evident in the early 1980s in public and political discourses. Consequently, it took some time before society realised that abuse of older people was an issue in Norway (Juklestad 2007, Stang and Evensen 1985). Firstly, in order to understand elder abuse in Norway, it is necessary to contextualise the environment within which it emerged. This discussion also incorporates research from Norway's neighbouring country, Sweden, which has similar cultural characteristics.

Like other Scandinavian countries, the Norwegian welfare system is based on the idea that needs in the population that cannot be solved by using a market mechanism will be met by the public service (Normann et al. 2009). Norway is not a member of the European Union (EU), but is affiliated to it by various agreements and treaties. In the past fifty years, social security has gradually increased and in 2006 Norway had the highest total social expenditure per capita in Europe. Despite this, social expenditure as a proportion of Norwegian gross national product is among the lowest in European countries as Norway is a wealthy country, mainly because of its oil production (Normann et al. 2009).

The main challenge for many countries is the demographic changes associated with an ageing population. Norway's population was over five million in March 2012 (Statistics Norway 2012); 15 per cent of the population are aged 65 years and older and this cohort will increase to 17 per cent in 2020 (Statistics Norway 2012). However, this represents a decrease from above 22 per cent in 2007 and it will take some decades before the numbers reach the same level (Normann et al. 2009). Life expectancy at birth is 83 years for women and 79 years for men. Immigrants and Norwegian-born with immigrant parents constitute about 12 per cent of the population with the largest proportion living in the capital city, Oslo (Statistics Norway 2012). A predominant expense for almost all European countries is that of retirement and survivor pensions, all with the exception of Norway and Iceland, where the costs of health and diseases constituted the biggest social spending (Normann et al. 2009). The official retirement age in Norway is 67 years, though it is possible for most of the working population to retire at 64.

Norway has a parliamentary democracy, with two administrative levels that regulate health and social policy. There are 430 municipalities governed by local authorities and the national government. In 2008, the government established four public health enterprises which are responsible for hospital services (Ministry of Health and Care Services 2008). Issues related to the control of health and social policies by local authorities or national government have always been contentious.

The national government aims to promote equality through national standards as well as specific action plans and a budget that commits health and social services at the frontline administrative level when important reforms or new services are implemented (Øverby 2009). Consequently, in 2012, a comprehensive coordination reform policy was implemented, entitled 'Proper treatment – at the right place and right time' (Ministry of Health and Care Services 2009). The aim of this reform is to increase the efficiency in the health care sector through better coordination of the service, in particular between the hospital service and the health care service in municipalities (Ministry of Health and Care Services 2009). The reform highlights two more challenges: the limited focus on preventing diseases, and the demographic and epidemiologic changes in the population. Policy changes are emphasised as necessary to sustain the Norwegian welfare system and an increasing number of the health services have been transferred to the municipalities, in particular in relation to aged health care.

In order to make services more efficient, especially with regard to the effective discharge and transition of patients from hospital, funding methods changed. In addition, several Acts that regulated the health care sector were transformed (Ministry of Health and Care Services 2011). However, such reforms created huge challenges, in particular for home nursing care, community care and residential care in relation to older people. Hospitals were more focused on the provision of specialised, acute services and this translated to additional health care work being allocated to primary care. However, due to the gap between the ability of primary care services to provide such care and the increased service demand, municipalities themselves have been forced to pay for patients that cannot be discharged from hospital. Consequently, this has increased the demands of informal care to older people by relatives and others although this is under-resourced (Dale et al. 2008). Unsurprisingly, researchers and professionals are concerned about the consequences of an insufficient capacity in primary care to handle the needs of frail, older people (Gjevjon and Romøren 2011). Thus, it has been claimed that the current policy reorientation constitutes a redistribution of tasks rather than a reform that promotes interaction and collaboration between different levels of the health care sector (Romøren 2011). Further-more, residential care for older people is also under pressure and access to such care is difficult particularly in townland areas (Fjelltun et al. 2009, Gjevjon and Romøren 2011).

Definition

Like most other countries, the definition of elder abuse has been debated for a long time in Norway (Wolf et al. 2002). In the 1980s, early researchers on the topic of elder abuse in Norway were critical of the broad definition that was used in the United States and Europe. Johns and Hydle (1995) claimed that the definition included too many types of abuse and that the definition did not have any objective criteria. The subjective and emotional component of such definitions were considered problematic in deciding the extent of elder abuse and in the context of developing responsive elder abuse inter-ventions (Johns and Hydle 1995). The debate on definitions was examined by the Council of Europe (1992) and resulted in clarification of the concepts family, violence and elderly people. The abuser was limited to someone in 'a trusted position' in the older person's family, such as relatives, partner or spouse. Violence included any act or omission or act that caused physical, psychological or financial harm to a person above national retirement age (Council of Europe 1992). Subsequently, Johns and Hydle (1995: 147) developed the following analytic definition:

> Abuse is a social act involving at least two actors, one of whom is violating the personal boundaries of the other. This is abuse insofar as it is interpreted and morally evaluated as illegitimate by a third party, the witness.

Johns and Hydle emphasised that suffering is caused in many situations without it being labelled as abuse. Such situations might come into existence, for example, when patients are treated for serious illness in hospital. The authors claimed that it is necessary to assess the different elements in the situation, such as culture, before it is possible to label an act as abuse. Although acknowledging that their definition was not objective, it was con-sidered of value in research and practice because it drew attention to who is labelling a situation as abuse and thereby strengthened the professionals' responsibility when they witness situations when someone is 'violating personal boundaries' of an older person (Johns and Hydle 1995).

The moral implication for the practitioner as a witness to abuse was also a concern for researchers in Sweden (Saveman et al. 1993). In defining 'elder abuse', Saveman et al. (1993) concurred with Johns et al. (1991) and argued that elder abuse has four dimensions. It constitutes a social act; it involves the abuser's power; it is an insult of the older person's boundaries and the witness's judgement is important in establishing the action as illegal.

The arguments for the definition outlined by Johns and Hydle (1995) were based on social anthropology and semiology, and could be considered complex to understand. One challenging issue was that the definition required the abusive actions to be observed by others and to be labelled as abuse. As most elder abuse occurs in private, the definition lacked the ability to comprehensively define elder abuse. Swedish researchers have attempted to overcome such limitations in an 'elder abuse anti-definition':

> Self-serving acts, lacking in compassion and unnecessary for improved life quality, that violate the right of the older person to be respected as a human being.
>
> (Erlingsson 2007: 58)

Erlingsson asserts that the 'anti-definition' includes all sorts of actions that offend and/or hurt an older person and claim that this definition does not necessarily require a witness. It is the older person's right to judge if an act is abusive. The definition emphasises human rights and does not limit the abuser to someone in a traditional 'position of trust'. Although the argument that older people have a right to determine the situation as abusive or not has some credence, it may pose difficulties. For example, a person who has, over time, been exposed to abuse will not necessarily be able to judge the situation because of the possible psychological consequences of the abuse. Moreover, a subjective element may be implied in advocating the practitioner's personal interpretation:

> The key that unlocks this definition is the ability to see a situation as if we were in it ourselves, experiencing the potential for disrespect, shame and unworthiness inherent in the act. The key to unlocking elder abuse is the ability for compassion.
>
> (Erlingsson 2007: 58).

The work by Swedish researchers at the Umeå University and the University of Calmar have been complemented by some Norwegian elder abuse researchers, and Norwegian and Swedish researchers have collaborated in some projects (Malmedal et al. 2009b, 2009a). This has been assisted by the fact that Norway and Sweden are geographically close, have similar cultures and understand each other's languages.

It is difficult to describe how the definition of elder abuse is understood through Norwegian policy, because governmental agencies who might take responsibility for providing definition and strategies to prevent and handle the problem do not exist (Sethi et al. 2011). Acknowledging this deficit in service and policy provision, the nationally funded research institute, the Norwegian Centre for Violence and Traumatic Stress Studies (NKVTS: www.nkvts.no) do refer to the Toronto Declaration's definition of elder abuse, which defines elder abuse as:

> a single or repeated act, or lack of appropriate action occurring within any relationship where there is an expectation of trust which causes harm or distress to an older person.
>
> (WHO 2002).

Abusive actions are considered to manifest in physical, psychological/emotional, financial/material and sexual abuse and also include intentional and unintentional neglect (WHO 2002).

Although the WHO definition does provide some clarity, Sandmoe (2011) questions the appropriateness of including unintentional neglect in the concept of elder abuse. Malmedal et al. (2009b) have used the term 'inadequate care' in nursing homes and drew upon the work of Fulmer and O'Malley (1987: 233) when defining inadequate care as 'the consequence, not only from abuse and neglect, but also from ignorance, lack of knowledge, lack of adequate service and lack of access to services'. Malmedal et al. (2009b) do not draw any distinction when it comes to the action as intentional or unintentional. Malmedal (1998) found that Norwegian health professionals working in nursing homes restricted the use of the term 'abuse' to severe and physical violence. The studies focused on nursing staffs' attitudes to reporting inadequate care in nursing homes, in addition to what they had observed and committed in practice (Malmedal et al. 2009b, 2009a). The questionnaire contained 20 statements about issues related to emotional abuse, inadequate care, neglect, physical abuse and theft (Malmedal et al. 2009b). The participants were not asked if they agreed with the definition of inadequate care, or how they understood the term. The statements included severe physical violence, but also actions such as 'Entering a resident's room without knocking' (Malmedal et al. 2009b: 235). Of course, it is important that the privacy of the patients is respected and failure to knock on the door might well be considered as inappropriate conduct.

Sandmoe and Kirkevold (2011a) found that nurse managers in community care generally understood the Norwegian word 'overgrep' ('abuse'), to mean physical abuse. A similar understanding of the term 'abuse' appeared when interviewing registered and auxiliary nurses in community care (Sandmoe and Kirkevold 2011b). The participants in the study experienced abuse as offences against an older person, but, if the intention to hurt was less apparent or the abusive actions were less severe, the findings indicated that cases were labelled as something other than abuse, such as for example 'difficult cases' (Sandmoe and Kirkevold 2011a, 2011b). Sandmoe et al. (2011) carried out a similar study of community care in Australia. One trend observed was that Norwegian participants were hesitant to categorise financial misuse of the client's money or property as abuse, whereas Australian participants more often understood such conditions to be abusive (Sandmoe et al. 2011).

We do not really know how older people themselves understand the term 'elder abuse', but elderly Norwegians can define abuse of older people as a family problem (Hjemdal and Juklestad 2006). However, Hjemdal and Juklestad assert that elderly people have relatively clear ideas of what elder abuse is, in particular that it is physical violence, but they also include economic and psychological abuse as well as neglect.

Policy

Acknowledgement of the problem of abuse of older people has been slow in Norwegian society (Juklestad, 2007), reflecting the situation in the other Scandinavian countries (Penhale 2006, Luoma and Koivusilta 2009). The Norwegian response to elder abuse began with a small project in the mid-1980s (Stang and Evensen 1985, Hydle 1993) and, as a result, a government-funded Protective Services for the Elderly (PSE) (in Norwegian 'Vern for eldre') was established. The PSE project was initially founded and located in Oslo (Juklestad 2007) and became a formal part of the municipal health and social service system in Oslo in 2000 (Protective Service for the Elderly 2010). From 2006 a second service has been available in Bærum (Hansen 2006). The population in Oslo and Bærum constitute about 700,000 people, or 14 per cent of Norway's 5 million inhabitants (Statistics Norway 2011). In the past ten years, two additional municipalities have tried to establish the service without success. Governmental initiatives to implement PSE in all municipalities have not been taken.

Both the Oslo and Bærum PSEs employ the Toronto Declaration (WHO 2002) as a framework for service delivery (Hansen, 2006, Protective Service for the Elderly, 2010). The PSE provides assistance for older people who are abused by someone they trust, and for those who allege that the health care system is neglecting their care needs. However, the annual report by the PSEs indicates that cases of self-neglect are also managed by the service, even though self-neglect is outside the scope of the definition in the Toronto Declaration (WHO 2002). The main target group for PSE is men and women aged 62 years and over who suffer from abuse or are at risk of suffering from abuse and are living in the municipality of Oslo or Bærum. The PSE is free and the concerned person may contact the service anonymously for advice and support.

Considerable effort has been made in the last ten years by the Ministry of Justice and the Police (2003, 2004, 2007, 2008, 2009) to raise public awareness of the issue of domestic violence and to improve support services to children and women experiencing abuse within the family. The White Paper 'Long term care: Future challenges' (Ministry of Health and Care Services 2006) included issues related to the abuse of older people, and emphasised that older abused people might have difficulties in getting assistance by established support services such as domestic shelters, health and social centres and the police. In addition, the report stressed that elderly victims of abuse often have needs outside the competence of the established health and social service. As a follow-up, the government established a three-year nationwide abuse helpline project, which has been operational since 2008, with an annual budget of NOK 1 million (130,000 euros) (Norwegian Directorate of Health 2008). In January 2012, the Ministry of Justice launched an action plan to combat domestic violence (including elder abuse) and proposed that the national helpline should be maintained as a permanent service feature (Ministry of Justice 2012). In 2012, the Government will present a White Paper about domestic violence (including elder abuse) to the Parliament followed by a new four-year action plan. It is anticipated that elder abuse will get more attention in these forthcoming plans and the Minister of Justice, Grete Faremo stated that:

> In recent years it has become widely accepted that domestic violence is a serious crime. Now it is time to break down the last taboo: Violence against the elderly.
>
> Faremo (2012)

Another method of government regulation of the health care system in Norway occurs through the policy of education via financing and the establishing of national curricula for universities, university colleges and the ongoing education of health personnel in the county. However, the Norwegian national curriculum regulations for nursing education do not include elder abuse as a mandatory course, nor do they require training in this topic (Ministry of Education and Research 2005), and few universities and colleges have incorporated elder abuse as a topic in elective courses (Sogn 2007). A White Paper about higher education and research promotes reform so that health and social care professionals are better able to meet the challenges in the welfare system (Ministry of Education and Research 2012). Demographic changes, particularly in relation to the ageing population, are emphasised. The report focuses on skills such as reflexive practice, respect for individual choices and freedom within the framework of the welfare state service, and the use of preventive measures to reduce health risk factors (Hedlund 2012). Such approaches are beneficial in the improvement of practice responses to elder abuse.

Legislation

There is no mandatory reporting of elder abuse in general and identified cases of abuse cannot be reported to the authorities by professionals without permission from the offended person (Ministry of Justice and the Police 2005), except where the life of the older person is threatened or it is very likely that such a situation might come into existence. The sentence for violence or threatening and inconsiderate behaviour was increased in the revised Criminal Code (Ministry of Justice and the Police 2005) and strengthened the individual's right to live in peace and privacy (Ministry of Justice and the Police 2010b). That implies that the police, when called in for domestic violence cases (including elder abuse), can now bring charges against the offender, without the consent of the victim.

As stated, the health and social service's obligation to report elder abuse cases is founded on criminal law and current provisions are located in legislation, such as the Municipal Health and Care Services Act (2011), and the regulation of the quality of the health care services (Ministry of Health and Care Services 2003). In addition, older people suffering from abuse have rights, through the Patients' Rights Act (Ministry of Health and Care Services 1999), to receive necessary health care services, which include preventive and health-preserving measures, adjusted to the individual's needs. However, an act amending the Patients' Rights Act came into force in 2009 and gave direction for the provision of necessary health care to adult people over 16 years of age without capacity to give consent (Ministry of Health and Care Services 2011). The amendment made it possible to intervene in situations where the older person suffers from dementia and resists necessary health care service intervention. In addition, the Guardianship Act (Ministry of Justice and the Police 2010a) makes it possible for the general practitioner (GP) to report the need for guardianship of a person, who is suffering from dementia and is legally mentally incapacitated, to the Public Guardian Office. Such regulation and legislation is particularly important when intervening in cases of physical, sexual and financial abuse.

Practice response

As explained above, issues related to elder abuse are not well acknowledged in Norwegian society. This is also true in the context of professional practice responses. Sandmoe and Kirkevold's (2011a) preliminary findings, when interviewing nurse managers, was that elder abuse was a poorly understood issue and that it was under-communicated among community care professionals, as only half of the 52 participants stated that they had identified cases in their departments during the previous year. However, closer analysis of the interviews indicated that abuse was experienced more often than was explicitly revealed by the participants. Additionally, several participants agreed that they had encountered abuse cases after receiving an outline of the WHO's (2002) definition of abuse. To describe a situation as 'abusive' challenges professionals to take actions, and, by avoiding the term, situations might be mistakenly considered to be less serious than they actually are.

Community care is not equipped with procedures or guidelines to assist in the process of identification of or intervention in elder abuse cases

(Sandmoe and Kirkevold 2011a, 2011b, Sandmoe et al. 2011). Without any procedures to assist the professionals, the response to suspected cases of abuse depends on the expertise and skill of individual professionals. In addition, the involvement and responsibility of managers in community care are important in coordinating and supporting the staff so that appropriate actions can be taken. Another finding in Sandmoe et al.'s (2011) study was that Norwegian community carer were less aware of the variety of external resources available to contact. Such services might include residential day-care, respite or long-term care, senior centre care, public health care centres, social services, mental health services and offices for the support of the family. Some residential care facilities also operate small units called safety-units (trygghetsavdeling) where older people in need of a place to feel secure due to health or social conditions can apply to stay for one or two weeks (Ministry of Health and Care Services 2006). These studies were conducted before the national elder abuse helpline was operational and, today, support provided by the helpline, which includes professionals who are qualified to identify suspected cases of abuse, might enhance the intervention processes in suspected cases of abuse. However, it seems likely that it will take time before health and social professionals in all Norwegian municipalities are aware of the helpline support. Several information campaigns have been launched and enquires to the helpline are increasing, though the total number of enquires outside Oslo is low (Protective Service for the Elderly 2012).

Professionals in the two municipalities where the PSE is established can contact the service for advice and practical help, without breaking case confidentiality. If the older person agrees, the professional/executive officer at the PSE can carry out meetings with that person, family members, health and social professionals and other relevant parties to clarify problems and to determine what sort of help the elderly person wants and needs. The PSE takes measures to protect the victim from the perpetrator and, where necessary, collaborates with relatives and other agencies and services as well as coordinating the measures taken. If the presenting case turns out to be something other than abuse, the executive officer may be helpful in referring the case to another more appropriate part of the health and social system or other relevant offices (Protective Service for the Elderly 2010).

Another option for abused older people is the provision of temporary residence at a domestic violence shelter and counselling by professionals. There are 51 domestic shelters in Norway and, since January 2010, municipalities have been required to provide shelters to people suffering from abuse, independent of gender and age (MCESI 2009). In 2010, there were 2,075 people who stayed at least one night at a shelter, some 2 per cent of whom were aged 60 years or older (Nersund and Govasmark 2011). This underuse might be due to these services not being prepared to meet the needs of elderly people because neither elderly victims nor professionals have acknowledged the services as being of benefit for older people

(Nersund and Govasmark 2011, Sandmoe et al. 2011); or it might be that health professionals consider these shelters to be less supportive for older people than for children and younger adults.

In addition, support by the domestic violence coordinator of the police department or the offices of Service for Victims of Crime (www.kriminalitetsofre. no) might be of value in cases involving physical violence. The latter service has offices in every county in Norway and its services are free to its clients. The Service for Victims of Crime also runs a nationwide helpline and provides information about free legal aid and economic compensation arrangements. In addition, the Norwegian Directorate of Health has published an instruction book for health care services for victims of partner abuse (Norwegian Directorate of Health 2007).

Research

To date, there have not been any national prevalence studies of elder abuse in Norway. Stang and Evensen (1985) conducted a four-month prevalence study of elder abuse among clients in a community care area in Oslo. Findings demonstrated a 1 per cent prevalence rate. Johnsen and Aschjem (1986) duplicated this study in two municipalities, Porsgrunn and Bamble, and found a higher elder abuse prevalence rate of approximately 3 per cent. Hydle and Johns (1992) also conducted a field study in the period 1988–91 which substantiated the need for a specialised service that could coordinate the support to elderly victims of abuse. Hydle and Johns (1992) concluded that, though there were resources in the existing health and social service, these services were difficult to access for older people. This body of research provided a significant catalyst for the establishment of the previously discussed Oslo PSE project which was later established as an ordinary service in the health care system. The PSE has not been evaluated, but Homelien (2011) interviewed seven elderly victims of abuse about the support they had received by the PSE and found that the comprehensive competence of the PSE professionals in individualising the intervention and building trust enhanced the victims' social support considerably and thereby their capacity to handle the situation.

Two more studies have been carried out with the objectives of clarifying the attitude and experiences of abused older people, what they have done to handle the situation and the support they have received from family, friends and professionals. Solhaug (2007) interviewed seven elderly victims of abuse. Findings emphasised that there are several barriers to seeking help, particularly if the abuser was an adult child of the elderly victim. The older parents were afraid that the situation for their son or daughter should deteriorate if they reported the problems and that they to a less degree defined themselves as victims of abuse. There were similar findings in another study, by Jonassen and Sandmoe (2012), where thirty victims of abuse, from the age of 62 years to 95 years, were interviewed. Results suggested that older people were reluctant to use the term 'abuse' if the abusive situation was caused by someone close to them, and in particular if the abuser was their adult child. The older parents' concerns were how to get support for the adult child's problem and usually they had been in touch with the ordinary health and social service several times without getting the support they needed (Jonassen and Sandmoe 2012). The turning point for all the older victims, regardless of who the abuser was, was contact with PSE and, for two of the victims, contact with staff at a domestic shelter (Jonassen and Sandmoe 2012).

Sandmoe's (2011) study revealed that nurse managers and registered and auxiliary nurses experienced the abuse of older people as complex and having contextual issues that challenged the individual health care professional and community care as service provider. Participants with access to PSE found the interdisciplinary collaboration as invaluable while participants without this support struggled to handle complex cases. The results indicate that community care services to older victims of abuse could be improved by training and educating staff in the phenomenon of elder abuse (Sandmoe 2011).

In 2007, the Government established five regional centres for violence, traumatic stress and the prevention of suicide as part of their plan of action to combat domestic violence (Ministry of Justice and the Police, 2004). Thus far, projects or publications addressing elder abuse have not been carried out by these regional centres (RVTS Vest 2010, RVTS Sør 2009).

An abuse resource centre was established in 1996 with parliamentary approval, and in 2004 the centre became part of the government-funded Norwegian Centre for Violence and Traumatic Stress Studies (NKVTS). The research activities of the Centre include examining abuse of older people, but prior to 2011 only one elder abuse research project (Hjemdal and Juklestad 2006) was carried out (NKVTS 2008, 2009, 2010). As already described in this section, the Centre conducted an elder abuse study in 2011 as directed by the Norwegian Directorate of Health (Jonassen and Sandmoe 2012).

In a multi-country research collaboration, the NKVTS had the opportunity to examine intercultural and inter-generational differences among elderly people in Norway (Hjemdal and Juklestad 2006). A postal survey with 20 statements about elder abuse was answered by 467 members of the Norwegian Association of Old Age Pensioners. Similar studies, though using different methods, were carried out in Finland, USA and Japan (Hjemdal and Juklestad 2006). The Norwegian results did not differ much from the other participating countries. The Norwegian participants agreed that elder abuse was unacceptable, though they were more reluctant to report the abuse to someone outside the family, such as the health and social service and the police. Thus, Norwegians viewed elder abuse as predominantly a private matter, which deviated from the findings of the other participating countries (Hjemdal and Juklestad 2006).

There have been several research projects about the use of restraint in nursing homes, completed by the Ageing and Health, Norwegian Centre for Research,

Education and Service Development (Kirkevold and Engedal 2004, 2006). These studies indicated that approximately 40 per cent of patients were subject to constraint and in particular patients who were suffering from dementia were exposed to physical restraint. If the patients had reduced mental and physical capacity, and particularly if the patients were aggressive, the quality of care was difficult to maintain and was also affected by the organization and staffing of the ward (Kirkevold and Engedal 2004, 2006). In addition, studies of inadequate care in nursing homes are important to enlighten health authorities and practitioners about elder abuse in residential care (Malmedal 1998, Malmedal et al. 2009a).

Conclusion

Norway took a lead among the Scandinavian countries in combating elder abuse in the 1980s and the 1990s and WHO gave Norway credit for parliamentary approval of the PSE project in Oslo and the establishment of the Norwegian Centre for Violence and Traumatic Stress Studies (Wolf et al. 2002). But on a national scale progression in the fight to combat elder abuse has faltered in the past ten years. Norway has made some admirable advances in measures taken to combat domestic violence, in particular how the society now addresses issues related to abuse of children and younger women, but abuse of older people appears to have been eclipsed by such efforts. This is in part due to a strong feminist discourse in Norway which has focused on 'traditional' domestic violence and has applied pressure on local and national authorities to implement remedial actions (Skjørten 2009). 'Elder abuse', as a specific social issue in Norway, has not been supported by any coordinated movement or organisation. Instead, the recent advances described in this chapter were a result of actions by a few enthusiastic health and social professionals and campaigners against elder abuse (Skjørten 2009, Juklestad 2007). But it is the responsibility of a welfare society such as Norway's to respond to 'silent' and marginalised groups of the population who find it difficult to promote their own rights (Normann et al. 2009). Acknowledging these challenges, the Norwegian Government has committed to action on elder abuse (Faremo 2012).

Recommendations

- It is recommended that the government initiate public awareness programmes that promote a national policy to combat elder abuse. The policy should include a strategy to develop national guidelines and procedures that are flexibly constructed to allow adjustment to local presenting circumstances. It is imperative that such elder abuse guidelines are incorporated into the health care service's quality assurance system and into other services that provide support to older people.

- Research projects should be supported to strengthen the implementation of procedures to identify and handle abuse cases in practice and to evaluate outcomes.
- Education on the topic of family violence is essential for interdisciplinary professionals. Such education should include general frameworks of family violence but also distinguish material pertaining to the case identification and case management of elder abuse.
- Disciplinary boundaries between health care and social services need to be reduced and mutual interdisciplinary collaboration promoted so that appropriate measures to deal with abuse problems can be planned and implemented together with the older client and/or their relatives. Barriers to effective interdisciplinary collaboration should be considered when developing national guidelines and further elaborated by each county and/or municipality when implementing such guidelines in the local health and social services.
- Finally, the PSE, currently available only in Oslo and Bærum, should be established in all counties. These services should be sensitive to the needs of older abused people and the support needs of professionals in health and social service, as well as other people involved.

References

Council of Europe (1992) Violence against elderly people. Strasbourg: Council of Europe Press.

Dale, B., Sævereid, H., Kirkevold, M. and Söderhamn, O. (2008) 'Formal and informal care in relation to activities of daily living and self-perceived health among older care-dependent individuals in Norway', International Journal of Older People Nursing, 3: 194–203.

Erlingsson, C. (2007) 'Elder abuse explored through a prism of perceptions: Perspectives of potential witnesses', unpublished thesis, Umeå University.

Faremo, G. (2012) Eldrevold: det siste tabu. [violence against the elderly: the last taboo] Oslo: Justis-og beredskapsdepartementet. Online. Available at <http://www.regjeringen. no/nb/dep/jd/tema/kriminalitetsbekjempelse/vold-i-nare-relasjoner.html?id=447110> (Accessed 22 February 2012).

Fjelltun, A.-M., Henriksen, N., Norberg, A., Gilje, F. and Normann, H. (2009) 'Nurses' and carers' appraisals of workload in care of frail elderly awaiting nursinghome placement', Scandinavian Journal of Caring Sciences, 23: 57–66.

Fulmer, T. and O'Malley, T. (1987) Inadequate care of the elderly: A health care perspective on abuse and neglect, New York: Springer Publishing Company.

Gjevjon, E. R. and Romøren, T. I. (2011) 'Vedtak om sykehjemsplass: Hvor høye er tersklene? (Granting nursing home placement: Are the thresholds insuperable?)', Demens and Alderspykiatri, 15: 36–7.

Hansen, M. (2006) 'Vern for eldre: Årsmelding 2005 (Protective Service for the Elderly: Annual Report 2005)'. Bærum kommune (the municipality of Bærum).

Hedlund, M. (2012) 'Norwegian health and social care', Public Service Review: European Science and Technology, 148–9.

Hjemdal, O. and Juklestad, O. (2006) En privatsak? Eldres oppfatning av vold og overgrep og om å melde fra om vold. (A private matter? Elders' attitude towards violence and abuse and reporting violence). Oslo: Norwegian Centre for Violence and Traumatic Stress Studies.

Homelien, S. (2011) 'Meningsdannende fellesskap ...: Om sosial støtte til eldre som utsettes for overgrep (Meaning making community ...: Social support for elderly victims of abuse)', unpublised minor thesis, Tønsberg: Høgskolen i Vestfold (Vestfold University College).

Hydle, I. (1993) 'Abuse and neglect of the elderly: A Nordic perspective report from a Nordic research project', Scandinavian Journal of Social Medicine, 21: 126–8.

——and Johns, S. (1992) Stengte dører og knyttede never: Når eldre blir utsatt for overgrep i hjemmet (Locked doors and clenched fists: When the elderly are abused in the home), Oslo: Kommuneforlaget.

Johns, S. and Hydle, I. (1995) 'Norway: Weakness in welfare', Journal of Elder Abuse and Neglect, 6: 139–56.

Johns, S., Hydle, I. and Aschjem, Ø. (1991) 'The act of abuse a twoheaded monster of injury and offence', Journal of Elder Abuse and Neglect, 3: 53–64.

Johnsen, J. and Aschjem, Ø. (1986) 'Rapport om eldremishandling i Telemark (Report on elder mistreatment in Telemark)'. Unpublished report, Porsgrunn, Norway.

Jonassen, W. and Sandmoe, A. (2012) Overgrep mot eldre i Norge: erfaringer og løsningsstrategier (Elder abuse in Norway: Experiences and solution strategies)'. Oslo: Norwegian Centre for Violence and Traumatic Stress Studies.

Juklestad, O. (2007) Report on current studies on elder abuse in Norway, including elder abuse-related activities. Oslo: Norwegian Centre for Violence and Traumatic Stress Studies.

Kirkevold, Ø. and Engedal, K. (2004) 'Prevalence of patients subjected to constraint in Norwegian nursing homes', Scandinavian Journal of Caring Sciences, 18: 281–6.

Kirkevold, Ø. and Engedal, K. (2006) 'The quality of care in Norwegian nursing homes', Scandinavian Journal of Caring Sciences, 20: 177–83.

Luoma, M.-L. and Koivusilta, M. (2009) 'Peanow – Prevalence study of abuse and violence against old women. Literature review: Finland and the Nordic countries'. National Institute for Health and Welfare: Finland.

Malmedal, W. (1998) '"Noen må følge bedre med": Om overgrep i sykehjem ("Someone must be more aware": abuse in nursing homes)', unpublished thesis. Trondheim: NTNU (Norwegian University of Science and Technology).

——, Hammersvold, R. and Saveman, B.-I. (2009a) 'To report or not report? Attitudes held by Norwegian nursing home staff on reporting inadequate care carried out by colleagues', Scandinavian Journal of Public Health, 37: 744–50.

——, Ingebrigtsen, O. and Saveman, B.-I. (2009b) 'Inadequate care in Norwegian nursing homes: As reported by nursing staff', Scandinavian Journal of Caring Sciences, 23: 231–42.

MCESI (2009) Lov om kommunale krisesentertilbod: Sist endret juni 2011 (The Municipal Domestic Shelter Act: Amendment June 2011). Oslo: Norwegian Ministry of Children, Equality and Social Inclusion.

Ministry of Education and Research (2005) Rammeplan for sykepleierutdanning (National curriculum regulations for nursing programmes) Oslo: Ministry of Education and Research.

——(2012) Melding til Stortinget nr 13 (2011–2012): Utdanning for velferd Samspill i praksis (Report to the Storting No 13 (2011–2012): Education for welfare Interaction in practice). Oslo: Norwegian Ministry of Education and Research.

Ministry of Health and Care Services (1999) Lov om pasient-og brukerrettigheter: Med endringer juni 2012 (The Patients' Rights Act: Amendments June 2012). Oslo: Norwegian Ministry of Health and Care Services.

——(2003) Forskrift om kvalitet i pleie-og omsorgstjenestene (Regulations of the quality of the health care service). Oslo: Norwegian Ministry of Health and Care Services.

——(2006) Stortingsmelding nr 25 (2005–2006): Mestring, muligheter og mening – Framtidas omsorgsutfordringer. (Report No 25 (2005–2006) to the Storting: Long term care – Future challenges: Care Plan 2015). Oslo: Norwegian Ministry of Health and Care Services.

——(2008) Fordeling av inntekter mellom regionale helseforetak (The distribution of income between regional health enterprises). NOU 2008:2. Oslo: Norwegian Ministry of Health and Care Services.

——(2009) St.meld. nr. 47 (2008–2009): Samhandlingsreformen, Rett behandling – på rett sted – til rett tid (Report No. 47 to the Storting (2008–2009): The Coordination Reform, Proper treatment – at the right place and right time). Oslo: Norwegian Ministry of Health and Care Services.

——(2011) Lov om kommunale helse-og omsorgstjenester m.m. (The Municipal Health and Care Service Act). Oslo: Norwegian Ministry of Health and Care Services.

Ministry of Justice (2012) Handlingsplan mot vold i nære relasjoner (Action plan domestic violence). Oslo: Norwegian Ministry of Justice.

Ministry of Justice and the Police (2003) Retten til et liv uten vold: Menns vold mot kvinner i nære relasjoner (The right to a life without violence: Men's violence against women in intimate relationships). NOU 2003:3. Oslo: Norwegian Ministry of Justice and the Police.

——(2004) Handlingsplan Vold i nære relasjoner (Action plan domestic violence) (2004–2007). Oslo: Norwegian Ministry of Justice and the Police.

——(2005) Lov om straff (Criminal code). Oslo: Norwegian Ministry of Justice and the Police.

——(2007) Handlingsplan mot vold i nære relasjoner 2008–2011: Vendepunkt (Action plan domestic violence 2008–2011: The turning point). Oslo: Norwegian Ministry of Justice and the Police.

——(2008) Vold i nære relasjoner: Veileder for utvikling av kommunale handlings-planer (Domestic violence: Guidelines for developing local action plans). Oslo: Norwegian Ministry of Justice and the Police.

——(2009) Regjeringens innsats mot vold i nære relasjoner (Government initiatives to combat domestic violence). Oslo: Norwegian Ministry of Justice and the Police.

——(2010a) Lov om vergemål (The Guardianship Act). Oslo: Norwegian Ministry of Justice and the Police.

——(2010b) Pressemelding nr 85–2010: I dag skjerpes straffene for vold og overgrep. (Press release No 85–2010: Intensifying penalties for violence and abuse). Oslo: Norwegian Ministry of Justice and the Police.

Nersund, R. and Govasmark, H. (2011) Rapportering fra krisesentrene 2010 (Report from domestic shelters 2010). Trondheim: Sentio Research Norge.

NKVTS (2008) Årsrapport 2007 (Annual report 2007). Oslo: Norwegian Centre for Violence and Traumatic Stress Studies.

——(2009) Årsrapport 2008 (Annual report 2008). Oslo: Norwegian Centre for Violence and Traumatic Stress Studies.

——(2010) Årsrapport 2009 (Annual report 2009). Oslo: Norwegian Centre for Violence and Traumatic Stress Studies.

Normann, T., Rønning, E. and Nørgaard, E. (2009) Utfordringer for den nordiske velferdsstaten: Sammenlignbare indikatorer (Challenges for the Nordic welfare state: Comparable indicators). Copenhagen: Nordisk Socialstatistisk Komité.

Norwegian Directorate of Health (2007) Overgrepsmottak Veileder for helsetjenesten (Abuse reception guidelines for the health services). Oslo: Norwegian Directorate of Health.

——(2008) Landsdekkende kontakttelefon for eldre som er utsatt for vold: Kunngjøring for tilskuddsordning (Nationwide contact phone for the elderly who are victims of violence: Announcing the grant scheme). Oslo: Norwegian Directorate of Health. Online. Available at <http://www.shdir.no> (accessed 31 July 2008).

Øverby, E. (2009) 'Internasjonale perspektiver på sosial politikk (International perspective on social policy)', in M. Stamsø (ed.) Velferdsstaten i endring: norsk sosialpolitikk ved starten av et nytt århundre (Changes of the welfare state: Norwegian social policy in the beginning of a new century), 2nd edn, Oslo: Gyldendal akademisk.

Penhale, B. (2006) 'Elder abuse in Europe: An overview of recent developments'. Journal of Elder Abuse and Neglect, 18: 107–16.

Protective Service for the Elderly (2010) Vern for eldre 2000–2009: Årsmelding 2009 (Protective service for the elderly 2000–2009: Annual report 2009). Oslo: Oslo kommune, Storbyavdelingen (the Municipality of Oslo).

——(2012) Årsmelding 2011: Vern for eldre (Protective Service for the Elderly: Annual report 2011). Oslo: Oslo kommune, Storbyavdelingen (the Municipality of Oslo).

Romøren, T.I. (2011) 'Samhandlingsreformen: Et kritisk blikk på en helsereform. (The coordination reform: A critical look at a health care reform)', Nordisk sykepleieforskning, 1: 82–8.

RVTS Sør (2009) Strategiplan 2009–2011 (Strategic plan 2009–2011). Kristiansand: RVTS (Regionalt ressurssenter om vold traumatisk stress og selvmordsforebygging) Sør, Sørlandet sykehus HF (RVTS (Regional Resource Centre on Violence, Traumatic Stress and Suicide Prevention) South). Online. Available at <http://www.rvts.no/sor> (accessed 21 Sept 2010).

RVTS Vest (2010) Årsrapport 2009 (Annual Report 2009). Bergen: RVTS (Regionalt ressurssenter om vold traumatisk stress og selvmordsforebygging) Vest, Klinikk for psykosomatisk medisin ved Psykiatrisk Divisjon i Helse Bergen HF.(RVTS (Regional Resource Centre on Violence, Traumatic Stress and Suicide Prevention) West). Online. Available at <http://vest.rvts.no/ > (accessed 21 Sept 2010).

Sandmoe, A. (2011) 'Older people at risk of being abused by someone close to them: A qualitative study of community care services in Norway and Australia' unpublished thesis, University of Oslo.

——and Kirkevold, M. (2011a) 'Identifying and handling abused, older clients in community care: The perspective of nurse managers', International Journal of Older People Nursing. Article first published online: 19 April 2011 (doi: 10.1111/j.1748–3743.2011.00279.x.) (Accessed 19 April 2011).

——(2011b) 'Nurses' clinical assessments of older clients who are suspected victims of abuse: An exploratory study in community care in Norway', Journal of Clinical Nursing, 20: 94–102.

——, Kirkevold, M. and Ballantyne, A. (2011) 'Challenges in handling elder abuse in community care: An exploratory study among nurses and care coordinators in Norway and Australia', Journal of Clinical Nursing, 20: 3351–63.

Saveman, B.-I., Hallberg, I. and Norberg, A. (1993) 'Identifying and defining abuse of elderly people, as seen by witnesses', Journal of Advanced Nursing, 18: 1393–400.

Sethi, D., Wood, S., Mitis, F., Bellis, M., Penhale, B., Marmoljo, I., Lowenstein, A., Manthorpe, G. and Kärki, F. (2011) European report on preventing elder maltreatment, Geneva: World Health Organization.

Skjørten, K. (2009) 'Partnervold blant eldre (Intimate partner abuse among elderly people)'. Tidsskrift for Psykisk Helsearbeid, 6: 120–27.

Sogn, H. (2007) Undervisning om vold ved universiteter og høgskoler (Education addressing violence at universities and university colleges). Oslo: Norwegian Centre for Violence and Traumatic Stress Studies.

Solhaug, A. (2007) 'Men det er vel egentlig ikke overgrep? En studie av eldre som er utsatt for overgrep i familien (But it is not really abuse? A study of elderly who are victims of abuse in the family)', unpublished minor thesis, Oslo: Det samfunnsvitenskapelige fakultet Universitetet i Oslo. University of Oslo.

Stamsø, M. (2009) Velferdsstaten i endring: Norsk sosialpolitikk ved starten av et nytt århundre (Changes of the welfare state: Norwegian social policy in the beginning of a new century), Oslo: Gyldendal Akademisk.

Stang, G. and Evensen, Å. R. (1985) 'Eldremishandling frem i lyset (Sheddding light on elder abuse)'. Tidsskrift for Den norske lægeforening, 105: 2475–8.

Statistics Norway (2011) Befolkning og areal i tettsteder (Population and land area in urban settlements). Oslo: Statistics Norway. Online. Available at <http://www.ssb.no/beftett/tab-2011-06-17-02.html> (accessed 5 March 2012).

——(2012) Statistical Yearbook of Norway 2011. Oslo: Statistics Norway. Online. Available at <http://www.ssb.no/english/yearbook/> (Accessed 20 February 2012).

WHO (2002) The Toronto declaration on the global prevention of elder abuse. Geneva: World Health Organization. Online. Available at <http://www.who.int> (Accessed 21 Sept 2010).

Wolf, R., Daichman, L. and Bennett, G. (2002) 'Abuse of the elderly', in E. Krug, L. Dahlberg, J. Mercy, A. Zwi and R. Lozano (eds) World report on violence and health. Geneva: World Health Organization.

10 Spain

Isabel Iborra, Yolanda García and Ester Grau

Introduction

There is general agreement among experts that levels of abuse and negligence will increase in the future due to specific demographic changes giving rise to an ageing population (caused by a decrease in infant mortality and an increase in life expectancy). During the mid-1990s in Spain the number of people over 65 reached 6 million, representing 15 per cent of the total population. By 2005, this per centage increased to almost 17 per cent (INE 2005). Changes in family size and structure, women's massive incorporation into the workforce and changes in social values have all contributed to a situation where fewer younger people are available to take care of their elderly relatives. Consequently, there has been an increase in the number of older people who live alone; in Spain this figure represents 16 per cent, although it is notably lower than in other western countries (UN 2002).

Definition

In Spain, there are three currently accepted definitions of what constitutes elder abuse. The first is the concept coined by Action on Elder Abuse (AEA 1995), which was ratified by the WHO in the Toronto Declaration (WHO 2002) and which defines elder abuse as 'a single, or repeated act, or lack of appropriate action, occurring within any relationship where there is an expectation of trust, which causes harm or distress to an older person'.

The second definition came out of the First National Conference on Elder Abuse, which then led to the Almeria Declaration (Kessel Sardiñas et al. 1996), stating that

> elder abuse means any act or omission suffered by a person of 65 or over which harms their physical, psychological, sexual and financial integrity, their autonomy or their individual basic rights; either subjectively or objectively evident, irrespective of intentionality or the setting in which it occurs (family, community or institution).

Thirdly, the Queen Sofía Centre defines elder abuse as

> any voluntary, i.e. non-accidental act, which harms or may harm an elderly person; or any omission that deprives an elderly person of the care they need for their well-being; as well as any violation of their rights. To be classified as elder abuse, such acts or omissions must take place within the framework of an interpersonal relationship in which one expects a certain trust, care, convivencia (positive coexistence) or dependency. The perpetrator may be a family member, a staff member from an institution (health sector or social services), a hired carer, a neighbour or a friend (Iborra 2008).

The age over which someone is considered to be elderly is 65 years.

In connection with the differing kinds of abuse, it is now commonly accepted that there are five categories of elder abuse (Iborra 2008, Bazo 2001, Pérez-Rojo et al. 2011, IMSERSO 2005, 2007, WHO 2011). This is the same typology traditionally used for child abuse (Sanmartín 2005) but with the obvious addition of financial abuse:

- Physical abuse: voluntary acts that cause or may cause physical harm or injury.
- Psychological abuse: acts (normally verbal) or attitudes that cause or may cause psychological harm.
- Neglect: failure to meet one's obligations in caring for a person.
- Financial abuse: the illegal or non-authorised use of a person's financial resources or property.
- Sexual abuse: any non-desired physical contact in which a person is used as a means to obtain sexual stimulation or gratification.

In addition to these categories some professionals include, for example, abandonment (where the person taking on the responsibility for an elderly person's welfare or having custody of an older person person physically abandons them) or the violation of basic rights (understood as depriving the older person of their basic legal rights in terms of their privacy, decision-making, religious opinion, etc.) (Pérez et al. 2011).

Policy and practice: response

Many diverse publications and projects, such as those devised by the WHO/ International Network for the Prevention of Elder Abuse (WHO/INPEA 2002), HelpAge International, the European Strategy to Combat Elder Abuse Against Older Women (EUSTaCEA) and Wellbeing and Dignity for Older People (WEDO) among others, are all evidence of the growing concern sparked by this problem both nationally and internationally.

In line with new European systems, Spain has developed a joint programme for the care of dependent adults with the collaboration of private and public organisations. The Spanish System for Personal Autonomy and

Care of Dependent Adults (SAAD) was developed in January 2007 after Law 39/2006 of 14 December for the promotion of personal autonomy and the care of dependent persons came into effect, and this has provoked an in-depth reform of the issues surrounding the protection of dependent adults.

Following on from this, the European Commission (2011) endorsed the Strategic Implementation Plan for the European Innovation Partnership on Active and Healthy Ageing. The final text adopted by the Steering Group structured the required work around three key areas: prevention, screening and early diagnosis; care and cure; and active ageing and independent living. By building on this model, and on the United Nations directives regarding prevention work, we have compiled the following list of actions for measures aimed at prevention and early diagnosis:

- Information and public-awareness measures for the general public.
- Educational programmes.
- Community and institutional policy programmes.

Information and public-awareness measures

- Information measures (Annex 1): These measures ensure information which is realistic and precise. Although information measures are necessary, they are however insufficient in creating a change in attitude (Moya Bernal and Barbero Gutiérrez 2005). These indirect measures are carried out by the Media (radio and television programme design, publicity campaigns, NGO support) as well as by schools (intergenerational education).
- Public-awareness programmes (Annex 2): There are diverse initiatives which aim to raise the general population's awareness of the existence of elder abuse and mistreatment, most notably:

  o   World Elder Abuse Awareness Day – an initiative created by the INPEA (International Network for the Prevention of Elder Abuse) and endorsed by the WHO;
  o   the campaign 'ponte en su piel' (put yourself in their shoes) (InfoElder), recognised by the INPEA;
  o   'maltrato a personas mayores' (elder abuse) from the Fisterra medical portal;
  o   Foundation Institute of Victimology (FIVE) – an independent, interdisciplinary organisation;
  o   the Alzheimer programme 'Juntos Podemos' (Together We Can) from the CEAFA (Spanish Confederation of Associations for Family Members of People with Alzheimer and other Dementias).

Educational programmes

The aim of educational programmes is to positively influence people's motivation, attitude and behaviour. They also include the creation of specific programmes to prevent and cope with the problem, and training programmes for professionals and informal carers.

Training for professionals

Spanish legislation highlights in diverse documents the need for training for professionals and carers (Article 36 in Law 39/2006 of 14 December and Royal Decree 1224/2009).

Some of the training programmes designed for professionals (see Annex 3a) are:

- 'Programa Desatar al anciano y al enfermo de Alzheimer' (Untie older people and patients with Alzheimer's), CEOMA: Spanish Confederation of Organisations for the Elderly;
- framework protocol for a coordinated approach to elder abuse. Government of Catalonia, Department of Social Action and Citizenship.

Non-professional carers – training, information and monitoring in the family setting

The dependency system cannot replace the informal care offered at home. Both types of care must reinforce and complement each other as they both involve a sharing of responsibility and risk control. The formal recognition of non-professional carers by the Social Security Agency is regulated by Royal Decree 615/2007, of 11 May.

State reference centres and other resources

Law 39/2006 (Article 16), includes State Reference Centres (SRC) in its 'Red de servicios del Sistema para la Autonomía y Atención a la Dependencia' (Network of system services for the autonomy and care of dependent persons). These centres are social service tools created by the Spanish Ministry of Health, Social Policy and Equality through the Institute of Social Services and the Elderly (Annex 3b):

- the Alzheimer SRC of Salamanca within the Institute for the Elderly and Social Services (IMSERSO).
- the SRC of Personal Autonomy and Technical Assistance (CEAPAT).
- the Queen Sofia Foundation Alzheimer Project.
- the Spanish Confederation of Relatives of Alzheimer Patients and Other Dementias (CEAFA): Memory Bank Project, Together We Can.
- the Grundtvig Lifelong Learning Programme.
- WISDEM: a global network of experts, carers, family members and people living with dementia.

- the Spanish Society of Geriatrics and Gerontology (SEGG), with funding from the Foundation BBK, has set up the 'Observatorio del Buen Trato a la Persona Mayor' (Observatory on the good treatment of the elderly).
- Foundation Pascual Maragall: ConemBeta Project, a research project of therapeutic advisory groups for carers of people with Alzheimer's; a project with the private Foundation ELISAVA University School.

Community-based programmes and institutional politics

These programmes combine resources from the public and private sector to deal with legal, healthcare and social issues:

- From a legal standpoint, the aim is to encourage the legal protection of the elderly and compliance with current regulations through things like the creation and mainstreaming of Adult Guardianship Agencies in certain Autonomous Communities in Spain. Adult Guardianship Agencies aim to respond to the legal, social and healthcare issues affecting older adults who are either disabled or in the process of applying for incapacity benefit and who are considered at risk at the time of being assessed by the legal authorities (Mas, 2004).
- In terms of healthcare the aim is to improve healthcare resources (home help services, providing more geriatric care posts, defining and developing abuse prevention protocols in health centres, social care centres, day centres and residential care homes, etc.). The 'Libro Blanco del Envejecimiento Activo' (White Paper on Active Ageing: IMSERSO 2010) has been compiled with this in mind and focuses on developing policies to improve older people's quality of life.
- The social aspect involves the creation and fostering of the necessary measures to enable caring for an older person in their own home, the coordination of social agencies to provide better cover, help-lines, the widespread installation of a teleassistance service, etc. Some relevant programmes are (Annex 4):

  o   'Cruz Roja Española: Social TV'. Cruz Roja (Red Cross);
  o   University Community Support Service (SACU) for the University of Seville in collaboration with the Regional Government of Andalusia;
  o   Programmes promoted by IMSERSO: 'Cerca de ti' (Near You) and 'Juntos en Navidad' (Together at Christmas).

Legal responses to elder abuse

This section provides an overview of existing legal resources for abuse in Spain, with an analysis of the specific legislation which may help address the problem dealt with in the next section.

One particularly innovative initiative is the recent 'Plan Mayor Seguridad' (elder security plan). Instruction 3/2010 from the Secretary of State for Security ratified the approval and launch of the Plan, which focuses on prevention and improving the security of older people in Spain. The law enforcement plan was drawn up by the Interior Ministry to improve the security of older people and remains in force until 31 December 2012. The aims of the Plan include preventing the financial or security abuse of the elderly, and developing information measures to highlight the potential risks for older people in residential care homes and day centres.

Other legal resources worth highlighting are (Annex 5):

- Living will (advance care directive): This document contains the instructions of an adult of sound mind regarding their future medical treatment and is activated should the person who signed it become incapable of expressing their intent. Each Autonomous Community regulates this in its legislation.
- The power of prevention: This document states in writing the provisions for how an individual's personal assets are to be managed if the person should suffer a future illness which impairs their decision-making ability.
- Self-guardianship: The self-guardianship document is signed with free will before a notary and names a guardian who will advocate for the elderly person's rights if at any time they are declared incapable. (Article 223 of the Civil Code, provided for by Law 41/2003 on asset protection for disabled people).
- Taking elderly people into care and mutual caring: It is essential that a care document is drawn up, overseen by a lawyer or notary, which outlines and regulates any action plan, and which provides security to a person entering the care system or a home care situation. The person receiving care lives in their own home with the carer or in the carer's home. It is a mutually beneficial home care situation.
- Dependent insurance and reverse mortgages: The regulation of dependent insurance and reverse mortgages is covered by Law 41/2007, of 7 December. A reverse mortgage functions differently to a normal mortgage in that the home owner receives a monthly sum from the lender until they die. The house is pledged as collateral and the owner continues to live there.
- Lifelong contract: This contract stipulates that a person promises to sell their property, but is allowed to live there until they die. They are paid an initial lump sum and then receive a monthly payment. When they die the house becomes the property of the co-signee of the lifelong contract.

Social care response to elder abuse

Social services departments need to develop joint actions which allow elderly people to remain in their own homes and maintain their family-based social environment whilst receiving professional care.

The National State Administration collaborates with Primary Care Social Services via the 'Plan Concertado de Prestaciones Básicas de Servicios Sociales' (partnership plan of basic social service benefits); care services for the elderly are included in specialised care services. These services are aimed at promoting active ageing (retirement homes and clubs, IMSERSO holiday programme, social thermalism, accessibility, home teleassistance, etc.) and at supporting family solidarity (help services and home care support, residential centres, day centres, etc.) (Libro Blanco del Envejecimiento Activo (White Paper on Active Ageing) : IMSERSO 2010).

Law 39/2006 stipulates the right of dependent adults and their families to access to help services. It establishes that care provision may be of a financial[1] or service[2] nature. It also includes the role provided by the Third Sector, with private, non-profit organisations from social or citizen initiatives which meet solidarity criteria whose aim is to defend social rights: volunteering and social cooperation, homes and clubs for older people, alternative housing services (assisted living facilities, family placement, shared housing, living units), etc. Some important examples are:

- The policy of subsidies for non-governmental social action organisations which provide personal attention programmes, family support programmes and housing adaptations, 24-hour cover and suitable residential places.
- The subsidies from IMSERSO given to NGOs dedicated to promoting and supporting the associative movement and to the social integration of older people. The I+D+I programme from IMSERSO stands out here; it is contained in the strategic health plan of the National Plan for Scientific Research, Development and Technological Innovation (2008–11).

Legislation

Spain does not yet have a specific law protecting older people from family abuse, as it does for children and women. However, it is referred to in the Criminal Code and in the Criminal Procedure Law.

Criminal code

There is no specific law in Spain that regulates elder abuse. Instead, it is covered by another criminal category referring to habitual violence between certain family members. In 1989 the crime of habitual family violence was created. At first it only applied to physical violence against a spouse or live-in partner, or against an antecedent or descendant, but in 1999 former spouses or live-in partners were then added as possible authors of the crime and it was widened to include psychological violence. In 2003, the Criminal Code was reformed and the crime of family violence, previously regulated in Article 153, was modified and is now found in Article 173, paragraph 2, which states:

Those who habitually exercise physical or psychological violence against someone who is or has been their spouse or against someone who is or has been linked to them by an analogous affective relationship, even without living together, or against descendants, ascendants ... or against someone forming part of the family unit in any other type of relationship ... as well as against people who because of their special vulnerability are under guardianship in public or private centres, will be punished with a prison sentence of between 6 months and 3 years

After the reform, it became obligatory for judges to impose restraining orders in cases of crimes occurring between people from the same family. This was very important because, prior to the reform, a restraining order could only be requested by one of the parties involved, i.e. the plaintiff, which prevented this measure from being applied or imposed if victims dropped the charges. Furthermore, the reform regulates what should be done with people under guardianship and in cases of institutional abuse (in both public and private centres). Other relevant Articles in the Criminal Code are those which typify the crime of abandonment of the family, minors or vulnerable persons (Articles 226 to 233) and those which typify the offense of bodily injuries (Articles 147 and 148).

Organic Law 1/2004 on Integrated Protection Measures against Gender Violence

Article 28 of Organic Law 1/2004 on Integrated Protection Measures against Gender Violence, covering access to public flats and residences for the elderly, establishes the following:

Women victims of gender-based violence will be considered a priority regarding access to protected housing and public residences for the elderly, under the terms of the applicable legislation.

Dependency law

Law 39/2006, of 14 December, for the Promotion of Personal Autonomy and Assistance to Persons in Situations of Dependence (Dependency Law), which came into effect on 1 January 2007, sets the groundwork for financing the services needed by dependent elderly people for their daily living activities (getting up, eating, bathing, etc.).

The Law is founded on: the universal and public nature of the services; and equal access to services. Situations of dependence are classified as follows:

- Grade I. Moderate dependence: When a person needs help at least once a day to carry out certain daily living activities.

- Grade II. Heavy dependence: When a person needs help two to three times a day to carry out certain daily living activities, but does not need the permanent presence of a carer.
- Grade III. Total dependence: When a person needs help several times a day to carry out certain daily living activities and due to their total loss of mental or physical autonomy also requires the continuous and indispensable support of another person.

The most important basic services established by this law are telephone help-lines, home-care services, household services, personal care, 24-hour centres, residential homes for the elderly and financial help.

Criminal procedure law

Finally, Article 263 in the Criminal Procedure Law underlines the responsibility of professionals who know of any case of abuse to report it to the authorities:

> Those, who by reason of their position, profession or line of work, learn about a public crime, are obliged to report it immediately to the Public Prosecutor, the competent Court, the investigating Judge or failing this, the municipal government or the nearest police officer, if and when it is a case of in flagrante delicto.

Civil procedure law

Article 762 is of particular interest in relation to the measures necessary to adequately protect the vulnerable person and their property (Perianes Lozano and Alia Ramos 2009). In Article 763, it establishes institutionalisation through involuntary commitment for mental disorders and in Article 247 the obligations of exercising guardianship are regulated. Once the incapacity assessment process is completed, the law establishes a series of fiscal measures under the control of the public prosecutor and the judiciary to ensure and monitor the proper protection of the person and their property.

Civil code

Articles 216 and 158 of the Civil Code (similarly to Article 727 in the Civil Procedure Law) establish a protection system of pertinent measures (preventive annotation on legal proceedings, naming of provisional administrator or guardian, naming of guardian ad litem, blocking of bank accounts, etc.). Additionally, it is important to refer to the right to sustenance as this recognises the right of any individual person in a state of necessity to claim from certain relatives what is considered essential for a dignified life. From a legal standpoint, sustenance is understood to mean not only food, but rather everything which is crucial for their subsistence, housing, clothing and medical attention.

This basic right is recognised and well accepted in cases of descending generations (parents to children or grandparents to grandchildren), but it is much more difficult to accept in respect of older generations. However, this is no reason to avoid demanding these basic rights if deemed necessary. This Civil Code right directly corresponds to Article 226 in the Criminal Code. It is included in the crimes against family rights and duties and it may incur the imposition of a part-time prison sentence of 8–20 weekends and the obvious obligation to provide all assistance, including financial assistance, which is constitutive of the essence and contents of this right.

Law 35/1995 for aid and support for victims of violent crime and crimes against sexual freedom

This law sets out a system of public aid to directly or indirectly benefit victims of intentional violent crimes which have resulted in death or serious bodily harm, or serious damage to health.

Research

Before examining the research into the incidence and prevalence of elder abuse, it is worth describing some of the findings of the research carried out by the Spanish Society of Geriatrics and Gerontology on elder abuse in Spain (IMSERSO, 2004). Among the interesting conclusions of the study, the report highlighted the following perceptions of older people themselves towards the concept of elder abuse:

- Older people seem to reserve the term 'abuse' for extreme cases of human rights violations, stereotypically those cases which reach the press. They do accept that events such as beatings, over-administration of sedatives or negligence when providing nourishment may occur in the family setting, but in their opinion this is only conceivable in settings which are clearly dysfunctional.
- There are two issues from the older generation's perspective which could explain this 'abuse' of an elderly person:

  o the stigmatisation of the social representation of the elderly by the young, with the elderly being passive, unproductive subjects, so therefore socially redundant and preconceived as a medium/short term responsibility. Older people perceive that their point of view is considered, almost by definition, as obsolete and scarcely relevant to the young;
  o the adverse global context which affects the functioning of traditional mechanisms to manage the needs of a dependent older person (based at home) without the creation of new, socially responsible systems to deal with the situation. This makes the possibility of an older person's

dignity and well-being dependent on the financial capacity and/or personal sacrifice of each individual (especially women) within their environment, turning into exceptional that which should be considered the norm.

- Older people consider that, while abuse is inconceivable in conventional settings, 'mistreatment' is more common than it appears, but its subtle and insidious nature makes it imperceptible to those who are not suffering it and difficult to disclose for those who are.
- The agencies identified by older people as being competent to detect and remedy situations of 'mistreatment' in the community are principally social services, which are backed up by the legal authority to intervene and the resources (although considered insufficient by older people) to deal with it. Health services are attributed an important role in terms of detection.
- Finally, older people identified six aspects of an elderly person's quality of life which are crucial to them and which act as areas of vulnerability where mistreatment might flourish: financial independence, social value, the community, the affective sphere (intimate partner and family), carer function and security.

We will now consider two national Spanish studies together with localised studies, preceded by a European study.

European study

Before analysing the situation in Spain it is worth noting the existence of a recent research study into abuse and health among the elderly in Europe (Soares et al. 2010). The study's investigation included the prevalence of elder abuse in seven countries (Germany, Greece, Italy, Lithuania, Portugal, Spain and Sweden). The results highlight the following across countries:

- Some 19.4 per cent of the elderly (60–84 years) were exposed to psychological abuse, 2.7 per cent to physical abuse, 0.7 per cent to sexual abuse and 3.8 per cent to financial abuse.
- Financial abuse occurred more often in Portugal (7.8 per cent) and Spain (4.8 per cent), psychological abuse occurred more often in Sweden and Germany, physical abuse in Sweden and Lithuania, and sexual abuse in Greece and Portugal.
- The pattern of abuse differed between countries. In contrast to Germany, the elderly in Greece, Italy, Portugal and Spain were at a lower risk of psychological abuse.

As for research on the incidence and prevalence of elder abuse, the main results of the most important studies carried out at the national and regional levels in Spain are now outlined.

National study of elder abuse in the family

There has been only one study on the incidence of elder abuse in the family in Spain at the national level (Iborra 2008).

Study sample

Two different groups were analysed at the national level:

- people over 64 years of age, of both sexes, living in private homes (2,401 interviews).
- carers of older people (789 interviews).

Method

First, a number of homes were randomly selected in the sampling points, stratified by size of locality and Nielsen area, to obtain a random representative sample. Second, subjects (older people and carers) were chosen within the homes in such a way as to obtain a final sample that was representative of age and sex. The questionnaires were administered in-person and at home.

Instruments

The Queen Sofia Centre designed two questionnaires, one for older people and the other for carers.[3] This permitted gathering information from the two different perceptions of this problem.

Results

Some 0.8 per cent of older people seemed to be victims of abuse in the family in Spain. This percentage is twice as high among dependent elders and four times as high among dependent elders with total disability (those requiring assistance at least five hours a day); 4.5 per cent of carers acknowledged having abused the elderly person in their care. As for the different types of abuse, psychological abuse has the highest prevalence, according to both victims and carer (see Figure 10.1).

National study of murder of elders by their relatives

Another national study looks specifically at the murder of elderly people at the hands of their own relatives in Spain (Iborra et al. 2011). The study followed these cases during the years 2000 to 2007 and it found that during this period 164 older people were killed by family members, making an average of 21 per year. In terms of gender, the average was 14 women a year (14.28) and 6 men a year (6.29). Table 10.1 outlines the incidence in terms of year and gender.

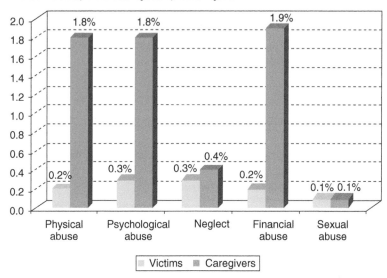

Figure 10.1 Prevalence of different types of abuse according to information source

Table 10.1 Incidence of older people killed by relatives

	2000	2001	2002	2003	2004	2005	2006	2007	*Variation 00–07*
Women	6	13	13	16	–	15	20	17	183.33 percent
Men	7	8	9	7	–	4	4	5	–28.57 percent
Total	13	21	22	23	20	19	24	22	69.23 percent

Source: Iborra, López and Sanmartín 2011

Basque Country

Sample

A total of 1,207 people aged 60 and over living in the family home and resident in the autonomous community of the Basque Country.

Method

Personal interview in the home by a trained analyst using a structured questionnaire. The information was gathered during May 2010.

Instruments

The Phototest (Carnero and Montoro 2004) was used to identify people with cognitive decline and to ascertain whether the older person was competent enough to complete the questionnaire by themselves. For suspicions of abuse, questions relating to mistreatment were used from the Elder Abuse Suspicion Index (EASI) questionnaire. Several questionnaires were used for risk factors associated with elder abuse: the Centre of Epidemiological Studies Depression Scale (CES-D8), the Goldberg Anxiety Scale, the CASP-19 quality-of-life measure, the Burden Interview and the Caregiver Abuse Screen.

Results

Some 0.9 per cent of the interviewed people aged 60 and over declared having been abused in some way. The interviewers identified suspicion of abuse in 1.5 per cent of cases, which in all instances was undeclared by the interviewee. That is to say, these cases are additional to those contained in the 0.9 per cent. The most frequent types of abuse perceived by the elderly are: psychological (0.5 per cent), negligence (0.2 per cent) and physical or sexual abuse (0.2 per cent). Some 25 per cent of victims declared having suffered more than one type of abuse (Pérez-Rojo et al. 2011).

Barcelona

Sample

A total of 219 people aged 70 years or over who were primary health care users from the Les Planes de Sant Joan Despí ABS.[4] Patients with cognitive disorders were excluded.

Method

Information was gathered at the health centre or at the patient's home using an interview and a questionnaire. Four previously trained physicians interviewed patients and administered the questionnaire.

Instruments

The questionnaire assessed the various socio-demographic variables, such as age, sex, marital status, educational level, profession, live-in situation, existence of a carer, social support.

A questionnaire of the Canadian Task Force and the American Medical Association was also used for the different types of abuse. It contains 9 questions (1 on physical abuse, 3 on psychological abuse, 1 on neglect and 1 on abandonment). One positive answer was considered an indication of possible abuse (suspected abuse).

Results

The prevalence of suspected abuse was 11.9 per cent (26 elderly people). The types of abuse were: psychological (20), physical (6), neglect (6, 3 of which were cases of abandonment) and sexual abuse (1). Nine individuals presented with more than one type of abuse (Ruiz Sanmartín et al. 2001).

Basque Country, Andalusia and Canary Islands

Sample

Home-care workers providing service to 2,351 dependent older people.

Method

The study was conducted in 5 metropolitan areas: Vitoria, Seville, Las Palmas, Telde and San Bartolomé de Tirajana. A questionnaire was administered to the Social Services home carers in the participating metropolitan areas. They all received an explanation of what the research study considered to be neglect and abuse.

Results

A total of 111 cases of abuse were detected, with a 4.7 per cent prevalence rate. Some 81 per cent of victims were women. The main type of abuse detected was neglect. The perpetrators in descending order were children and children-in-law (55 per cent), spouses (12 per cent) and siblings (7 per cent) (Bazo 2001).

Other investigations into suspicion of abuse

There have been an additional series of studies in Spain on the prevalence of the suspicion of abuse in the elderly population (Risco et al. 2005, Pérez-Cárceles et al. 2009, Pérez-Rojo et al. 2008 and Garre-Olmo et al. 2009) among others, which showed abuse suspicion rates of between 2.1 per cent and 52.6 per cent, depending on where the sample was taken, the instrument used and the person interviewed, etc.

Conclusion

Elder abuse is the latest 'discovery' in the phenomenon of domestic violence and as such is not backed up by a corresponding body of scientific evidence as is the case with children and women (Bazo 2004, Bennet et al. 1997). This is also the case regarding social awareness of the problem. What is true is that society has recently become more aware of the impact of elder abuse. There has been growing media reporting in recent years condemning the situation suffered by some older people in certain residential homes, as a consequence of the existence of illegal institutions which do not comply with current regulations and which do not provide adequate care for their elderly residents. Although many experts coincide in affirming that elder abuse is much more common in the family than in institutions, the former is still considered 'the great unknown', at least in Spain. This lack of social awareness, along with the invisibility of the phenomenon in the media, has contributed to the absence of legislation and specific support resources for this group even though other groups with similar rates of violence do have these resources.

It is therefore necessary to work on the three action areas of prevention of elder abuse. At the primary prevention level it is vital to increase visibility of the phenomenon and raise social awareness of the problem. At the secondary prevention level protocols are needed for detection and action applied to different areas (health, social, etc.) and their standard use needs to be promoted (as occurs in other instances of domestic violence). Finally, at the tertiary prevention level, it is essential to mobilise intervention support resources, both for the victims (aiming at reducing the negative consequences of abuse and preventing revictimisation) and for the aggressors (aiming at avoiding recidivism). The intervention itself will also need to pay special attention to maintaining the balance between the respect for the victim's autonomy and their protection in situations of risk.

Notes

1 In this case, financial aid is to cover the costs incurred through caring for a dependent person in the family setting, support for non-professional carers and personal assistance.
2 Specifically teleassistance, home help, day centre or residential attention.
3 To download the questionnaire, in either English or Spanish, go to: http://www.centroreinasofia.es/informes/Maltrato_Elder.pdf
4 ABS is the Área básica de salud, the primary health care area.

References

AEA (1995) Definition of elder abuse, Action on Elder Abuse Bulletin, No. 11, May–June 1995. Published by AEA, Astral House, 1268 London Rd, London SW16 4ER.

Bazo, M.T. (2001) 'Negligencia y malos tratos a las personas ancianas en España', Revista Española de Geriatría y Gerontología, 36, 1: 8–14.

——(2004) 'Perfil de la persona mayor víctima de violencia', in J. Sanmartín (ed.) El laberinto de la violencia. Barcelona: Ariel, Estudios sobre Violencia Series.

Bennet, G., Kingston, P. and Penhale, B. (1997) The dimensions of elder abuse: Perspectives for practitioners. London: MacMillan Press.

Carnero, C. and Montoro, M. (2004) 'El test de las fotos', Revista de Neurología, 39: 801–6.

European Commission (2011) 'Strategic implementation plan for the European innovation partnership on active and healthy ageing steering group working document'. Online. Available at <http://ec.europa.eu/research/innovation-union/pdf/active-healthy-ageing/steering-group/implementation_plan.pdf#view=fitandpagemode=none> (accessed 10 October 2011).

Garre-Olmo, J., Plana-Pujol, X., López-Pousa, S., Juvinya, D., Vila, A. and Vilalta-Franch, J. (2009) 'Prevalence and risk factors of suspected elder abuse subtypes in people aged 75 and older', Journal of American Geriatrics Society, 57: 815–22.

Iborra, I. (2003) 'La protección del mayor. Violencia y maltrato físico y psíquico a los mayores', in J. Soldevilla and M. Nicolás (eds) El envejecimiento del envejecimiento. Madrid: X Congreso Nacional de la SEEGG and I Congreso de la AMEG.

——(2005) Violencia contra personas mayores. Barcelona: Ariel, Estudios sobre Violencia Series, n. 11.

——(2006) 'Maltrato de personas mayores', Diario de campo, 40 (Nov./Dec.): 53–60.

——(2008) Maltrato de personas mayores en la familia en España. Valencia: Queen Sofía Center, Documentos Series n. 13. Online. Available at <http://www.centroreina sofia.es/informes/Maltrato_Elder.pdf> (accessed 12 January 2009).

——(2009) 'Factores de riesgo del maltrato de personas mayores en la familia en población española', Zerbitzuan, 45: 49–57.

——(2010a) 'Maltrato de personas mayores en la familia', in J. Sanmartín, R. Gutiérrez, J. Martínez and J. Vera (eds), Reflexiones sobre la violencia. Mexico City: Siglo XXI.

——(2010b) 'Introducción al maltrato de personas mayores', in M. Javato (ed.) Violencia, abuso y maltrato de personas mayores: Perspectiva jurídico-penal. Valencia: Tirant lo Blanch.

——, López, M.J. and Sanmartín, J. (2011) Ancianos asesinados por familiares en España (2005–2007). Saarbrücken: Editorial Académica Española.

IMSERSO (2004) Vejez, negligencia, abuso y maltrato : La perspectiva de los mayores y de los profesionales. Madrid: IMSERSO.

——(2005) Malos tratos a personas mayores: Guía de actuación. Madrid: Observatorio de Personas Mayores, Colección Manuales y Guías. Personas Mayores Series.

——(2007) 'Maltrato hacia personas mayores en el ámbito comunitario'. Boletín sobre el envejecimiento: Perfiles y tendencias, 31.

——(2010) Libro blanco del envejecimiento activo. Madrid: Ministerio de Sanidad y Política Social. Online. Available at <http://www.csd.gob.es/csd/estaticos/planintegral/ Resumen_extracto_LIBRO_BLANCO_envej_activo_20101014.pdf> (accessed 15 October 2011).

INE (2005) National Statistics Institute website. Available at http://www.ine.es/jaxi/ tabla.do.

Kessel Sardiñas, H., Maturana Navarrete, N. and Marín, N. (1996) 'Almeria Declaration about elder abuse', Revista Española de Geriatría y Gerontología 31: 367–72. Available at <http://www.imsersomayores.csic.es/documentacion/biblioteca/registro. htm?id=50814> (accessed 13 November 2012).

Mas, J. (2004) 'El ejercicio de la tutela por parte de las Instituciones la sumisión al tratamiento ambulatorio y curatela sanitaria', Psicopatología Clínica, Legal y Forense, 4: 81–9.

Moya Bernal, A. and Barbero Gutiérrez, J. (eds) (2005) Malos tratos a personas mayores: Guía de actuación. Madrid: Ministerio de Trabajo y Asuntos Sociales, IMSERSO. Online. Available at <http://www.imsersomayores.csic.es/documentos/ documentos/imserso-malostratos-01.pdf> (accessed 13 July 2011).

Pérez-Cárceles, M.D., Rubio, L., Pereñiguez, J.E., Pérez Flores, D., Osuna, E. and Luna, A. (2009) 'Suspicion of elder abuse in south eastern Spain: The extent and risk factors', Archives of Gerontology and Geriatrics, 49: 132–7.

Pérez-Rojo, G., Izal, M., Montoro, I. and Penhale, B. (2008) 'Risk factors of elder abuse in a community dwelling Spanish sample', Archives of Gerontology and Geriatrics, 17–21.

Pérez-Rojo, G., Sancho, M., del Barrio, E. and Yanguas, J.J. (2011) 'Estudio de pre-valencia de malos tratos a personas mayores en la Comunidad Autónoma del País Vasco'. Donostia-San Sebastián: Servicio Central de Publicaciones del Gobierno Vasco. Online. Available at <http://www.gizartelan.ejgv.euskadi.net/r45contss/es/contenidos/informacion/publicaciones_ss/es_publica/adjuntos/ESTUDIO%20DE%20PREVALENCIA_CAST.pdf> (accessed 21 November 2011).

Perianes Lozano, A. and Alia Ramos, M.J. (2009) Medidas jurídicas de prevención y protección: Personas mayores vulnerables: maltrato y abuso. Madrid: Consejo General del Poder Judicial.

Risco, C., Paniagua, M.C., Jiménez, G., Poblador, M.D., Molina, L. and Buitrago, F. (2005) 'Prevalencia y factores de riesgo de sospecha de malos tratos en la población anciana', Medicina clínica 125(2), 51–5.

Ruiz Sanmartín, A., Altet Torner, J. and Porta Martí, N. (2001) 'Violencia doméstica: Prevalencia de sospecha de maltrato en ancianos', Atención Primaria, 27, 331–4.

Sanmartín, J. (2005) 'Concepto, tipos e incidencia', in J. Sanmartín (ed.) Violencia contra niños (3rd edn). Barcelona: Ariel, Estudios sobre violencia Series.

Soares, J.F., Barros, H., Torres-Gonzalez, F., Iannidi-Kapolou, H., Lamura, G., Lindert, J., de Dios Luna, J., Macassa, G., Melchiorre, M.-G. and Stankunas, M. (2010) Abuse and health in Europe. Kaunas: Lithuanian University of Health Sciences Press.

UN (2002) Report of the second world assembly on ageing. Madrid: United Nations. Online. Available at <http://www.c-fam.org/docLib/20080625_Madrid_Ageing_Conference.pdf> (accessed 15 August 2011).

WHO (2002) Declaración de Toronto para la prevención global del maltrato de las personas mayores. Online. Available at <http://www.who.int/ageing/projects/elder_abuse/alc_toronto_declaration_es.pdf> (accessed 15 August 2011).

——(2011) European report on preventing elder maltreatment. Denmark: World Health Organization. Report edited by Sethi, Wood, Mitis, Bellis, Penhale, Iborra, Lowenstein, Manthorpe and Ulvestad.

WHO/INPEA (2002) Missing voices: Views of older persons on elder abuse. Geneva: World Health Organization.

Annexes Resource Guide

Information and public-awareness measures

Annex 1: Information Measures

- 'Portal Mayores' (portal specialising in gerontology and geriatrics): <http://www.imsersomayores.csic.es/>
- Programme for care in the home volunteering, 'Instituto Provincial de Bienestar Social de Córdoba' (social welfare organisation in Cordoba): <http://www.ipbscordoba.es/paea/vouluntariado-y-personas-que-viven-solas-en-atenciones-domiciliarias>
- Intergenerational Program for Community Development. Active ageing (IMSERSO): <http://pedagogia.fcep.urv.cat/revistaut/revistes/desembre07/article07.pdf>
- 'Proyectogeneraciones@conectadas' (project connecting generations) (Fundació Viure i Conviure): <http://www.reyardid.org/proyectos_detalle.php?id=10>
- 'Programa Persones grans, grans persones' (Older people, Great People Programme), Catalonian Government, Ministry of Social Welfare and Family:

<http://www.imsersomayores.csic.es/recursos/programas/registro.htm?iPos=18&id= 302&irPag=1&clave=er8mO5fb4O&pos= 0>

Annex 2: Public awareness-raising campaigns

- World Elder Abuse Awareness Day (INPEA): http://www.imsersomayores.csic.es/ documentos/documentos/inpea-community-01.pdf
- The campaign 'ponte en su piel' (put yourself in their shoes), InfoElder: <http:// ponteensupiel.infoelder.com>
- Fisterra 'Maltrato a personas mayores' (elder abuse): <http://www.fisterra.com/ formacion/bioetica/anciano.asp>
- Fundación Instituto de Victimología (FIVE) (Institute of Victimology): <http:// www.fundacionfive.com>
- Programa Alzheimer 'Juntos Podemos' ('Together We Can') by the CEAFA: Spanish Confederation of associations of relatives of people with Alzheimer's: <http://www.ceafa.es/ceafa>

Educational programmes

Annex 3 (a): Training programmes designed for professionals

- Programa Desatar al anciano y al enfermo de Alzheimer. (Untie older people and patients with Alzheimer's) by CEOMA: Spanish confederation of organisations for the elderly: <http://www.imsersomayores.csic.es/documentos/documentos/ceoma-memoriadesatar-01.pdf
- Framework protocol for a coordinated approach to elder abuse. Catalonian Government, Dept. of Social Action and Citizenship: <http://www.imsersomayores. csic.es/documentos/documentos/catalunya-protocol-01.pdf

Annex 3 (b) State reference centres and other resources

- State Reference Centres (SRC): <http://imserso.es/imserso_01/centros/cre/index.htm>
- The SRC for Alzheimer in Salamanca (IMSERSO); The SRC for Personal Autonomy and Technical Aids (CEAPAT); The Alzheimer Project at the Queen Sofia Foundation. <http://www.fundacionreinasofia.es/proyectoalzheimer/visita-nueva/proyecto-ides-idweb.html>
- Spanish Confederation of Relatives of Alzheimer Patients and Other Dementias (CEAFA): Memory Bank Project. 'Together We Can': <http://www.ceafa.es/ceafa>
- Grundtvig Lifelong Learning Programme: <http://www.oapee.es/oapee/inicio/pap/ grundtvig.html>
- Wisdem: <http://www.wisdem.org/>
- Spanish Society of Geriatrics and Gerontology (SEGG)-Fundación BBK: 'Observatorio del Buen Trato a la Persona Mayor' (Observatory on the good treatment of the elderly): <http://www.segg.es/noticia/la/segg/crea/observatorio/del/buen/trato/ persona/mayor>
- Pascual Maragall Foundation: 'ConemBeta' project – research project by therapeutic groups supporting carers of Alzheimer patients, joint project with the private Foundation Elisava University School: <http://www.fpmaragall.org/es_index.html>

Community-based programmes and institutional politics

Annex 4: Community-based programmes and institutional policies

- Cruz Roja Española: Social TV. Red Cross: <http://www.cruzroja.es/portal/page?_pageid=619,12289367and_dad=portal30and_schema=PORTAL30andP_Codigo=10482>
- Programme offering university students free housing with the disabled, older people and parents with dependent children: <http://www.sacu.us.es/es/07_04.asp>
- Programme 'Cerca de ti' ('Near You') (IMSERSO): <http://www.imserso.es/imserso_01/envejecimiento_activo/cercadeti/index.htm>
- Programe 'Juntos en Navidad' ('Together at Christmas') (IMSERSO) <http://portalmayores.csic.es/recursos/programas/registro.htm?id=1306>

Legislation

Annex 5: Relevant Spanish legislation

- Law 35/1995, of 11 December, on aid and support for victims of violent crime and crimes against sexual freedom (BOE 12 December 1995): <http://www.boe.es/aeboe/consultas/bases_datos/doc.php?id=BOE-A-1995-26714>
- Organic Law 14/1999, of 9 June, amendement of the Criminal Code of 1995, on the protection of victims of abuse and the Criminal Procedure Law (BOE 10 June 1999): <http://www.boe.es/boe/dias/1999/06/10/pdfs/A22251-53.pdf>
- Law 41/2003, of 18 November, on protecting the assets of disabled people, amendement of the Civil Code, the Civil Procedure Law and the relevant tax legislation (BOE 19 November 2003): <http://www.boe.es/boe/dias/2003/11/19/pdfs/A40852–63.pdf>
- Organic Law 1/2004, of 28 December, on integrated protection measures against gender violence (BOE 29 December 2004): <http://www.boe.es/boe/dias/2004/12/29/pdfs/A42166–97.pdf>
- Law 39/2006, of 14 December, on promoting the personal autonomy and care of dependent adults (BOE 15 December 2006): <http://www.boe.es/boe/dias/2006/12/15/pdfs/A44142–56.pdf>
- Organic Law 3/2007, of 22 March, on effective equality for men and women (BOE 23 March 2007): <http://www.boe.es/boe/dias/2007/03/23/pdfs/A12611–45.pdf>
- Law 41/2007, of 7 December, which amends Law 2/1981, of 25 March (Mortgage Act), other regulations of the mortgage and finance systems, the regulation of reverse mortgages and care insurance, and certain tax legislation (BOE 8 December 2007): <http://www.boe.es/boe/dias/2007/12/08/pdfs/A50593–50614.pdf>

11 United Kingdom

Bridget Penhale

Introduction

In recent years there has been an increasing emphasis within many societies on dealing with situations of violence and abuse. In the United Kingdom, following an initial focus on child abuse in the 1970s and domestic violence in the 1980s, the abuse and neglect of older people began to elicit concern during the 1990s. The predominant focus was on abuse and neglect of elders in the domestic setting although increasingly there has been a move towards consideration of abuse and neglect occurring within institutional settings (Glendenning and Kingston 1999, Stanley et al. 1999). This chapter will discuss abuse and neglect occurring in the UK. It aims to provide a brief overview of current knowledge concerning elder abuse followed by a discussion of some of the issues relating to the prevention of abuse and neglect from a UK perspective.

Elder abuse and neglect are not new phenomena (Stearns 1986) and literary and historical documents exist to confirm this. Nevertheless, it is effectively only since 1988 that the problem has really begun to be identified and examined within a UK context. Although the phenomena were initially recognised by English doctors in the mid-1970s, it was not until the late 1980s that the issue was really taken seriously within the different countries that comprise the UK and this was at different points in time. The focus that developed in England was largely due to a national conference in London in 1988 organised by the British Geriatrics Society (a group of physicians concerned with older people).

The amount of research and material published about the subject in the UK has been increasing quite steadily. However, in many ways, it is still comparatively early in the identification of the problem and the development of responses to it. For example, it was not until 1993 that there was any clear sign from the UK government that elder abuse was perceived as a problem in need of attention (DoH 1993), although there has been a consistent, if rather slow approach from successive governments since that time (DoH 1999, DoH 2000, WAG 2000). The abuse of older people in institutions is an area where there has been even less research and attention paid. While there has been a long history across the UK of scandals in institutional care, these tend to have been investigated and treated as separate inquiries into standards and quality of care rather than as concerns relating to abuse and abusive situations.

Undoubtedly elder abuse and neglect are complex and sensitive areas to explore. This was also the case with child abuse and domestic violence against younger women. There have been difficulties as well in establishing a sound theoretical base. This is partly due to the lack of agreement concerning definitions, but also due to problems in researching the topic (Ogg and Munn-Giddings 1993, Penhale 1999). Since the 1990s, however, issues concerning violence towards older people in the UK have been raised on a consistent basis and the taboo associated with elder abuse has been challenged and has gradually diminished, although in relation to some areas, such as sexual abuse, the taboo is still evident within society, which mirrors an initial reluctance to discuss and consider child sexual abuse when this was discovered as an issue in the 1980s.

Differing forms of abuse

Although there is an absence of agreed or standard definitions of abuse, commented on by McCreadie (1996) and others, a number of definitions of elder abuse have emerged. Early attempts at defining abuse in the UK context were relatively specific as seen, for example, in the following: 'A single or repeated act or lack of appropriate action occurring within any relationship where there is an expectation of trust, which causes harm or distress to an older person' (Action on Elder Abuse 1995).

This definition was later adopted by the International Network for the Prevention of Elder Abuse (INPEA) and the World Health Organization (WHO). However, subsequent definitions used in the UK tend to have been more widely drawn, as seen in the English government document, No Secrets, concerning the abuse of vulnerable adults, in which the following definition is given: 'Abuse is a violation of an individual's civil or human rights by any other person or persons' (DoH 2000: 9).

Given the lack of consensus concerning definition, which may not lead to any major difficulty as long as key stakeholders are aware of and recognise that differing definitions exist (Penhale 1993), it is at least reassuring to find that most people concerned with the issue agree on the different types of abuse that can occur. The usual types of abuse included within most definitions are physical abuse, sexual abuse, neglect, financial abuse (including exploitation and misappropriation of an individual's property and possessions), psychological abuse and emotional abuse. In England and Wales, the category of discriminatory abuse was added in the policy guidance that was issued (DoH 2000, WAG 2000). Institutional abuse is also usually included within policy documents produced at the local level, and considerations of societal level abuse may also appear in such documents.

When considering neglect, separate stand-alone definitions do not usually appear, and neglect is often considered almost as a sub-type of abuse. Thus, in an early Department of Health document the definition of elder abuse is described as 'physical, sexual, psychological or financial. It may be intentional or unintentional or the result of neglect' (DoH 1993: para. 2.1). More recently, draft guidance issued by the Social Services Inspectorate indicated that abuse might occur 'as a result of a failure to undertake action or appropriate care tasks. It may be physical, psychological, or an act of neglect' (DoH 1999: para. 2.7). Neglect and acts of omission are then further described as: 'including ignoring medical or physical care needs, failure to provide access to appropriate health, social care or educational services, the withholding of the necessities of life, such as medication, adequate nutrition and heating' (DoH 1999: para. 2.8).

To these may be added such categories as enforced isolation and deprivation of other necessary items for daily living (warmth, food or other aspects, such as teeth). However, in general, situations of self-neglect by an older person would not be considered within the UK perspective on elder abuse. Although many health and social care practitioners work with older individuals who self-neglect, usually this is not considered within an elder abuse or indeed an adult protection or safeguarding framework, but rather as part of health and social care practice.

There are a number of different types of setting and institutions in which abuse and/or neglect may take place. These are: nursing or residential care homes, day care settings of all types and hospital settings. Abusive or neglectful situations may happen in any of these places. Practitioners therefore need to be aware of this possibility when visiting service users or patients in such locations as these. As guidance from the UK government states:

> Abuse can take place in any context. It may occur when a vulnerable adult lives alone or with a relative, it may also occur within nursing, residential or day care settings, in hospitals, custodial situations, support services into people's own homes, and other places previously assumed safe, or in public places.
>
> (DoH 2000: para. 2.14)

Abuse within institutions also covers situations that arise because of the regime or system that may operate in the unit as well as individual acts of abuse that occur in such settings. It is also possible to find abusive situations that occur between a resident and a member of the care staff, but instigated by the older person as protagonist, so there may be dual directionality of abuse, or even uni-directional abuse from resident towards staff member (McCreadie 1996).

As well as different types of abuse and different settings in which abuse and neglect can happen, individuals need to be aware that there can be a range of different participants involved in abusive situations and within different locations, depending on the setting. This includes residents, staff, relatives, friends, neighbours or volunteers. It is also necessary to acknowledge that a change of setting (from home to institution, perhaps) does not necessarily mean that any pre-existing abuse will necessarily cease. A different type of abuse might then occur or the nature of the abuse could be transformed somewhat between the individuals involved. As indicated in the UK government guidance: 'Assessment of the environment, or context, is relevant, because exploitation, deception, misuse of authority, intimidation or coercion may render a vulnerable adult incapable of making his or her own decisions' (DoH 2000, para. 2.16).

Different responses and interventions to alleviate or prevent institutional abuse and neglect (rather than abuse and neglect in the domestic setting) may be necessary, depending on the type of abuse that is happening within the institutional setting and the numbers of individuals involved. The location of the abuse, for example, whether the situation is occurring in a private or a public area of the unit, is also relevant to consider in relation to such aspects.

Prevalence of abuse

For many years there was an absence of reliable data about prevalence of elder abuse in the UK. Initially, the UK research most widely referred to (Ogg and Bennett 1992, as described in Ogg and Munn-Giddings 1993) drew some conclusions about the prevalence of abuse but contrasted the difficulty of determining UK prevalence figures, particularly when compared to the situation in the United States.

Ogg and Bennett's (1992) study used questions as part of a broader survey of 2,000 older people living in the community. However, as the authors acknowledged, this excluded those living in residential settings and very likely many of those who were very frail. A comprehensive picture was therefore not obtained. However, the study provided a useful baseline from which more comprehensive research on prevalence could be developed. In the Ogg and Bennett study, the most prevalent type of abuse was psychological (5 per cent) followed by physical (2 per cent) and financial (2 per cent) types of abuse (Ogg and Bennett 1992).

The Health Select Committee report of a Hearing on Elder Abuse, held in late 2003 (House of Commons Health Select Committee, 2004) drew attention to Action on Elder Abuse's (AEA) analysis of calls to its Helpline in 1997–1999 (ibid.: paras 19–20). This study showed an approximate estimate of elder abuse incidence (Bennett et al. 2000). From the analysis, the most commonly reported type of elder abuse found was psychological abuse, as in the Ogg and Bennett study, followed by physical abuse and then financial abuse (Bennett et al. 2000). The analysis also found that reports of domestic abuse were more frequent than institutional abuse although reported incidents of physical abuse and neglect in institutional settings were more frequent than in domestic settings (Bennett et al. 2000). Once again, as a further recent analysis of the Helpline acknowledged (Action on Elder Abuse/Help the Aged 2004), drawing conclusions from these figures requires caution. Further data from an AEA study of adult protection referrals to local authorities has recently become available (DoH 2005) but this too has its limitations since thresholds were varied, definitions were inconsistent and data collection systems were under-developed.

From the late 1990s it was generally agreed that research into the prevalence of abuse in the UK has been limited and out-dated and that there needed to be a more comprehensive prevalence study. In 2005, a prevalence study funded by the charity Comic Relief and the English Department of Health was commissioned and findings were reported in 2007. This nationally representative population-based study of 2,100 people living in community settings and aged 66 years or older established a base prevalence rate of 2.6 per cent (of all types of abuse, experienced in the past 12 months) across the UK (O'Keeffe et al. 2007). For the purposes of this study, perpetrators of mistreatment were confined to those individuals in a 'position of trust': relatives and family members, care workers and friends. If the definition was broadened to include neighbours and acquaintances the prevalence rate increased to 4 per cent. Neglect was the most commonly cited form of mistreatment, followed by financial abuse and the victims in the study were predominantly women. Those older women who lived alone were more likely to experience neglect, while those who had poor health, poor quality of life or reported loneliness were more likely to experience interpersonal abuse. The most likely perpetrators were partners, family members or neighbours, followed by care workers and then friends. The study did not include those individuals who were impaired by cognitive or major/severe health problems or those living in institutions, which thus limits the applicability of the findings to the whole population, and it also arguably represents an under-estimate of the extent of abuse and neglect as those who might be considered most vulnerable to abuse were excluded and did not participate

A framework for protection

There are many different pieces of legislation used by professionals working in the field of elder abuse in the UK. This includes social workers, social care staff and allied professionals from healthcare settings. Attaining a fundamental knowledge of legislation is necessary for all practitioners in this type of work and this should form part of qualifying training. It may often be the case that social workers are primarily and predominantly involved in application of the law, although, depending on the exact nature of the circumstances, other professionals may also need to have essential knowledge of the law. Social workers protect individuals from others, from themselves, from circumstances and from various types of disadvantage in life. They also in some ways protect society from danger and harm by regulating individuals' lives. As will become apparent, in order to do this a wide range of law and policy is needed. Within the UK setting, the general approach taken to issues of protection is that of adult safeguarding, concerning the abuse of vulnerable adults in general. Such an approach covers the needs of those older adults who experience situations of elder abuse and neglect.

Legislation to protect

Older people with impairments or disabilities, (physical and/or cognitive) or complex health problems may be vulnerable and at risk of abuse from other people in a variety of contexts. They may also put others at risk of harm by their actions. It is important to note, however, that there is no single piece of legislation that specifically (and uniquely) concerns the protection of vulnerable adults (of any age) in England, Wales or Northern Ireland, although following a review of the policy guidance (in 2008–11) this may develop in future. Instead of a single law, there are a number of different pieces of legislation, different parts (or specific 'sections') of which may be used by individuals who are in need of protection. At times another person, for example a professional practitioner, can use legislation on behalf of an individual.

There is legislation designed to protect people with mental illness from harm or harming others (Mental Health Acts 1983 and 2007, Supervised Discharge Procedures 1995). The legislation concerning mental health also extends to adults with severe learning disabilities, and includes such provision as guardianship and arrangements for the Court of Protection to assist in the management of a person's finances. The Mental Health Act was reviewed and updated in 2007, including some revision of the Court of Protection to include personal and welfare decisions as well as finances (Lord Chancellor's Office 1999). The Mental Capacity Act 2005 (MCA) covers those older adults who lack the capacity to take decisions (as well as other adults who also lack decision-making capacity) and this includes some provision relating to protection from abuse, specifically in the creation of a specific offence of ill-treatment or wilful neglect of an adult who lacks capacity (Section 44 of the MCA), with punishment relating to a fine, or imprisonment. While legislation relating to domestic violence was extended to include adults experiencing elder and adult abuse (see for example the Family Law Act 1996), the Domestic Violence, Crime and Victims Act 2004, which covered elder abuse in the domestic setting, including being killed by family members, included a new offence of familial homicide. Additionally, the government agenda for the modernisation of social services also included explicit recognition of the need to both promote independence and increase measures of protection for vulnerable individuals (DoH 1998). These changes were gradually implemented over the period 2000–2006. For example, the Public Interest Disclosure Act 1998 was introduced to provide protection for individuals who whistle-blow about abusive situations within organisations (such as care homes or hospitals).

In terms of previously existing legislation in England, Wales and Northern Ireland, adults with a range of needs are largely protected from a range of difficulties in life experiences by entitlement to an assessment and services to meet identified needs to assist them to remain living in the community with support. This is provided within the National Health Service and Community Care Act 1990, which was implemented in April 1993. The Sexual Offences Act 1957 offers protection to people from unwanted sexual advances or sexual abuse, whereas the Protection from Harassment Act 1997 may offer protection from bullying, stalking and harassment of individuals, including sexual harassment.

Additionally, Part IV of the Family Law Act 1996 affords individuals some protection from violence that takes place in the domestic setting. This legislation provides a range of measures that might be used, including non-molestation and ouster orders (concerning abusers/perpetrators) in certain situations. The scope of this legislation was widened when it was introduced in order to include a broader range of individuals living together, not just spouses or those people in a cohabitation relationship. There is also the possibility of a third party such as a professional practitioner taking action on behalf of an individual, so it can therefore be used in situations concerning the safety and protection of vulnerable older people.

As stated, in most of the UK there is no legislation comparable to the Children Act 1989, which specifically concerns the abuse of adults. In England, Wales and Northern Ireland, current legal remedies to the abuse and harm of a vulnerable adult include use of the above-mentioned laws, and may include use of legislation to remove the person in need of protection to a place of safety (see also the National Assistance Act 1948, section 47). Of course, general legal measures, using both the criminal and the civil law, may also be used to protect older individuals. These would concern such situations as assault or theft. However, in relation to financial abuse, although general legislation concerning theft is often applicable, but it would seem that it is not often used. Additionally, it is important to acknowledge that within the UK as a whole there is no mandatory reporting law concerning elder abuse or, indeed, adult safeguarding in more general terms. Although such reporting is a requirement concerning matters of child safeguarding, this is not the case concerning the safeguarding of adults who might be considered vulnerable to abuse due to their situations or circumstances (Penhale and Parker 2008).

In Scotland specific legislation relating to adult protection was developed and enacted in 2007. The Adult Support and Protection (Scotland) Act was implemented across the country (Scotland) from the autumn of 2008. This followed an earlier consultation exercise led by the Scottish Law Commission during the late 1990s and a subsequent decision to introduce specific, unified legislation to protect adults at risk of harm (Scottish Office 1997). This law is based on a fundamental set of principles: that any intervention must be of benefit to the individual, that this benefit could not have been attained without the intervention and that the intervention must be the option that is least restrictive of the individual's rights and freedom. The statute's purpose is to provide the means by which intervention can prevent harm from continuing, to develop stronger measures to protect individuals at risk of harm and to improve inter-agency co-operation and inter-disciplinary practice.

The key aspects of the Act are:

- a duty on local authorities and their key partners, health boards, police, education and voluntary organisations to work together to support and protect adults at risk of harm (including attendance at adult protection board meeting held at local level);
- a duty on a range of agencies to investigate suspected abuse;
- new powers to carry out assessments of the person and their circumstances in private where necessary, including a power of removal for a temporary period;
- a range of options for intervention to address and manage instances of abuse;
- any intervention under the Act must benefit the adult and be the least restrictive option.

A useful guide to relevant legislation that exists in the UK context was developed in response to one of the recommendations from the consultation and review processes for the policy guidance in both England and Wales and provides helpful additional information on this aspect (Mandelstam 2011).

Protection and risk: important considerations in the UK

The previous section concerning the appropriate use of legislation is important to the development of good management systems, particularly within social and health care professions. This may perhaps be particularly the case within the area of protection, when it is essential that individuals are not further disadvantaged or disempowered by the systems that are designed to assist them. Health and social care organisations should not just be concerned with the provision of direct care and protection to individuals. It must be recognised that the delivery of such care must be based upon clear and effective policies, procedures and guidance. These should be explicitly designed to ensure that the services and care provided are the most appropriate for individuals and that resources are used effectively and represent good value for money.

It is therefore essential for health and social care practitioners to have a good working knowledge of the policies and procedures of whichever agency they work for and the legislation that underpins these. In any policy there should be clear lines of responsibility and accountability, so that decisions that are made within that policy framework are checked and authorised by those persons with the training and experience necessary to make them.

Thus it is crucial that social workers and others in the helping professions begin to learn protective practice during qualifying training. This should include training in the assessment and management of risk and risky situations and the development of risk enablement strategies for individuals in need for support and assistance. This was emphasised for social workers by the Central Council for Education and Training in Social Work (CCETSW) in their revised Paper 30 (CCETSW 1995), which was subsequently adopted by the General Social Care Council (GSCC). At the present time, social workers need to be competent in six key areas, each of which has a number of practice requirements attached. These requirements include competence in protective practice as it relates either to work with children at risk or to work with adults who may be vulnerable to abuse. The General Social Care Council was previously responsible for the registration and licensing of social work and social care practitioners as well as having functions relating to the education and training of social work and social care practitioners. Following a review undertaken during 2010 by the coalition government to reduce the extent of bureaucracy, the functions of the GSCC transferred to the appropriate regulator, the Health and Care Professions Council (HCPC) from July 2012 and the organisation was dismantled.

The general approach taken in this area appears premised on the notion that the provision of regulation and a clear regulatory framework can provide the foundations on which professional practice can be developed and, furthermore, that this will also serve to protect vulnerable individuals if or as necessary. However, to further illustrate the complexity of this area and the attention paid by the government in England and Wales to matters of regulation and the provision of a regulatory framework, it is necessary to know that there is a section of the government known as the Care Quality Commission, which has powers in relation to health, social care and mental health, following an amalgamation of three separate commissions. The key functions of this organisation, of relevance here, are to inspect the provision of services by local authority social services and health services (which are publicly run) as well as having registration and inspection functions concerning the provision of residential and nursing home care and domiciliary care provided within the independent and private sectors.

National guidance, local approaches

Guidance from government in relation to adult safeguarding does not generally appear to have been a priority area for concern until comparatively recently. Nevertheless this is likely to be an important aspect of prevention of abuse, violence and neglect towards older adults. The initial guidance concerning elder abuse was published in 1993 by the Department of Health, from the Social Services Inspectorate, England. Guidance in connection with adults with learning disabilities was also first issued in 1993 (ARC/NAPSAC 1993). Both of these documents were limited, however, in their approaches. The document concerning elder abuse was clear that it only applied to situations occurring within the domestic setting, while that relating to learning disabled adults predominantly focused on situations of sexual abuse. The establishment of guidance in these areas, even if limited, is, of course, necessary and important. Professionals do not operate in a vacuum from the wider society and must therefore have the direction of national government and their employing bodies in order to ensure that standards of practice are clear and take place at appropriate levels.

In 1998, the English Department of Health (Social Services Inspectorate) began work to rectify the lack of guidance concerning other vulnerable adults (e.g. adults with physical disability, sensory impairment or mental health difficulties who might also have needs relating to vulnerability and protection) in order to produce necessary guidance on what was then called adult protection for authorities and organisations to adopt in their work. The guidance development process was understandably lengthy given the need for involvement and working party participation across the broad spectrum of adult protection. In late 1999, a draft guidance document was produced for consultation purposes (DoH 1999), and a final document, entitled No Secrets was published during 2000 (DoH 2000). The final document produced guidance concerning the roles and responsibilities of differing organisations and disciplines and the processes that should take place in relation to abuse. Social services departments were designated as the lead agency for co-ordinating responses within adult protection in each local authority area, and the guidance itself had sufficient status that it was a requirement for the guidance to be implemented by authorities, although the requirement rested with local authority social services departments rather than with other or all organisations involved at the local level. The guidance was implemented in autumn 2001. A similar process took place in Wales with the development and introduction of policy and procedural guidance over roughly the same time period, the document bearing the title In Safe Hands was also introduced in 2000 and covered broadly similar areas to its English counterpart.

In Northern Ireland, the comparable policy document, Safeguarding vulnerable adults: Regional adult protection and policy procedural guidelines, was introduced some years later, in 2006 (NISSB 2006). This guidance document laid out the relevant policy framework for adult protection in Northern Ireland and included discussion of definitions, principles as well as emphasising the importance of inter-agency working. Rather more recent developments have included a Protocol for Joint Investigation of Alleged and Suspected Cases of Abuse of Vulnerable Adults by the Regional Adult Protection Forum, which is a partnership body, with representation from Health and Social Care Trusts and Board, Police Service for Northern Ireland, the Regulation and Quality Improvement Authority and the voluntary sector. This protocol outlines roles and responsibilities of the respective agencies and provides guidance about joint working arrangements and processes of investigation (Health and Social Care Board).

Similar to other jurisdictions in the UK, the policy guidance has been subject to review in recent years. In November 2009, Reforming Northern

Ireland's adult protection infrastructure, a consultation document produced by the Department of Health, Social Services and Public Safety (DHSSPS 2009) and the Northern Ireland Office (NIO) with the support of other relevant government departments was issued. Following the consultation process, the new Northern Ireland Adult Safeguarding Partnership (NIASP) and five Local Adult Safeguarding Partnerships (LASPs) were established and also reflected a change in terminology, comparable to England's, from protection to safeguarding. Good practice guidance Safeguarding vulnerable adults: A shared responsibility was also launched (Volunteer Now 2010). This guidance set out eight key safeguarding standards and the associated criteria to achieve these standards, as well as inclusion of additional helpful resources for practitioners working in this area.

Many local authorities began work in the area of adult protection/ safeguarding some time ago and did not wait for national initiatives to improve practice in this area. Successive surveys throughout the 1990s indicated that an increasing number of health and social care organisations implemented policies and procedures in adult protection. A large number of these authorities had initially begun work in the area of elder abuse and then expanded their focus and remit. However, it is now generally agreed that the frameworks developed should be inter-agency in nature and that the same approach should be taken to developing responses at the local level (Pritchard 1999). Policies and procedures can be shared across agencies or separate procedures developed by agencies, who then work to a shared, over-arching policy that is multi-agency in nature and scope.

It is essential here to recognise that policies and procedures are necessary and important tools to be used to inform practitioners of the actions that should be taken at particular points in the process of responding to potentially abusive or neglectful situations. Yet, policies and procedures on their own cannot ensure that good practice follows. It is absolutely fundamental here to consider how these are actually put into practice and operationalised (Penhale 1993). Most policies and procedural documents detail what should happen from the initial referral or alert concerning alleged abuse of an adult and the subsequent stages of investigating or assessing the circumstances within that situation and determining whether abuse has occurred or not. There will then be a further stage during which decisions will be taken about whether there is a need for any ongoing work or monitoring and review of the situation. However, specific strategies of intervention and how these are applied are unlikely to be entirely prescribed by procedures. Good practice in this area needs to evolve further beyond merely the development of regulation and documentation designed to guide practitioners through a sequence of processes. This will include developing our knowledge and understanding about what sorts of interventions are most appropriate for specific types of abuse, together with a thorough evaluative framework for interventions, including those designed and targeted to prevent abuse (WHO 2011).

Multi-disciplinary approaches within protection

Within the difficult, complex and sensitive situations that often arise within situations of elder abuse, and across the range of different types of abuse that can occur, it is essential that there is effective collaboration between agencies. This is an approach that has been taken across all nations in the UK. It is vital that there is successful multi-disciplinary working within situations of adult protection as even within a relatively discreet area such as elder abuse it is apparent that no single profession or specialism has sufficient expertise to deal with all potential situations. Consequently, there is a need for both participation and collaboration between the different specialisms from within social work and also on an inter-disciplinary basis with other organisations, such as the police and other criminal justice agencies, health organisations and third sector and NGO representatives. Thus, for instance, when exploring a situation of potential sexual abuse of an older adult, it may be highly appropriate for a social work practitioner to request guidance and assistance from colleagues from the field of child safeguarding, as well as from professionals from health, police, housing, victim support and other voluntary agencies.

This is where a co-ordinated approach to adult safeguarding, including the establishment of a specific co-ordinator or managerial post, is likely to be of particular value. This type of role often encompasses the provision of in-service training of staff and/or consultation concerning specific cases which practitioners are dealing with. This can be of particular value since the UK has not seen the development of US-style Adult Protective Services teams. The safeguarding co-ordinator can also put practitioners in contact with each other or suggest other possible options to explore, as well as providing advice and information and assisting in the overall co-ordination and direction of a situation. This is likely to be in addition to the involvement of the practitioner's normal processes of line management. The co-ordinator may come from any disciplinary background within the helping professions or even from within criminal justice agencies, as police forces have been developing skills and expertise in the area of public protection (including domestic violence and adult safeguarding) in recent years. The need for awareness, understanding and clear communication skills in dealing with professionals from across the range of professions, is therefore paramount. Since the implementation of No Secrets guidance from 2001, an increasing number of local authorities have developed co-ordinator posts. It is not, however, at this stage a mandatory requirement by government and not all authorities have full-time manager or co-ordinator positions (Perkins et al. 2007, Braye et al. 2010). Adult safeguarding units are also a fairly recent development in the UK, but some local authorities have well-established and experienced units and these may provide advice and guidance to other authorities concerning how to create and promote such approaches. A national network for co-ordinators within regional branches has also been developed in recent years which provides support and allows for information exchange between co-ordinators in the development of their work.

Specialist input from different disciplines is likely to be valuable throughout the process of assessment and investigation of a situation. This may be in the form of a specialist contribution to an assessment or an assessment conducted jointly between different relevant agencies. For instance, an older adult with a chronic debilitating and degenerative illness will profit from both specialist nursing and health and social care involvement in community care assessment and subsequent care management. This may also include potential needs for protection and safety planning, depending on the nature of their circumstances. In other situations, involvement of police, housing and voluntary organisations is likely to be useful in addition to contributions from health care professions. Under the National Service Framework for Older People (DoH 2001) complex assessments, to which a number of professionals may contribute, also included specific consideration of issues relating to safety and protection.

Multi-disciplinary input at the stage of a strategy meeting or a case conference can also be crucial in relation to (potentially) abusive situations. In situations where there are a number of disciplines involved with a person, contributions from as many of these as possible at the strategy meeting and/ or case conference stage will help to ensure that the fundamental elements of an individual's care are fully considered. A case conference is likely to be the accumulation of events, quite possibly encompassing several incidents and escalating risks, and it is not likely to be used in all situations. However, the majority of situations will benefit from regular and systematic meetings and liaison between those professionals involved in assessment, service delivery, monitoring and review. Strategy, network and safety planning meetings can all be used to good effect within adult safeguarding, including elder abuse, even if at different points in the process. A number of inquiry reports into failures of care or serious untoward incidents confirm the importance of inter-disciplinary communication in the effective management of abusive situations. This is the case in relation to older adults just as much as situations concerning children.

Considering developments concerning case conferences within child protection systems, the issue of service-user involvement and participation in the process is also relevant here. There has been much useful work relating to parental involvement undertaken within child protection (see e.g. Thoburn et al. 1995). From this, useful lessons are apparent about ways to increase engagement with and participation in protection processes and these lessons should be transferred to work with older and other vulnerable adults. Moreover, the increasing amount of information and knowledge about the sexual abuse of young women and children means that useful information concerning, for instance, the use of disclosure interviews is increasingly being used with vulnerable adults who have been sexually abused, the majority of whom are women (Draucker 1992).

The involvement of the police is also of major importance within many (if not all) situations of alleged abuse. Many established domestic violence units (DVUs) within police forces have widened their scope over the past 5–10 years and are now also concerned with children and adults who experience abuse, violence and exploitation. Some units have been renamed as family or public protection units, while others retain the title DVU. Many of these units will consider the needs of vulnerable individuals beyond a narrow interpretation of either family or domestic setting. It is usually beneficial to involve the police in processes as early as possible. This includes securing advice and guidance, if not direct involvement and attendance at case conferences. This is therefore increasingly necessary as a central part of the process in dealing with abusive situations. Contact with the police at an early stage is particularly helpful in order to clarify whether a situation may benefit from police involvement or if active involvement and investigation of situations by the police is likely to be necessary or not.

Of course, obtaining clear legal advice concerning situations is also quite likely to be necessary in a good number of circumstances. As suggested earlier in this chapter, professionals working with older and vulnerable adults should acquire a basic understanding of legal frameworks in relation to protection. They may also need ready access to expert assistance where necessary. In the UK, for social care professionals, this may often be appropriately acquired through access to local authority legal sections.

However, individuals themselves may also require assistance to gain access to appropriate legal support and also increasingly independent advocacy. This is an aspect that can add unnecessary stress to an already difficult situation. The provision of appropriate advice from professionals in such situations can help to ease situations for those individuals experiencing such distress.

Good practice issues

Despite the recognition of elder abuse since the latter decades of the twentieth century, the development of appropriate responses to situations of both elder and adult abuse appears to be at comparatively early stages of formation in most of the UK, although Scotland has been developing more rapidly since the introduction of legislation. In general, however, most work seems, so far, to have taken place concerning the establishment of procedural systems for professionals to follow. This is particularly in relation to the assessment and investigation of situations that are held to be abusive. There is broad agreement that councils with social services responsibilities (formerly known as social services departments) should have a lead co-ordinating role within this area and that assessment should take place within the context of overall systems for assessment and care management (DoH 1993) and increasingly personalisation of care. Assessment needs to be holistic (in accordance with earlier guidance in relation to community care for adults: DoH 1991a, 1991b), but within situations relating to potential abuse and/or neglect, it should also be 'abuse-focused' as a fundamental part of this process (Bennett et al. 1997).

Good practice in the safeguarding of vulnerable adults should include such elements as a distinction between initial referral (or alert) and subsequent investigation, the careful co-ordination of the investigation and separate, sensitive and suitable arrangements for interviews. The use of case conferences in order to determine a protection plan for an individual, where this is necessary and as an effective means to promote shared decision making, is also indicated as good practice. Involvement of the individual service user within such meetings is also an area under development, with many authorities developing good practice in this area (Penhale et al. 2007). It is also apparent that a balance between the needs of the service-user for support and protection and the need for sanction or treatment for the abuser should be found in many situations. The protection (or safety) plan that is developed should ideally include attention to the needs of the service-user for safety, support and service provision (or treatment), together with careful consideration of issues relating to the ongoing management of risk and increasingly risk enablement within more personalised and individualised approaches to care and support.

The modernising agenda for social services as outlined in 1998 (DoH 1998) appeared to relate more to institutional and service settings as key areas where attention was needed in order to protect vulnerable service-users. However, emphasis was also given to partnership and collaborative working to improve protection for individuals as a crucial prerequisite to the development of effective responses (Penhale et al. 2000). Research has been conducted to explore the nature and extent of partnership working in this area (Penhale et al. 2007, Braye et al. 2012). Effective inter-agency working is absolutely essential within many situations, which may be assisted through the development of clearly defined inter-agency working arrangements and shared protocols covering, for example, such aspects as information-sharing at local levels.

Concluding comments

We do not yet know or understand enough about elder abuse and neglect in the UK, irrespective of the setting in which this occurs. More needs to be done to improve the recognition of such situations and some of the causes, as well as to increase understanding about which approaches to prevention and intervention are most successful and effective within situations. Professional standards, and also to an extent personal values, for individuals working in such situations, need to be acknowledged, explored and developed. It is essential to continue to work on establishing effective systems of public accountability, including developing clear lines of support for individuals, as well as expectations of what is required of professionals and paraprofessionals working in this area. Interventions need to be appropriate and sensitively tailored in order to meet the needs of the individuals involved as fully and effectively as possible. There is also a need to further explore and develop the different levels at which prevention may be targeted in the UK context.

It is very important to increase awareness and knowledge about this problem, including at the level of the general public, where this is still very much needed. Public awareness campaigns form one obvious element of this and the continued development of World Elder Abuse Awareness Day now this has achieved UN recognition (since November 2011) will also assist with this. However, in order to really acquire increased knowledge and awareness of the issue, systems and approaches to education and training must be further developed, consisting, perhaps of a more integrated approach to such provision. This would then act as the framework from which appropriate and effective responses to prevention can further develop. In conjunction with this, there is also a critical need for more research in this area as a whole so that we can improve both our knowledge and understanding of abuse and neglect and, ultimately, how to prevent it. We need both commitment and action on the part of individuals and governments to pursue this agenda as far as is needed in the coming years and the continued impetus from within and across countries is a fundamental element of continuing progress in this most complex of areas.

References

Action on Elder Abuse (1995) 'New definition of abuse', Action on Elder Abuse Bulletin, May–June 1995, issue no. 11.

Action on Elder Abuse/Help the Aged (2004) Hidden voices: Older people's experience of abuse. London: Action on Elder Abuse/Help the Aged.

ARC/NAPSAC (1993) It could never happen here, Bradford: Thornton and Pearson.

Bennett, G., Kingston, P. and Penhale, B. (1997) The dimensions of elder abuse: Perspectives for practitioners. Basingstoke: Macmillan.

Bennett, G.C.J., Jenkins, G. and Asif, Z. (2000) 'Listening is not enough: An analysis of calls to the elder abuse response helpline'. Journal of Adult Protection, 2, 1: 6–20.

Braye, S., Orr, D. and Preston-Shoot, M. (2010) The governance of adult safeguarding: Findings from research into adult safeguarding boards. Brighton: University of Sussex.

Braye, S., Orr, D. and Preston-Shoot, M. (2012) 'The governance of adult safeguarding: Findings from research', Journal of Adult Protection, 14, 2: 55–72.

CCETSW (1995) Rules and requirements for the diploma in social work, London: CCETSW.

DoH (1991a) Care management and assessment: The practitioner's guide. Department of Health. London: HMSO.

——(1991b) Care management and assessment: The manager's guide. Department of Health. London: HMSO.

——(1993) No longer afraid: the safeguard of older people in domestic settings. Department of Health. London: HMSO.

——(1998) Modernising social services. Department of Health. London: HMSO.

——(1999) 'No secrets: The protection of vulnerable adults – guidance on the development and implementation of multi-agency policies and procedures'. Department of Health (consultation document). London: TSO.

——(2000) No secrets: The protection of vulnerable adults – guidance on the development and implementation of multi-agency policies and procedures. Department of Health. London: TSO.

——(2001) National service framework for older people. Department of Health. London: TSO.

——(2005) Action on elder abuse: Report on the project to establish a monitoring and reporting process for adult protection referrals made in accordance with 'No secrets'. London: Department of Health.

DHSSPS (2009) Reforming Northern Ireland's adult protection infrastructure, Belfast: Department of Health, Social Services and Public Safety.

Draucker, C.B. (1992) Counselling the victims of childhood sexual abuse. Newbury Park: Sage.

Glendenning, F. and Kingston, P. (eds) (1999) Elder abuse and neglect in residential settings: Different national backgrounds and similar responses, New York: Haworth Press.

Health and Social Care Board (2009) *Protocol for Joint Investigation of Alleged and Suspected Cases of Abuse of Vulnerable Adults*, Belfast: Regulation and Quality Improvement Authority.

House of Commons Health Select Committee (2004) Elder abuse, Second Report of Session 2003–4, Vol. 1. Report, together with formal minutes. London: The Stationery Office.

Lord Chancellor's Office (1999) Making decisions, London: TSO.

McCreadie, C. (1996) Elder abuse: an update on research, London: TSO.

Mandelstam, M. (2011) Safeguarding adults at risk of harm: A legal guide for practitioners, London: Social Care Institute for Excellence.

NISSB (2006) Safeguarding vulnerable adults: Regional adult protection policy and procedural guidelines. Ballymena: Social Services Directorate, Northern Ireland Social Services Board.

O'Keeffe, M., Hills, A., Doyle, M., McCreadie, C., Scholes, S., Constantine, R., et al. (2007) UK study of abuse and neglect of older people. Prevalence survey report. London: King's College London and National Centre for Social Research.

Ogg, J. and Bennett, G. (1992) 'Elder abuse in Britain'. British Medical Journal, 305: 998–9.

Ogg, J. and Munn-Giddings, C. (1993) 'Researching elder abuse', Ageing and Society, 13, 3: 389–414.

Penhale, B. (1993) 'The abuse of elderly people: Considerations for practice', British Journal of Social Work, 23, 2: 95–112.

——(1999) 'Research on elder abuse: Lessons for practice' in M. Eastman and P. Slater (eds) Elder abuse: Critical issues in policy and practice. London: Age Concern Books.

——and Parker, J. (2008) Working with vulnerable adults, London: Routledge.

——, Parker, J. and Kingston, P. (2000) Elder abuse: Approaches to working with violence. Birmingham: Venture Press.

——, Perkins, N., Pinkney, L., Reid, D., Hussein, S. and Manthorpe, J. (2007) Partnerships and regulation in adult protection: Final report. Sheffield: University of Sheffield.

Perkins, N., Penhale, B., Reid, D., Pinkney, L., Hussein, S. and Manthorpe, J. (2007) 'Partnership means protection? Perceptions of the effectiveness of multi-agency working and the regulatory framework within adult protection in England and Wales', Journal of Adult Protection, 9, 3: 9–23.

Pritchard, J. (1999) (ed.) Elder abuse work: Best practice in Britain and Canada, London: Jessica Kingsley Publishers.

Scottish Office (1997) Scottish Law Commission Report No 158: Report on vulnerable adults. Blackwell: Edinburgh.

Stanley, N., Manthorpe, J. and Penhale, B. (1999) (eds) Institutional abuse: Perspectives across the lifecourse, London: Routledge.

Stearns, P. (1986) 'Old age family conflict: The perspective of the past', in K.A. Pillemer and R.S. Wolf (eds) Elder abuse: Conflict in the family. Dover, MA: Auburn House Publishing Company.

Thoburn, J., Lewis, A. and Shemmings, D. (1995) Paternalism or partnership? Family involvement in the child protection process, London: HMSO.

Volunteer Now (2010) Safeguarding vulnerable adults: A shared responsibility, Belfast: Volunteer Now.

WAG (2000) In safe hands: Implementing adult protection procedures in Wales, Cardiff: Welsh Assembly Government.

WHO (2011) European report on preventing elder maltreatment, Rome: World Health Organisation.

12 United States of America

Joy Swanson Ernst and Patricia Brownell

Introduction

The United States is grappling with how to address the needs of the growing population of older adults. By 2030, 20 percent of the US population will be age 65 and older. As the cohort of baby boomers ages, the percentage of older adults who are aged 85 and older will continue to grow as well, with the population of the oldest elders (90+) growing at the fastest rate (He and Muenchrath, 2011). The population is also changing with respect to racial and ethnic composition. Non-white older adults now account for about 20 percent of the older population; in 2050, this number is projected to be about 42 percent (Vincent and Velkoff 2010).

These shifts in population will have an impact on public and private resources. While many older adults are living longer in greater health, aging-related health changes, increased frailty, and dementia will affect many of the oldest elders, who will need care. The US must determine how to provide care for dependent older adults when families are stressed by multiple caregiving demands, the short- and long-term impact of the economic downturn, and shrinking public resources. Protecting the independence and self-determination of older adults who may live in the community and be mistreated by dependent family members and fall victims to targeted crimes by strangers is also of concern to practitioners, policymakers and law enforcement. The increase in the number of older adults will mean an increase in the number who are at risk of being abused, neglected and financially exploited. While the efforts by the US to address elder mistreatment have increased over the past two decades, the realities of a growing older population and shrinking resources suggest that older adults will continue to be at risk of being mistreated.

This chapter explains the context in which policy is created in the US and provides an overview of policy and practice related to elder abuse in the US. Once a largely hidden problem, elder abuse has garnered more public attention lately particularly due to media coverage such as the highly publicized case of actor Mickey Rooney. The March 2011 Senate testimony by the 92-year-old actor Mickey Rooney about his exploitation by relatives

(Pham 2011) is a recent example of the increased awareness of a problem for which the policy response is still inadequate.

Definitions

According to the World Health Organization (WHO 2002: 3), elder abuse can be defined as "a single, or repeated act, or lack of appropriate action, occurring within any relationship where there is an expectation of trust which causes harm or distress to an older person." Elder abuse can take various forms such as physical, psychological, or emotional, sexual and financial abuse. It can also be the result of intentional or unintentional neglect. Although efforts to standardize definitions have increased in recent years, no universally accepted definition of elder mistreatment exists within the US, and definitions used for research and in the agencies that respond to abuse vary.

The US National Committee on the Prevention of Elder Abuse (2008) defines elder abuse broadly as "any form of mistreatment that results in harm or loss to an older person". This definition encompasses physical abuse, sexual abuse, financial exploitation, psychological abuse, neglect, self-neglect, and domestic violence as forms of elder mistreatment.

The research community has taken steps to develop standardized research definitions of elder mistreatment, but legal responses to elder abuse are shaped by laws developed at state level. In 2003, the Panel to Review Risk and Prevalence of Elder Abuse (Bonnie and Wallace 2003) addressed the inconsistency of definitions used in research. The Panel defined elder mistreatment as being perpetrated by a person in a "trust relationship" with the older adult, which excludes crimes perpetrated by strangers. The perpetrator is someone with whom the older person has an ongoing, committed partnership, familial, or other type of trust relationship. This definition excludes self-neglect. However, when addressing elder abuse policy in the US it is important to include self-neglect in the discussion because self-neglect accounts for the majority of cases reported to Adult Protective Services. Crimes perpetrated by strangers against older adults who are targeted because of their age and vulnerability is another category of elder abuse that is identified by law enforcement, including prosecutors.

Policy response to elder abuse

Government in the United States

The structure of government in the US and the history of the government's response to addressing social problems have left the US with an uncoordinated approach to elder abuse on a national level. To understand elder abuse policy in the US, it is necessary to understand how federal, state, and local levels of government are involved in efforts to prevent, identify, and respond to elder abuse. The response to elder abuse – prevention, identification, response, treatment – is shaped and constrained by laws, policies, and practices at the federal, state, and local levels of governments.

In the US, policy direction on elder abuse comes from the federal government but is left to the states to carry out. This bifurcation of responsibility is the result of an ongoing debate, continuing since the 1930s (the New Deal), of whether social welfare and other policy issues affecting the family are the responsibility of the federal government or the governments of the now 50 states. The US response reflects the complex, multifaceted nature of elder abuse and is shaped by the structure of the government and how the US has historically provided social services. The response is also shaped by political battles over the size of the federal government, state budgets constrained by economic recession, and existing entitlement programs (Medicare and Medicaid), which will continue to claim a larger share of federal and state budgets.

Traditionally, the provision of social services has been left to state and local governments. The Social Security Act, passed in 1935, provided grants to the states for social services, which the states used to meet needs as specified by those states, within the broad constraints of the legislation. Title XX of the Social Security Act, passed in 1974, provided block grants, which are sums allocated on the basis of each state's population to use for social services, that included protective services to adults as one of the categories for which states could use money. States developed or enhanced adult protective services programs to respond to reports of abuse, neglect, and exploitation of older adults (and dependent adults aged 18–59). However, it is important to note that Adult Protective Services (APS) has had to compete with other programs funded by Title XX (see above) funds, including domestic violence residential and non-residential programs, child day care and vital programs for children.

No federal laws or policies, therefore, direct how protective services should be delivered, and state statutes differ in terms of the definitions of abuse and what types of abuse are covered (Brandl et al. 2006). While localized control means that states and counties can determine the response that best fits the needs and resources of their communities, one result is that the US does not collect uniform data that would help determine trends in reporting. There is insufficient evidence-based research and dissemination of best practices to APS agencies, which have limited information on evidence-based practices that would help them address complex cases (US Government Accountability Office 2011).

The localized response also means that there are distinctions among state laws and policies that determine the response to elder abuse. One distinction is whether reporting suspected elder abuse in the community to APS is mandated or not. Currently, 4 of the 50 states (Colorado, New York, North Dakota, and South Dakota) do not have mandated reporting of elder abuse in the community (all states have mandated reporting of elder abuse in institutional settings). One issue associated with mandated reporting includes the question of who is mandated to report and who is to receive the report, with some states sanctioning licensed professionals such as doctors, nurses and social workers for failure to report, and some requiring all citizens to report but do not penalize would-be reporters for not doing so. Another issue related to mandated reporting is the consequences associated with failure to report. The definitions of elder abuse in state statutes vary as well, with self-neglect included as a form of abuse in some states but not in others.

Federal legislation related to elder abuse

In the US, three significant federal laws address elder abuse in different ways. Through amendments passed in 1987, the Older Americans Act (OAA), first passed in 1965, became the first federal law that specifically identified elder abuse as a social problem of national concern. Amendments to the 1994 Violence Against Women Act (VAWA) that were passed in 2000 and 2006 specifically addressed the needs of older women. The Elder Justice Act, passed in 2010 as part of the Affordable Care Act, is the first national law specifically addressing elder abuse.

The OAA passed into law in 1965 as part of a broad social rights-based movement in the US that included the Civil Rights Act, which sought to empower and mainstream formerly legally marginalized groups such as Americans of African descent, older adults, and ultimately children and women. While the earlier Social Security Act (SSA) of 1935 through its Title One defined indigent vulnerable older adults (age 65 years and above) as needing protection, the Older Americans Act of 1965 redefined older adults (age 60 years and above) as vital members of society who have the right to live with dignity and independence in their communities as long as possible. Title Seven of the Older Americans Act, which was included as an amendment to the Older Americans Act in 1994 and again in 2000, added a service category related to legal education and services for older adults in the community, including those who may be experiencing family abuse. However, little federal funding has ever been allocated to the implementation of this title of the Older American Act, and legal services have never been defined as core services for the national, state, and county-based aging service network. As a result, state and county aging programs authorized by the Older Americans Act may provide some public education on elder abuse and may be represented on state and county elder abuse coalitions; however, they are seldom considered to be significant providers of elder abuse services to older adults living in the community.

The second significant federal law is the Violence Against Women Act (VAWA), passed as part of an omnibus crime prevention act in 1994. During the reauthorization of VAWA in 2000, and again in 2006, a section was added specifically to address abuse of older women (defined by the domestic violence advocacy community as age 50 and over to signify these

are women past the age of procreation). Appropriations to implement programs nationwide for this provision totaled 5 million dollars in 2000 and
10 million dollars in 2006. States that applied for these funds could use them
primarily for pilot projects and to fund agencies providing services to older
battered women who have experienced abuse that rises to a the level of a
crime as defined by state penal codes and have reported this to the police. The
allocations to date fund only 11 projects nationwide serving older battered
women.

The Elder Justice Act (EJA) is the first national law that specifically addresses
elder abuse. Some provisions of this Act, which was first introduced into
Congress in 2002, passed into law as part of the Affordable Care Act in
2010. While provisions that passed into law primarily focused on elder
abuse in nursing home settings, services provided to older adult victims of
abuse provided by state APS programs were also addressed, providing
recognition of the need for direct service intervention at the state and county
level for protective services for older adults living in the community who are
victims of elder abuse and neglect. To date, however, no appropriations have
been allocated to fund authorized services.

Practice response

Over the past thirty years, awareness of elder abuse as a significant social
problem has increased. Due to the multifaceted nature of elder abuse, there
is no uniform practice response. The aging, health, and criminal justice systems
have developed ways to prevent elder abuse and to intervene when it occurs.
All states have APS programs to respond to allegations of abuse or neglect,
but these programs vary from state to state. As mentioned above, the
response to elder abuse is shaped by federal and state laws, and the practice
response has been fragmented. However, over the past few years, more efforts
have been made to create a comprehensive response to elder mistreatment that
relies on cooperation among different service systems.

Aging service systems

Service systems serving older adults that provide primarily preventive services
include the Older Americans Act programs, through state offices for the
aging and county- and regional-based area agencies on aging. These can serve
as both prevention and early intervention programs, by both providing
community-based services such as senior community and nutrition centers,
case management and information and referral services, transportation, and
in-home meals and home care services to assist older adults 60 years of age
and older to remain independent in the community as long as possible.
Aging service systems also address spouse and partner abuse when spouse/
partners are 60 years of age and older, have mental capacity, and for whom the
abuse may not rise to the level of a crime, using public service announcements,

videos, and educational programs with older adults in the community to raise awareness about abuse.

Intervention models such as education, public awareness and caregiver support groups are found in the aging service system in the US. This service system assumes that older adults are vital, productive members of society and have the right to live independently and safely with dignity in the community as long as possible. Abuse experienced by older adults as perpetrated by loved ones is assumed to be able to be ameliorated by education, increased community support, and intervention by other service systems as a last resort.

Health and aging systems

In 2000, an amendment to the Older Americans Act provided authorization and funding for caregiver support programs and other caregiver support related activities, including those available to family members of older adults suffering from Alzheimer's disease, a health problem that has a significant social component. The recently promulgated National Association of Social Workers (NASW) Standards for Social Work Practice with Family Caregivers of Older Adults represent an example of a preventive strategy to ensure that family caregivers for frail elderly maintain a robust level of well-being in spite of potential stressors related to caregiving, and mitigate against elder abuse and neglect related to caregiver stress (National Association of Social Workers, 2010). Other interventions to support caregivers and provide early intervention for elder abuse have been developed in collaboration with universities and aging and health care systems. For example, findings from research into communication patterns between abusive older patients with Alzheimer's disease and their caregivers have led to the development of intervention strategies that help caregivers anticipate and manage confusion and anxiety on the part of loved ones with Alzheimer's disease. These strategies have been found to diminish violent behavior of patients toward their caregivers and defensive and retaliatory behavior by the caregivers (Vandeweerd and Paveza 2005).

Doctors and other health professionals have been reluctant to report suspected elder abuse to APS (Halphen et al. 2009). The medical professions, through publications and training, have made efforts to raise awareness of the signs of elder abuse and to increase reporting (Daly 2011, Lachs and Pillemer 2004). The routine use of elder abuse screening tools in medical settings, such as the emergency room, has become more commonplace though more evaluation of the tools is needed (Fulmer et al. 2004).

Criminal justice and domestic violence systems

Intervention models such as multi-disciplinary teams based in district attorneys' offices, law enforcement, domestic violence crisis intervention and psycho-educational support groups are found in the law enforcement/ domestic violence service systems and assume that abuse of older adults has risen to the level of a crime as defined by a state penal code and that the perpetrator is using power and control dynamics. These models assume that the victims have the capacity to make decisions about their relationships with their abusers and must ultimately choose to end the relationship with the abusers, with the abusers subject to punishment by law enforcement.

Service systems providing interventions through the criminal justice system and within the domestic violence service network include law enforcement, prosecutors' offices, crime victims service programs, and domestic violence residential and non-residential programs. Residential programs include domestic violence shelters and non-residential programs include victim and perpetrator psycho-educational support groups, and legal services for the elderly. While elder abuse victims are identified and served in these systems, for example law enforcement (Brownell, 1998), there is very little funding in these systems for programs specifically for older adult victims of crimes and family abuse and their abusers. The federal Department of Justice has provided funding to counties for training curricula for law enforcement, judges and court personnel, and district attorney's offices to assist professionals and workers in these systems to understand and be more aware of the issues related to older adult victims and their perpetrators. The National Clearinghouse on Abuse in Later Life is a federally funded initiative of the State of Wisconsin Coalition Against Domestic Violence and provides advocacy, education, and intervention models for replication to states and localities interested in serving older adult victims of family abuse who do not meet the eligibility requirements for protective services for adults (Raymond and Brandl 2008). An identified gap in elder abuse research is that of elder abuse and law enforcement (Brownell 1998). The most extreme form of abuse in this framework is homicide. Some limited research has been conducted on homicides of older women using secondary data (Brownell and Berman 2004). Interventions within this framework could be defined as prevention if homicide is one possible negative outcome. Insufficient research has been conducted to date to determine the correlates of elder mistreatment that culminate in homicide, and prevention and intervention strategies to address risk factors.

Protective service systems

Intervention models such as case management including mental health and intensive case management interventions, guardianships, and other involuntary services are found in the protective service systems for adults. These models assume that victims lack the capacity to care for themselves or protect themselves from harm, whether the harm is coming from their own inability to care for themselves (self-neglect) or from others (abuse or neglect), and most state elder abuse mandatory reporting systems are modeled after child protective service statutes and based on the premise that older adults need protection by the state if they are being harmed by others, are unwilling to accept services, and meet some predetermined criteria for diminished capacity to make informed decisions on their own behalf.

Service systems representing protective services for older adult victims have to date been state- and county-based in the US, enabled by state laws that differ from state to state. These service systems are based on case management models, generally operated or funded by government, and serve older adults who are living in the community with limited mental and physical capacity, with no one willing or able to assist them in meeting their needs in the community, and in need of immediate assistance to remain in the community. The protective service system for adults evolved in the 1970s, along with the deinstitutionalization movement for the mentally ill, and was designed to assist self-neglecting single adults. Older adults served by this system are largely involuntary in that they often are not willing to accept help or they are unaware that help is needed. In most states with mandatory reporting of elder abuse, it is the adult protective service system that is designated to respond to these reports. Intervention options include case management services, crisis intervention, and access to law enforcement, mental health, court-based guardianship programs, and – in limited cases – removal to a hospital or skilled nursing home, possibly without the consent of the victim. This service system would benefit from funding that has not yet been appropriated for the Elder Justice Act that was passed by the US Congress as part of the health reform legislation in 2010.

As noted above, most states have mandatory reporting laws. Training of persons who are designated as mandated reporters and of individuals who come into contact with vulnerable older adults on a regular basis, whether mandated to report or not is part of the effort to address elder mistreatment. The range and type of training available has expanded in response to growing concerns about abuse (Gironda et al. 2010). However, many cases are still underreported. Lack of knowledge, ageism, and the cognitive impairment and/or physical limitations of older adults in their care can lead those who work with older adults, even those working with APS, to not recognize signs and symptoms of abuse. A survey of APS workers in the state of Georgia revealed that they need more training in recognizing and responding to abuse; researchers recommended that states need to do a better job of defining minimum training standards and preparing their workers in the areas of collecting evidence and distinguishing signs of physical abuse from normal aging (Strasser et al. 2011).

A literature review of education efforts for physicians, other hospital-based personnel, and aging service providers concludes that promising practices include training that utilizes "patient cases and hands-on active learning with real or standardized patients appear to result in improved knowledge and perceived ability to manage and appropriately refer elder abuse cases" (Alt et al. 2011: 228). Training must be tailored to specific groups of professionals. For example, the Center of Excellence on Elder Abuse and Neglect at the University of California, Irvine, offers training to pharmacists, certified nursing assistants, home health aides, and individuals associated with the courts, among others (see http://www.centeronelder abuse.org/education_overview.asp).

Intervention for older adult victims of abuse in the United States

While this chapter has discussed intervention within legislative frameworks, another way of viewing interventions is through a public health theoretical framework (Rapp-Paglicci and Dulmus 2005, Gordon 1987, Gordon 1983). Gordon (1983, 1987) identifies three categories of preventive interventions:

- universal preventive interventions targeted to the general public or a whole population group that has not been identified on the basis of individual risk;
- selective prevention interventions targeted to individuals or subgroups of the population who are at high risk of experiencing a problem; and
- indicated preventive interventions targeted to high risk individuals.

An additional series of interventions could be identified that would target an individual who has been identified as experiencing a problem, such as elder abuse, based on an assessment of psycho-social factors that includes environmental as well as psychological and social dimensions (Brownell and Podnieks 2005). For example, older individuals who are healthy and well-functioning members of their community but who are experiencing abuse by family members or loved ones may benefit from psycho-educational support groups, informational seminars, or counseling using a model such as the "Staircase Model" developed by Breckman and Adelman (1988). This is a form of cognitive therapy in which a professional guides a therapeutic client through the stages of pre-cognition, cognition, and ultimately decision to act upon cognition of abuse: this is similar to therapeutic treatment for younger victims of domestic violence. However, if the older victim is suffering from depression, a not uncommon correlate of experiencing abuse by a loved one or trusted other, assessment and treatment of depression may be a necessary precursor of action on the part of the victim (Berman and Furst 2011). Professionals working with victims of elder abuse must continue to assess level of dangerousness in this process (Van Wormer and Roberts 2009). Older victims of abuse who are assessed as not having the ability to understand or to make informed decisions about the circumstances of their situations may need interventions that are involuntary, such as law enforcement, guardianships, and even institutionalization. In summary, interventions must include assessment, if necessary investigation, and then the least intrusive intervention necessary starting with prevention (Brownell and Giblin 2009). All assessments, investigations and interventions must include a cultural component (Brownell 1997).

Research

Over the past decade, steps have been taken to improve the quantity and quality of research in order to gain reliable estimates of the extent of the problem, to understand the characteristics of victims and perpetrators, and to evaluate models of practice. However, research on elder abuse and neglect in the US has lagged behind research on other forms of domestic violence (Bonnie and Wallace 2003).

Incidence and prevalence

A number of studies in recent years have added to our knowledge of incidence and prevalence of elder abuse in the US. While measurement of incidence and prevalence is a unique challenge, incidence is the number of new cases within a certain timeframe, usually the past year, and prevalence is the number of cases in existence at a certain time, no matter what the stage of development (Thomas 2000). These studies have used different methodologies, but they provide some knowledge about the extent of elder mistreatment and have established an estimated prevalence rate between 2 percent and 10 percent of adults over the age of 60 years of age. Some population-based studies (Acierno et al. 2010, Laumann et al. 2008) have excluded respondents who are cognitively impaired. Studies have also excluded different types of mistreatment. For example, one study of the prevalence of elder mistreatment asked respondents about physical and verbal aggression, but not about neglectful behaviors such as leaving a bed-bound person alone and ignoring basic duties of care including feeding, toileting, and bathing (Laumann et al. 2008).

The most widely cited population-based study, a random sample survey of older adults in Massachusetts (Pillemer and Finkelhor 1988), found that the overall mistreatment rate was 32 per 1,000. A study using a nationally representative sample (Acierno et al. 2010) found that during the previous year prevalence of all types of mistreatment studied was 11.4 percent; the prevalence of potential neglect was 5.1 percent, financial mistreatment, 5.2 percent, emotional mistreatment, 4.6 percent, physical abuse, 1.6 percent, and sexual abuse, 0.6 percent. In contrast, a study conducted in New York State that combined a population-based survey of community-dwelling older adults with a study of cases reported to agencies charged with serving community-based elder abuse victims found a starker difference between rates for reported and unreported mistreatment. The New York State population-based study found that the total cumulative incidence rate (i.e. number of new cases in the past year) of self-reported elder abuse, including neglect, financial exploitation, psychological/verbal abuse, or physical abuse was 76 per 1,000, with major financial exploitation the most common form of mistreatment (41.1 per 1,000), physical abuse (22.4 per 1,000), activities of daily living (ADL) and independent ADL neglect (18.2 per 1,000) and psychological/verbal abuse (16.4 per 1,000) (Lifespan of Greater Rochester et al.

2011). This study also uncovered a total cumulative prevalence rate (any elder abuse event at any time since turning age 60) of 141.2 per 1,000.

In contrast, the study of reported cases in New York State revealed a dramatic gap between the rate of elder abuse events reported by older New Yorkers and the number of cases referred to and served in the formal elder abuse service system. Overall the study found an elder abuse prevalence rate in New York State that was nearly 24 times greater than the number of cases referred to social service, law enforcement, or legal authorities who have the capacity as well as the responsibility to assist older adult victims. Emotional abuse was the most common form of mistreatment reported by agencies providing data on elder abuse victims. This finding stands in contrast to the results of the self-reported study in which financial abuse was the most prevalent form of mistreatment. The dramatic gap may be attributed in part to the adequacy of the documentation system to provide elder abuse case data and the inability of some service systems and individual programs to report on their involvement in elder abuse cases (Lifespan of Greater Rochester et al. 2011).

Other studies of elder abuse that have relied on cases reported to APS or cases known to the aging service sector provide additional information about the extent of the problem and also reveal the extent to which APS agencies must address cases of self-neglect. The National Elder Abuse Incidence Study estimated that in 1996 there were 450,000 non-institutionalized older adults who were abused, neglected, or exploited, and that there were five unreported cases for every reported case; an additional 100,000 older adults experienced self-neglect (National Center on Elder Abuse 1998). The 2004 survey of state Adult Protective Services, which reported results for 32 of the 50 states, revealed that there were 253,426 incidents involving elder abuse (including self-neglect) in 2003 (Teaster et al. 2006).

Risk factors for elder abuse

Risk factors for elder abuse have been identified in many studies and include poor physical health and cognitive impairment of the abused person, mental health and/or substance abuse problems in the caregiver, and social isolation (Bonnie and Wallace 2003). A telephone survey of nearly 6,000 elderly individuals conducted by Acierno et al. (2010) found that, for cases of elder physical mistreatment reported, the majority (57 percent) of perpetrators of physical abuse were partners or spouses. Half of perpetrators were using drugs or alcohol at the time of the mistreatment; 30 percent of the perpetrators had a history of mental illness, over one-third were unemployed, and 40 percent were socially isolated.

Forensic markers of abuse

A study that compared the bruises of non-abused older adults with adults whose abuse was substantiated by APS found that abused older adults were more likely to have bruises on the head and neck, the back, and the lateral right arm (Wiglesworth et al. 2009). In contrast, 90 percent of the bruises found on non-abused adults were on the arms and/or legs. Burgess et al. (2008) found that markers of sexual abuse (i.e. signs that triggered reports to APS or law enforcement) included strong ambivalence of the older person towards suspected offenders, victim's distress during personal care, signs of physical trauma, and sexually transmitted diseases. Sexual behaviors or statements made by suspected offenders also triggered investigation.

Research on services

Older women who experience domestic violence face barriers in receiving help from domestic violence (DV) agencies (e.g. shelters for abused women) if those agencies do not have the expertise to respond to their age-related needs (Kilbane and Spira 2010). A study of 1,057 older individuals, mostly women, who accessed DV services in Illinois from 1990 to 1995 (0.84 per-cent of all cases) found that over one-third were abused by their current or ex-husband and another one-third were abused by male relatives, with the majority reporting physical abuse. The most widely mentioned needs were for emotional support and legal assistance, much like the population of younger service users; researchers were not able to derive the exact types of support needed from the data (Lundy and Grossman 2004). Research that compared younger and older women who accessed domestic violence ser-vices in Illinois (Lundy and Grossman 2009) found that older women were less likely than younger women to be physically abused and more likely to be abused by a male or female relative than their husband/intimate partner. Older women were less likely than younger women to be self-referred, referred by a friend, or an abuse hotline, and more likely than younger women to be referred by the State's Attorney's office. Older women received significantly more hours of help for criminal legal advocacy but fewer hours of individual and group counseling.

Results of the Domestic Violence against Older Women Study, which looked at data from focus groups with 134 older women, revealed that older women face both internal and external barriers to accessing services from DV agencies. Internal stressors included the need to protect their families, including the abuser, and a sense of self-blame and shame that had increased over the course of a long marriage. Family members (non-perpetrators) are often non-supportive, and clergy failed to refer the women to DV agencies or the justice system. The participants questioned the efficacy of restraining orders and anger management classes for abusers, and were reluctant to go to shelters where they would have to co-exist with mothers with small children or to services that would advocate their separation from their abusers. Some also voiced fears of being ridiculed or mistreated by the justice system (Beaularier et al. 2008).

Studies have revealed barriers to service for victims of sexual abuse as well and that the service system that deals with the report of sexual abuse will determine what happens following a report. A comparison of cases of sexual abuse of elders by whether they were reported to APS or the criminal justice system found that victims reported to APS were less likely to receive a physical exam and their offenders were less likely to be convicted even though they were more likely to be identified by the victim; perpetrators in these cases were more likely to be older and related to the victim (Burgess et al. 2008).

Intervention models evaluated for effectiveness

A recent meta-analysis of evaluations of intervention models published in the literature identified only eight studies that reviewed outcomes of interventions and met a standard of pre-post tests that included experimental or quasi-experimental design, comparison group, and data on outcomes (Ploeg et al., 2009). Of these most found no statistically significant differences pre- and post-interventions between intervention and control group members. Some evaluations resulted in negative findings: targeted participants experienced poorer outcomes than control group participants. Intervention evaluations are difficult, time consuming, and expensive to implement, and, if undertaken in an academic setting, are difficult to get approved by University Institutional Review Boards (IRBs), according to Paveza (2010). Most recently there has been considerable interest in multidisciplinary team approaches to elder abuse intervention (Brandl et al. 2006, Wiglesworth et al., 2006). Further research is needed to determine if this intervention strategy, which has the advantage of linking different service systems in assessing and serving complex elder abuse case situations, is more successful than single system and method approaches (see e.g. Ernst and Smith 2012).

One study funded by the John A. Hartford Foundation that used measures of mental health, health, and wellbeing to evaluate outcomes of a pilot elder abuse psycho-educational support group model found no statistically significant difference among participant and control group members on pre- and post-tests (Brownell and Heiser 2006). However, self-satisfaction post-test evaluations have found that older women participants may feel less alone and isolated, develop new problem-solving and coping skills, learn about their rights under the law, find a place to relax and feel safe, gain a sense of hope, and focus on issues of more interest and concern to their age group (Raymond and Brandl 2008).

Conclusion

The US has a well-organized system of services for individuals living in the community and who need protection, and a fairly comprehensive system of long-term care. However, policies and practices shaped by individual states, have led to inconsistencies in the way that the US addresses this very serious and costly social problem. Advocates continue to press for greater leadership from the federal government and for research that will help practitioners and policy makers understand the characteristics of victims and perpetrators and the best ways to address the problem.

References

Acierno, R., Hernandez, M.A., Amstadter, A.B., Resnick, H.S., Steve, K., Muzzy, W. and Kilpatrick, D.G. (2010) 'Prevalence and correlates of emotional, physical, sexual, and financial abuse and potential neglect in the United States: The National Elder Mistreatment Study', American Journal of Public Health, 100: 292–97.

Alt, K.L., Nguyen, A.L. and Meurer, L.N. (2011) 'The effectiveness of educational programs to improve recognition and reporting of elder abuse and neglect: A systematic review of the literature', Journal of Elder Abuse and Neglect, 23: 213–33.

Beaularier, R.L., Seff, L.R. and Newman, F.L. (2008) 'Barriers to help-seeking for older women who experience intimate partner violence: A descriptive model'. Journal of Women and Aging, 20: 231–48.

Berman, J. and Furst, L.M. (2011) Depressed older adults: Education and screening, New York: Springer Publishing Company.

Bonnie, R.J. and Wallace, R.B. (eds.) (2003) Elder mistreatment: Abuse, neglect, and exploitation in an aging America, Washington, DC: The National Academies Press.

Brandl, B., Dyer, C.B., Heisler, C.J., Otto, J.M., Stiegel, L.A. and Thomas, R.W. (2006) Elder abuse detection and intervention: A collaborative approach. New York: Springer Publishing Company.

Breckman, R.S. and Adelman, R.D. (1988) Strategies for helping victims of elder mistreatment. Thousand Oaks, CA: Sage.

Brownell, P. (1997) 'The application of the Culturagram in cross-cultural practice with elder abuse victims', Journal of Elder Abuse and Neglect, 9: 19–33.

Brownell, P. and Giblin, C.T. (2009) 'Elder abuse', in A.R. Roberts (ed.) Social workers' desk reference (2nd edn). New York: Oxford University Press.

Brownell, P. and Heiser, D. (2006) 'Psycho-educational support groups for older women victims of family mistreatment: a pilot study', Journal of Gerontological Social Work, 46: 145–60.

Brownell, P. and Podnieks, E. (2005) 'Long-overdue recognition for the critical issue of elder abuse and neglect: A global policy and practice perspective', Brief Treatment and Crisis Intervention, 5: 187–91.

Brownell, P.J. (1998) Family crimes against the elderly: Elder abuse and the criminal justice system. New York: Garland.

Brownell, P.J. and Berman, J. (2004) 'Homicides of older women in New York City: a profile based on secondary data analysis' in A.R. Roberts and K.R Yeager (eds) Evidence-based practice manual: Research and outcome measures in health and human services. New York: Oxford University Press.

Burgess, A.W., Ramsey-Klawsnik, H. and Gregorian, S.B. (2008) 'Comparing routes of reporting in elder sexual abuse cases', Journal of Elder Abuse and Neglect, 20: 336–52.

Daly, J.M. (2011) 'Elder abuse prevention'. Journal of Gerontological Nursing, 37: 11–17.

Ernst, J.S. and Smith, C.A. (2012) 'Assessment in Adult Protective Services: Do multidisciplinary teams make a difference?' Journal of Gerontological Social Work, 55: 21–38.

Fulmer, T., Guadagno, L., Dyer, C.B. and Connolly, M.T. (2004) 'Progress in elder abuse screening and assessment instruments', Journal of the American Geriatrics Society, 52: 297–304.

Gironda, M.W., Lefever, K., Delagrammatikas, L., Nerenberg, L., Roth, R., Chen, E. A. and Northington, K.R. (2010) 'Education and training of mandated reporters: Innovative models, overcoming challenges, and lessons learned', Journal of Elder Abuse and Neglect, 22: 340–64.

Gordon, R. (1983) 'An operational classification of disease prevention', Public Health Reports, 98: 107–9.

——(1987) 'An operational classification of disease prevention' in J.S. Sternberg and M.M. Silverman (eds) Preventing mental disorders. Rockville, MD: US Department of Health and Human Services.

Halphen, J.M., Varas, G.M. and Sadowsky, J.M. (2009) 'Recognizing and reporting elder abuse and neglect' Geriatrics, 64: 13–18.

He, W. and Muenchrath, M.N. (2011) American Community Survey Reports: 90+ in the United States. Washington, DC: Government Printing Office.

Kilbane, T. and Spira, M. (2010) 'Domestic violence or elder abuse? Why it matters for older women', Families in Society, 91: 165–70.

Lachs, M.S. and Pillemer, K. (2004) 'Elder abuse', Lancet, 364, 1263–72

Laumann, E.O., Leitsch, S.A. and Waite, L.J. (2008) 'Elder mistreatment in the United States: Prevalence estimates from a nationally representative study', Journal of Gerontology: Social Sciences, 63B: S248–54.

Lifespan of Greater Rochester, Weill Cornell Medical School of Cornell University and New York City Department for the Aging (2011) Under the Radar: New York State Elder Abuse Prevalence Study. Online. Available at <http://www.lifespan-roch.org/documents/UndertheRadar051211.pdf> (Accessed 29 June 2011).

Lundy, M. and Grossman, S. (2004) 'Elder abuse: Spouse/intimate partner abuse and family violence among elders', Journal of Elder Abuse and Neglect, 16: 85–102.

——(2009) 'Domestic violence service users: A comparison of older and younger women victims', Journal of Family Violence, 24: 297–309.

National Association of Social Workers (2010) NASW standards for social work practice with family caregivers of older adults. Washington, DC: National Association of Social Workers.

National Centre on Elder Abuse (1998) National elder abuse incidents: Final report. Washington, DC: Administration for Children and Families, Administration on Aging, US Department of Health and Human Services. Online. Available at <http://www.aoa.gov/eldfam/Elder_Rights/Elder_Abuse/ABuseReport_Full.pdf> (accessed September 9 2007).

Paveza, G.J. (2010) 'Elder abuse and Alzheimer's disease'. Presentation at the CoNGO Committee on Ageing, United Nations, 3 June.

Pham, S. (2011) 'Government report finds elder abuse on the rise'. The New Old Age. Online. Available at <http://newoldage.blogs.nytimes.com/tag/elder-abuse/> (accessed 12 January 2012).

Pillemer, K. and Finkelhor, D. (1988) 'The prevalence of elder abuse: A random sample survey', The Gerontologist, 28: 51–7.

Ploeg, J., Fear, J., Hutchison, B., Macmillan, H. and Bolan, G. (2009) 'A systematic review of interventions for elder abuse', Journal of Elder Abuse and Neglect, 21: 187–210.

Rapp-Paglicci, L.A. and Dulmus, C.N. (2005) 'Prevention across the adult lifespan', in L.A Rapp-Paglicci and C.N. Dulmus (eds) Preventive interventions for adults. Hoboken, NJ: John Wiley and Sons.

Raymond, J.A. and Brandl, B. (2008) In their own words: Domestic violence in later life. Madison, WI: National Clearinghouse on Abuse in Later Life/Wisconsin Coalition Against Domestic Violence.

Strasser, S.M., Kerr, J., King, P.S., Payne, B.K., Beddington, S., Pendrick, D., Leyla, E. and McCarty, F. (2011) 'A survey of Georgia Adult Protective Services staff: Implications for older adult injury prevention and policy', Western Journal of Emergency Medicine, 12: 357–64.

Teaster, P.B., Dugar, T.A., Mendiondo, M.S., Abner, E.L., Cecil, K.A. and Otto, J. M. (2006) The 2004 survey of state Adult Protective Services: Abuse of adults 60 years of age and older. Washington, DC: National Center on Elder Abuse and National Adult Protective Services Association. Online. Available at <http://www. elderabusecenter.org/pdf/2-14-06%20FINAL%2060+REPORT.pdf> (accessed 31 August 2007).

Thomas, C. (2000) 'The first national study of elder abuse and neglect: Contrast with results from other studies', Journal of Elder Abuse and Neglect, 12: 1–11.

US Government Accountability Office (2011) Elder justice: Stronger federal leadership could enhance national response to elder abuse. Washington, DC: Government Printing Office.

US National Committee on the Prevention of Elder Abuse (2008) 'What is elder abuse?'. Online. Available at <http://www.preventelderabuse.org/elderabuse/> (accessed 15 December 2012)

Van Wormer, K. and Roberts, A.R. (2009) Death by domestic violence: Preventing the murders and murder-suicides, Westport, CT: Praeger.

Vandeweerd, C. and Paveza, G.J. (2005) 'Verbal mistreatment in older adults: A look at persons with Alzheimer's disease and their caregivers in the state of Florida', Journal of Elder Abuse and Neglect, 17: 11–30.

Vincent, G K. and Velkoff, V.A. (2010). The next four decades: The older population in the United States – 2010 to 2050 population estimates and projections. (Current population reports.) Washington, DC: US Census Bureau.

WHO (2002) The Toronto declaration on the global prevention of elder abuse. Geneva: World Health Organisation.

Wiglesworth, A., Austin, R., Corona, M., Schneider, D., Liao, S., Gibbs, L. and Mosqueda, L. (2009) 'Bruising as a marker of physical elder abuse'. Journal of the American Geriatrics Society, 57: 1191–6.

Wiglesworth, A., Mosqueda, L., Burnight, K., Younglove, T. and Jeske, D. (2006) 'Findings from an elder abuse forensic center'. Gerontologist, 46: 277–83.

13 Concluding thoughts

Amanda Phelan

The topic of elder abuse is one which has generated considerable debate. Since its initial formal articulations (Baker 1975), elder abuse has emerged in different ways in various countries. This book has presented insights into how the topic has been constructed and addressed in various states and jurisdictions around the globe. One striking observation within these chapters is that the authors have chartered varying ways of addressing this issue in their related societies. Undoubtedly, an ageing global population is an important impetus for increasing social and political discourses on elder abuse. Such demographic change has focused governments' attention on the needs of older people in general (albeit with a varying degree of importance for each country) and heightened awareness of the social challenge of elder abuse. In particular, it has been noted that the increase in the 'older old', those over 80 years of age, has impacted on dependency levels and posed challenges for both governments and families in the context of the provision of care. Such challenges are particularly evident in recessionary times where both human and financial resources are scarce in many countries.

The emergence of elder abuse in some countries has been hindered by a belief that it was not an issue in traditional societies. In the chapters on Kenya, Ireland, China and Israel, the authors remark that the lack of action and apathy in the area of elder abuse may be due to a societal perception that it did not occur due to cultural, religious or other traditional beliefs. Often, it is due to evidence by research or media scandals which have provided the impetus for public discussion and resultant action in terms of official responses. Acknowledgement of elder abuse has also been hindered by ageist perspectives, which have made society more tolerant of abuse towards older people and promoted a lack of recognition of abuse. Even when abuse has been recognized, Kurrle notes that older people fear not being believed, not being supported and may experience a lack of knowledge by helping professionals

The definition of elder abuse has evolved since 1975. Many countries reviewed in this book cite a relationship to the Toronto Declaration on Elder Abuse (WHO 2002) or other international definitions. However, even within some countries, such as Australia, the United States and Spain, for example, several definitions may exist, although fundamental similarities are apparent. Elder abuse is frequently described as occurring within a 'relationship of trust'. Such understandings echo the domestic violence literature, which also frequently cites abuse within intimate relationships and kinship relationships. However, conversely, the third domain of family violence, child protection, has a broader focus on perpetrator type, which can include both kinship and those outside a traditional relationship of trust. As such, a debate on extending the definition of elder abuse is required. Even when using the term 'expectation of trust' as a parameter for elder abuse perpetrators, one must be cautious as this ultimately draws upon traditional social constructions of the family, where trust relationships between kin are taken for granted as being altruistic. Equally, those not in the traditional relationship of trust such as neighbours may engender more trust from the older person than his/her own family member.

Definitions can also be influenced by professional discipline. For example, discrepancies may be apparent when the same case is considered from a legal, healthcare professional and researcher point of view. In this volume, Penhale suggests that the presence of different definitions may not pose a problem, if the stakeholders are aware of such variations in disciplinary understandings. However, in the context of multi-disciplinary and multi-agency collaboration, definitional diversity may lead to obvious problems in case management. Thus, additional consideration of a wider understanding of elder abuse is useful. In chapter three, McDonald describes research which has developed definitional consensus. Moreover, the legal perspective in Canadian common law can include abuse by strangers, grooming of an older person for abuse and exploitation. Such perspectives have the advantage of allowing the act itself to primarily constitute abuse without reference to who perpetrates that act.

Many definitions are enshrined in policy and as such can render the subjective understanding of elder abuse by older people silent. For instance, studies which have considered older people's interpretations of abuse demonstrate a greater association with societal abuse rather than simple didactic abuse. This depersonalization of elder abuse may be influenced by older people not seeing themselves as being affected by the types of elder abuse. For example, in studies cited in the chapters on Spain, Canada and Norway, older people may indicate yes to questions referring to traditional examples of abuse, but can be reluctant to position themselves as victims of abuse. This represents a personal disassociation of self from the context of abuse, which is compounded by possible kinship ties with the abuser. It may also be difficult for 'well' older people to contextualize themselves as being abused as dependency may be associated with such abuse. Brownell and Joy state that this cohort of abused older people benefit from psycho-social support, although for this to work, initial assistance needs to focus on other possible presenting issues such as depression.

The way society treats older people is seen as important and this can be directly related to the experience of older people. In chapter 6, (Draichman and Giraldo) present insights into Latin America's identification of structural abuse which is linked to issues of the marginalization of older people and social exclusion. However, political support of this form of elder abuse may be challenging as it fundamentally targets policy and service provision by governments themselves. Another important issue is the experience of elder abuse within a gender perspective. Older women may be doubly marginalized, through age and gender, as described by Draichman and Giraldo. In Latin America, older women have poorer health, poorer education status and are the inevitable caregivers.

Most of the chapters in this book consider abuse within a framework of the typologies of elder abuse. These are physical, sexual, financial and psychological abuse and neglect. The issue of self-neglect remains contentious, with some countries, such as the Unites States including this under the definition of elder abuse, while other countries exclude this typology. However, even in countries where self-neglect is not specified or is explicitly excluded in policy definitions, self-neglect is often accounted for in official statistics (see for example Ireland and Norway). Consequently, further research is required to examine this definitional quagmire as such uncertainty exacerbates standardized understandings. Consideration of self-neglect as a form of elder abuse also involves some debate on issues of self-determinism, autonomy and mental capacity. Moreover, as self-neglect activities may have a negative influence on the rights of others, (for example in relation to a safe environment), each case requires careful consideration in the context of a balancing of rights.

Cultural aspects of definition are vital and are likely to become more important as ethnic and cultural diversity increase. Although standardized definitional statements have the advantage of some uniformity in a global consensus on elder abuse, such statements have been criticized as neglecting the cultural context. In China, Tiwari and colleagues observe how common (and generally western) definitions can be insensitive to the Chinese culture. Equally, in chapter seven (Abodoerin & Hatendi), strong cultural realities related to the abuse of older people are located in witchcraft beliefs and the resultant persecution of older people thought to practice witchcraft. Such beliefs are engendered in a community's tacit support of the labeling and subsequent intimidation of older people who are 'generally blamed' for various misfortunes of the community. Furthermore, Lowenstein and Doron, and Brownell and Joy emphasise the need for additional research related to cultural interpretations as the demographics of Israel and the United States show diverse ageing populations. In addressing elder abuse within a cultural framework, it is necessary that definitions are flexible enough to acknowledge cultural perspectives but strategic enough to target the conditions upon which such perspectives are based to ensure the appropriate safety for older people.

Changes in modernity have also seen tensions between older people's cultural interpretation of abuse as compared to younger generations. In China, the tradition of Confucian piety has engendered particular expectations of filial responsibility which can be at odds to the reality of such duty's performance by younger generations. For example, traditional caregivers (daughters and daughters in law) may now be employed and the reduction in extended families due to urbanization and employment mobility reduces the time available to provide expected family care.

The phenomenon of elder abuse is predominantly one which occurs in the community setting. One challenge in this environment is how to publically regulate the private space of family. Families have traditionally been seen as being private entities and it is only in recent years that issues of family violence has forced public intervention into the abuse of family members. Some major barriers present themselves. Firstly, access to the older person can be hindered by a gatekeeper and healthcare professionals must often make extensive attempts to gain and sustain access (Phelan 2010). Even when entry is allowed, it can be difficult to identify elder abuse as the older person may not be left alone to enable disclosure and families can 'stage manage' their social presentation, which also makes it difficult to identify the abuse. The identification of abuse is also complicated by issues of health as physical and/or cognitive decline can impact on the older person's access to a helping person (either a professional or family/friend/neighbor). Isolating the person is one of the key actions by perpetrators. Such was the context of one of Kurrle's case descriptions in Chapter 2, where the older person was isolated from the General Practitioner and others and the suspicion was only raised when a neighbour reported observing the older person frequently distressed in his garden. Even when abuse is suspected action can be hampered by the older person being reluctant to take intervention due to issues of family ties, embarrassment or apathy regarding the situation.

In terms of legislation, many countries cite generic laws as being applied to situations of elder abuse. Although discussions on such laws identify gaps in relation to elder abuse, almost all chapters detail a developing legislative protection system. Some countries do have specific legislation for older people in general and elder protection specifically. A major legal instrument employed in many jurisdictions is that of guardianship legislation for older people with mental capacity challenges. This appears to be considered appropriate in ensuring the beneficence of the older person. However, some legislation remains archaic. For example, the witchcraft laws of Kenya and the Lunacy Regulation Act in Ireland require urgent attention to ensure that the legislation matches contemporary needs, rather than sustaining societal cannons from a different century. Moreover, in Kenya the debate linking elder abuse and witchcraft has generally been absent, although it is often the older family member who is the target of persecution.

In particular, the chapter on Israel charts legislative progression from a paternalistic and intervention approach to a more contemporary empowerment approach. This reflects an acknowledgement of the rights of older people and a move from hierarchical, professional decision making to a participatory framework, which values the older person's engagement, self-determination and autonomy. Similarly, in the United Kingdom, the Scottish Adult Support and Protection Act 1997 emphasizes that interventions must be of benefit to the older person and promote the rights and freedom of individuals. Advances in Spain include a focus on issues of an Elderly Security Plan, which attempts to prevent abuse and improve the safety of older people. Another piece of noteworthy legislation is the recent Elder Justice Act in the United States, which allows direct service intervention for older people who are subject to abuse and neglect.

A striking issue in both legislation and service provision is the use of a domestic violence lens to address elder abuse. Although, such legislation is useful to a point, it does not have the capacity to address the finer issues in relation to the complexities of abuse in older people. In terms of the use of domestic violence shelters, it has been observed in the United States and Norway that, although there is not an age limit in service use, older people do not use such services very much. Possible reasons suggested for this are that the service is not typically considered by either the public or health care professionals as a helping mechanism. Older people themselves may be reluctant to attend such shelters due to the high population of younger age groups using this service and may consider leaving their own home as inappropriate.

The merit of establishing mandatory reporting is debatable. Standards for mandatory reporting can vary between and within countries. Although the function of mandatory reporting is to ensure the observer of elder abuse reports it so that early intervention may be initiated, statistics on reporting do not demonstrate a strong argument that this works in practice (see e.g. Chapters 4 and 12, on Chinese societies and the United States). Furthermore, issues arise in relation to who is mandated to report, who is responsible for reporting and what penalty is appropriate for non-reporting.

A service response to elder abuse varies from having no specific service which addresses the problem (Kenya) to cases being managed in general older person services (e.g. Australia) or an adult protective service (e.g. the United States and the United Kingdom) to services which are specific for elder abuse (Ireland). Education of multi-agency professionals is important so that prevention, identification and amelioration of elder abuse exists in all services that interface with older people. Furthermore, the need for multi-disciplinary and multi-agency collaboration is in evidence in many chapters. This is particularly relevant due to the complexity of elder abuse and the fact that it transcends a single disciplinary domain. Multi-disciplinary teams require named key workers and core participants. Such teams should also have access to various agencies depending on the presenting and emerging aspects of each individual case. Thus, case responses are carefully tailored to the needs of each older person.

Such response services need a number of structures to be in place to support robust reactions to elder abuse. Firstly, policy needs to be culturally acceptable and realistic as well as being resourced properly. However, policy on its own is limited without 'legislative teeth'. As Penhale observes (Chapter 11), policy also requires clear lines of responsibility and accountability as well as the effective operation of policy principles. Service provision requires constant quality improvement mechanisms which are realised through stakeholder review, case review, reflective practice and clinical government mechanisms. Evaluation of intervention through research is fundamental to improving service and also promotes financial rectitude.

An important aspect of assessment in possible elder abuse cases is the ability to correctly distinguish the older person's presenting symptoms. Rather than taking an ageist approach that symptoms are due to physiological decline, careful assessment of forensic markers of abuse can assist case identification. Professionals need to be able to differentiate the signs of ageing from the consequences of elder abuse. This can improve the identification of abuse and also provide important legal evidence.

The use of help lines and resource centres, such as those in Spain and Australia, allow older people to independently gain information and support in the experience of elder abuse. As such, they are important 'springboards' to access intervention. Some authors argue that intervention should be placed in the context of an ecological approach which acknowledges the multiple impacts on the abuse of that individual and also examines the life-course or chronological context. Such an approach has the advantage of integrating macro, meso and micro elements of the abuse to the individual and appropriate action may, for example, incorporate the different meaning people attribute to violence and its consequences and how strategies are deployed (if any) to address the abuse. McDonald (Chapter 3) states that issues such as a history of child abuse can be influential in the experience of abuse throughout the lifetime of an individual.

In the context of ongoing research, many countries are pursuing 'home grown studies'. The major advantage of such studies is that they allow the development of knowledge specific to particular populations. Many countries have conducted prevalence studies and these provide an important insight into 'local' elder abuse as well as a powerful impetus to lobby government for action. It is acknowledged that prevalence studies underestimate the problem and a recent study in New York has suggested that only one case in 24 comes to the attention of formal services (Lifespan of Greater Rochester Inc. et al. 2011). This implies that a particular focus is required to improve case finding in elder abuse. Certainly, public information campaigns have been described in many chapters in this book. These have the advantage of opening up society's understanding of abusive actions, emphasising that abuse is unacceptable and helping to remove the taboo status of abuse, particularly in the context of the family. Indeed, the use of the media has been crucial in generating public support and the need for action (see e.g. Chapters 2 and 5, on Australia and Ireland). However, while drawing on international knowledge is advantageous, cultural variations may mean not all findings are universally appropriate. In addition, comparisons are hampered by differing methodological approaches, different age references, varying definitions of elder abuse and some differences in inclusion typologies (such as neglect, sexual abuse).

Only a small proportion of older people live in residential care, sheltered housing or other forms of assisted living. Yet, even when admitted to residential care, abuse can occur. Research into institutional abuse of older people remains inadequate. Studies indicate a higher prevalence of abuse in care facilities. For example, Lowenstein and Doron (Chapter 8) detail a 2002 study in Tel-Aviv (Katzman and Litwin 2002), which demonstrated that some form of abuse was perpetrated on over half of the residents in a care unit. The dynamics of institutional abuse are different from abuse in the home. Issues such as systems of care, multiple formal caregivers and the profit-making focus can all influence the standard of care. Therefore, an alternative perspective is required to address elder abuse in institutions. In Chapter 3, McDonald suggests that using a theory of complex organisations may provide new insights into institutional abuse as it can accommodate intrinsic and elusive understandings of maltreatment in this setting. Another important development in some countries is the establishment of care standard authorities (see Chapters 5 and 11, on Ireland and the United Kingdom), which have made a particular impact on standards in residential care settings and facilitate action if systems of care are demonstrated to be lacking.

This book has provided an insight into elder abuse in multiple countries and jurisdictions around the globe. While much progress has been presented in terms of definition, research and practice, each country has developed separate ways of addressing the issue. In each chapter, the authors have reiterated that gaps remain and that more research and education is needed as well as further improvements in legislation and policy. Central to this is the need to value the older person, ensure that interventions do not infringe on individual rights, guarantee full participation and engagement of older people and protect self-determination and autonomy. It is difficult when self-determination means older people choose risky environments and future debate should centre on issues of how such risks can be balanced to ensure the safety of the person. Ultimately, as Tiwari and colleagues argue (Chapter 4), zero tolerance is essential. This fundamentally involves multiple foci through an ecological lens. It requires a societal mind shift, a comprehensive service within evidence-based interventions and substantive legislative responses so that all older people can be empowered as valued citizens.

References

Baker, A.A. (1975) 'Granny bashing', Modern Geriatrics, 8: 20–24.

Katzman, B. and Litwin, H. (2002) Protecting the elderly and preventing violence against them. Jerusalem: The National Insurance Institute (Hebrew).

Lifespan of Greater Rochester Inc., Weill Cornell Medical Centre of Cornell University and New York City Department for the Aging (2011) Under the Radar: New York State elder abuse prevalence study. New York: New York Department for the Aging.

Phelan, A. (2010) 'Discursive constructions of elder abuse: Community nurses' accounts'. Unpublished thesis, University College Dublin.

WHO (2002) The Toronto declaration on the global prevention of elder abuse. Geneva: World Health Organisation.

Index

Locators in *italics* refer to tables and figures.